Manual of
Emergency
Medicine
Fifth Edition

Manual of Emergency Medicine
Fifth Edition

Michael Eliastam, M.D., M.P.P., F.A.C.E.P.

Director of Emergency Services
Associate Professor of Surgery and Medicine
Stanford University Medical Center
Stanford, California

George L. Sternbach, M.D., F.A.C.E.P.

Deputy Director, Department of Emergency Services
Clinical Associate Professor of Surgery
Stanford University Medical Center
Stanford, California

Michael Jay Bresler, M.D., F.A.C.E.P.

Associate Director, Department of Emergency Services
Clinical Associate Professor of Surgery
Stanford University Medical Center
Stanford, California

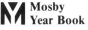

Mosby
Year Book

St. Louis   Baltimore   Boston   Chicago   London
Philadelphia   Sydney   Toronto

A Year Book Medical Publishers imprint of Mosby-Year Book, Inc.

Mosby-Year Book, Inc., 11830 Westline Industrial Drive, St. Louis, MO 63146.

4   5   6   7   8   9   0   MC   93   92

Library of Congress Cataloging-in-Publication Data

Manual of emergency medicine.
    Includes bibliographies and index.
    1. Emergency medicine—Handbooks, manuals, etc.
I. Eliastam, Michael. II. Sternbach, George L., 1946–
III. Bresler, Michael Jay.   [DNLM: 1. Emergencies.
WB 105 M2944   1989]
RC86.8.M37   1989   616′.025   88-33841
ISBN 0-8151-3059-7

Sponsoring Editor: David K. Marshall
Assistant Director, Manuscript Services: Frances M. Perveiler
Production Project Manager: Gayle Paprocki
Proofroom Manager: Shirley E. Taylor

Publisher's Note

The authors and publisher of this book have made every effort to ensure that the recommended drug dosage schedules presented are accurate and in accord with sound medical practice. Because new research and experience may lead to changes in drug therapy, however, the reader is advised to verify drug dosage schedules in the manufacturer's product information insert prior to administration of the drug. This is particularly important for new or infrequently used drugs. It remains the responsibility of the physician to ascertain the suitability of the drugs and dosage regimens.

20 / Facial Injuries   275

21 / Otolaryngologic Emergencies   293

22 / Ophthalmologic Emergencies   313

23 / Acquired Immunodeficiency Syndrome and Oncological and Hematologic Emergencies   325

24 / Pediatric Emergencies   357

25 / Allergic Emergencies   377

26 / Dermatologic Disorders   389

27 / Environmental Trauma   405

28 / Anesthesia   419

29 / Poisoning, Overdose, and Envenomation Management   441

30 / Psychiatric Emergencies   501

Index   529

Contents

Preface to the Fifth Edition   vii

Preface to the Fourth Edition   ix

Preface to the First Edition   xi

1 / Shock   1

2 / Trauma Care   11

3 / Cardiac Emergencies   17

4 / Electrolyte and Acid-Base Disorders   51

5 / Respiratory Emergencies   75

6 / Thoracic Injuries   97

7 / Neurological Emergencies: Altered Level of Conciousness   117

8 / Syncope   137

9 / Headache   141

10 / Dizziness and Vertigo   145

11 / Convulsive Disorders   149

12 / Neurological Trauma   155

13 / Acute Abdominal Emergencies   167

14 / Genitourinary Tract Disorders   185

15 / Obstetrics and Gynecology   199

16 / Soft-Tissue Infections   213

**17 / Peripheral Vascular
    Emergencies**   229

18 / Bone and Joint Trauma   241

19 / Hand Injuries   259

Preface to the Fifth Edition

We are very pleased to present this review of the *Manual of Emergency Medicine*. Each chapter has been carefully reviewed and updated. In addition, based on suggestions from readers and reviewers, we have added a number of chapters (Trauma Care, Dermatologic Disorders, Acquired Immune Deficiency Syndrome [AIDS] and Oncologic and Hematologic Emergencies, and Soft Tissue Infections).

The focus of this book is not confined to life-threatening emergencies only, but recognizes that the emergency department is a site for care for people with less urgent conditions as well. We received many helpful suggestions and criticisms from readers of the Fourth Edition, and many of their ideas were incorporated in the current revision. We urge readers of this volume to continue this tradition.

We want to acknowledge the very important contributions of Dolly Kagawa and Jackie Traeger, who managed us well, and without whom we would not have completed this revision.

Michael Eliastam, M.D., M.P.P., F.A.C.E.P.
George L. Sternbach, M.D., F.A.C.E.P.
Michael J. Bresler, M.D., F.A.C.E.P.

Preface to the
Fourth Edition

John Schneewind, M.D., published the first edition of this book in 1963. His untimely death in 1972 was a tragic loss not only to his family but to the practitioners involved in emergency care. Consider that, when the first edition was published, very few people understood the concept of emergency medical services; and sophisticated prehospital care was not yet developed. Emergency departments were generally the orphans of the hospital system, and of course emergency medicine as a specialty did not even exist. The first edition was one of the earliest attempts by any physician or surgeon to pull together a pocket manual containing the essential information necessary to manage patients coming through an emergency "room." One of us (M.E.) had the good fortune to serve as John Schneewind's intern at Rush Presbyterian-St. Luke's Hospital in Chicago, where Dr. Schneewind practiced as a hand surgeon. His devotion to his patients, exemplified by the meticulous attention he paid to operative technique and postoperative management, made a tremendous impression on all who worked with him.

The first edition was written in a style that very much reflected Dr. Schneewind's personality. We have attempted wherever possible to retain the original text because in its own special way the text is very successful at imparting the message. Obviously, the revisions could not be carried out in his original style, and we apologize to the readers for the inconsistency of style only to the extent that we are not able to duplicate the material in the original form.

Preface to the First Edition

This manual was designed originally for use at the University of Illinois Hospitals and was privately printed and distributed through two editions for that purpose. The present volume has been broadened as much as possible so that it might be of value to hospitals which are not university affiliated and which have no interns or residents. This has been accomplished by the addition of new sections on Resuscitation and Anesthesia, Medical Emergencies, Emergencies in Otolaryngology and Ocular Emergencies. Many of the original sections have been revised, including those on Pediatrics, Poisons, Fractures, and so on, and illustrations have been added in appropriate places. Also new is Part III, Preparation for Disaster.

Some subjects, such as cardiac arrest, are discussed in more than one section, but the management is essentially similar. We realize that many controversial points of therapy are presented without extensive discussion, but believe that this is unavoidable in a manual of this kind.

The editor expresses his indebtedness to the faculty members whose contributions made this manual possible.

John H. Schneewind, M.D.

1

Shock

I. Definition

A. Shock is a clinical state resulting from inadequate tissue perfusion.

B. There are several major types of shock (Table 1–1).

1. Hypovolemic shock is caused by the loss of blood, plasma, or body water. This chapter will address hypovolemic shock primarily.

2. Cardiogenic shock is caused by failure of the heart as a pump (see Chapter 3).

3. Septic shock is caused by vasodilation, increased capillary permeability, and myocardial depression due to systemic infection or endotoxemia.

4. Anaphylactic shock is due to vasodilation and capillary leakage caused by immunologically mediated vasoactive substance release (see Chapter 25).

5. Spinal shock is due to vasodilation secondary to the withdrawal of neural influence (see Section IV of this chapter).

6. Obstructive shock may also occur secondary to mechanical obstruction of the venous return to the heart such as in cardiac tamponade and tension pneumothorax. Cardiac outflow may be obstructed due to dissection of an aortic aneurysm (see Chapter 3).

TABLE 1–1.
Clinical Findings in Shock

Type	Skin	Chest	Neck Veins	Vital Signs	Other
Hypovolemic	Cold, clammy, pale, mottled	Clear	Flat	Tachypnea, tachycardia, hypotension	Thirst
Cardiogenic	Cold, clammy, diaphoretic	Clear or may have findings of congestive heart failure	May be engorged	Tachypnea, hypotension, tachycardia, or bradycardia	Cardiac gallop; rubs or murmurs may be audible
Anaphylactic	Urticaria, maculopapular rash or angioedema	May have wheezing, cough, cyanosis	Flat	Tachypnea, tachycardia, hypotension	Conjunctival infection, nausea, vomiting, abdominal pain, diarrhea

Septic	Warm and flushed or cool and pale or cyanotic	Clear unless findings of pneumonia are present	Flat	Tachypnea, tachycardia, hypotension	Signs of focal infection or disseminated intravascular coagulation
Spinal	Warm and flushed	Clear	Flat	Bradycardia, hypotension	Neurological deficit, urinary retention, priapism
Obstructive (cardiac tamponade or tension pneumothorax)	Cold, clammy, pale, or cyanotic	Distant heart sounds or unilateral absent air entry sounds and tracheal and mediastinal shift	Engorged	Tachypnea, tachycardia, hypotension	Increased pulsus paradoxus

II Hypovolemic Shock

A. Causes.
   1. Blood loss.
      a. This may be external such as via an open wound.
      b. Internal bleeding may cause hypovolemic shock if such hemorrhage is into the thorax, abdomen, retroperitoneum, or thigh.
   2. Plasma loss is commonly the result of burns, crush injury, or peritoneal inflammation.
   3. Water loss may be due to excessive gastrointestinal, urinary, or other loss with inadequate replacement.
B. Clinical findings.
   1. Mental status.—Alterations in the sensorium are characteristic of the shock state. Anxiety, restlessness, fear, apathy, stupor, or coma may be present. These abnormalities reflect diminished cerebral perfusion.
   2. Vital signs.
      a. Blood pressure.—The earliest change in blood pressure due to hypovolemia is a narrowing of the pulse pressure. This is the result of an elevated diastolic pressure due to sympathetically mediated vasoconstriction. Systolic blood pressure may be maintained at normal levels until a volume loss of 15% to 25% has occurred. Postural and thereafter supine hypotension will occur. A postural difference greater than 15 mm Hg is significant.
      b. Pulse.—Postural and eventually supine tachycardia is characteristic of shock. A postural change greater than 15 beats per minute is significant. There is a decrease in the pulse amplitude. Tachycardia may be absent in the patient taking β-blockers.
      c. Respirations.—Tachypnea is characteristic, and

respiratory alkalosis is common in the early stages of shock.

3. Skin.
   a. The skin may be cool, pale, and mottled. It generally blanches easily.
   b. The veins of the extremities display a low pressure—the so-called collapse of the peripheral veins. There is no jugular venous distention.
4. Symptoms.—The patient may complain of nausea, weakness, or fatigue. Profound thirst is common.

C. Treatment.
   1. Monitoring.—The following parameters should be monitored during stabilization and treatment: heart rate, respiratory rate, blood pressure, central venous pressure, and urine output. A urine output of less than 30 mL/(or 0.5 ml/kg/hr) indicates inadequate renal perfusion.
   2. Respiratory management.—The patient should be given high-flow oxygen via mask or cannula. A clear airway should be maintained by proper head and mandible positions and a thorough suctioning of blood and secretions. Arterial blood gas determinations should be performed as indicated to assess ventilation and oxygenation. If these are inadequate on the basis of clinical or blood gas criteria, the patient should be intubated and ventilated with a volume-cycled ventilator. Tidal volume should be set at 12 to 15 ml/kg, respiratory rate at 12 to 16 min. Oxygen should be administered to maintain the Po_2 in excess of 100 mmHg. If the patient is "bucking" the ventilator, sedative or muscle-paralyzing agents should be administered (see Chapter 12). If this regimen fails to provide adequate oxygenation or if pulmonary function deteriorates, 3 to 10 cm of positive end-expiratory pressure should be added.
   3. Fluid administration.
      a. Fluid replacement should begin with the rapid administration of lactated Ringer's solution or

normal saline. The rate of administration and the number of intravenous lines necessary vary with the severity of shock. Generally, at least 1 to 2 L of Ringer's solution should be infused within the first 45 to 60 minutes, or more briskly if necessary. If hypotension is corrected and the blood pressure remains stable, it is an indication that blood loss has been minimal. If hypotension persists despite fluid administration or if the blood pressure rise is transient, severe or persistent blood loss is indicated. Blood should be transfused in these patients as soon as possible, and the rate and amount administered should be guided by the response of the monitored parameters (see Section IV, A).

(1) O-negative or uncrossmatched blood may be administered initially if shock persists and there is not sufficient time (about 45 minutes) to wait for crossmatching to be accomplished.

(2) Immediately after crossmatch is accomplished, type-specific blood should be administered.

(3) Dilutional coagulopathy may develop in the patient who receives massive transfusions. Banked blood is devoid of viable platelets and clotting factors V and VIII. One unit of fresh frozen plasma should be administered for every 5 units of whole blood infused. Platelet count and coagulation status should be followed in patients receiving massive transfusion therapy.

(4) Hypothermia is also a consequence of massive transfusion. Blood should be warmed by a warming coil and the patient's core temperature monitored.

    b. Military antishock trousers (MAST)—External counterpressure with the MAST suit is useful as an adjunct to fluid replacement. The MAST suit is applied to the legs and abdomen of the patient, and each of the three individual compartments (extremity and abdominal) may be inflated. The suit redistributes blood from the lower extremities to the central circulation and reduces the arterial flow in the legs by reducing vessel diameter.

      (1) Contraindications to use.

        a Concomitant pulmonary edema.

        b Pregnancy.—This applies only to the abdominal compartment.

      (2) Precautions.

        a The MAST suit may increase the hemorrhage of supradiaphragmatic injury.

        b Prolonged (24 to 48 hours) application over an injured leg may contribute to the development of the fascial compartment syndrome.

4. Vasopressors.—The use of vasopressors in the treatment of hypovolemic shock has fallen into disfavor in the past decade. The reason for this is that these may further reduce tissue perfusion. In most cases, vasopressors should not be used; however, they may be useful in some instances. They may be administered as a temporary measure to increase the blood pressure until adequate fluid replacement can be instituted. This may be especially beneficial in older patients with significant coronary or cerebral vascular disease. Agents to use are norepinephrine, 4 to 8 mg in 500 mL 5% dextrose in water (D_5W), or metaraminol, 5 to 10 mg in 500 mL D_5W, which are predominantly vasoconstrictors with minimum cardiac effect. The dose should be titrated against blood pressure.

III. Septic Shock

A. Causes.
1. The most common cause of septic shock is bacteremia with gram-negative enteric organisms namely, *Escherichia coli, Klebsiella, Enterobacter, Proteus, Pseudomonas,* and others.
2. Less frequently, gram-positive bacteria, viruses, fungi, and rickettsiae are responsible for the infection that causes septic shock.
3. Many patients have a predisposing factor to their severe infection. This may be a chronic illness—diabetes, malignancy, alcoholism, cirrhosis—immunosuppression, or recent surgery or urinary tract instrumentation.

B. Clinical findings.
1. Mental status.—Impaired mental status is the result of reduced cerebral perfusion and consists of confusion, obtundation, or coma.
2. Vital signs.—Fever is frequently present, although the temperature may be normal or below normal. The onset of septic shock is frequently attended by a chill and rapidly rising fever. Tachypnea, tachycardia, and hypotension are usually present.
3. Skin.—The skin is warm and may be flushed in the early stages of the disease—reflecting arterial vasodilation. Later in the course, if vasoconstriction occurs, the skin will be cold and pale.
4. Other signs and symptoms.—The patient may have findings that indicate a source of the infection such as a cough or meningeal signs. Signs of gastrointestinal tract irritation such as vomiting and diarrhea may be present. If disseminated intravascular coagulation (DIC) appears as a complication of sepsis, there may be abnormal bleeding from the gastrointestinal tract, in the urine, from venipuncture sites, or from other sources.

C. Laboratory studies.

1. The only laboratory test diagnostic of septic shock is a blood culture that grows the infecting organism. Due to the seriousness of septic shock, treatment should be instituted as early as possible after the diagnosis is considered.

2. The white blood cell count usually indicates a leukocytosis with a shift to the left, but a leukopenia may also be seen. Increased amounts of serum glutamic oxaloacetic transaminase and amylase are common.

3. If the findings of DIC are present, the platelet count, fibrinogen level, partial thromboplastin time (PTT), and prothrombin time (PT) should be determined. Thrombocytopenia, hypofibrinogenemia, and prolonged PT and PTT are found in persons with DIC.

D. Treatment.

1. Parameters as outlined in Section IV, A should be monitored.

2. Volume replacement should be initiated as indicated to replace fluid sequestered in the body. Care must be taken to watch for the clinical signs of congestive heart failure and to monitor the central venous pressure.

3. Since the infecting organism is rarely known at the time of the initial evaluation, antibiotic coverage should be empirical. After blood cultures and cultures of other appropriate factors—urine, sputum, wound, cerebrospinal fluid—are performed as indicated, antibiotic administration should be begun. Gentamicin or tobramycin, 5 mg/kg/day intravenously (IV), and ampicillin, 2 gm IV every 6 hours are recommended. If an anaerobic organism is suspected, clindamycin, 20 mg/kg/day IV, or chloramphenicol, 4 gm/day IV, or cefoxitin, 8 gm/day IV, in divided doses is indicated. If *Pseudomonas* is considered a likely in-

fecting organism, carbenicillin, 500 mg/kg/day IV, in divided doses should be added.

4. Adrenal corticosteroids may be administered, but their use in septic shock is controversial, and it is not clear that their use significantly alters patient outcome.

5. If volume replacement fails to reverse hypotension, vasoactive medications are indicated. Dopamine, 2 to 20 μg/kg/min, is recommended.

6. Fresh frozen plasma should be administered if DIC is present.

E. Toxic shock syndrome.

1. A form of staphylococcal endotoxic shock characterized by fever $\geq$38.9° C, hypotension (systolic blood pressure $\leq$90 mm Hg), a diffuse macular erythroderma that subsequently desquamates, and involvement of at least three organ systems.

2. Most cases are reported in menstruating women, some related to tampon use.

3. Management is similar to that of septic shock. The addition of an antistaphylococcal antibiotic such as naficillin, 1 Gm IV every 4 hours may be warranted in cases in which a definite source of staphylococcal infection is identified.

IV. Spinal Shock

A. Causes.—This entity is the result of spinal cord injury, with peripheral vasodilation due to withdrawal of neural vasoconstrictor influence below the injury site.

B. Clinical findings.—These are outlined in Table 1–1. Note the presence of bradycardia, a finding relatively exclusive to this type of shock.

C. Treatment.—This should be as outlined in section II, C, except that the heart rate is not a reliable resuscitation parameter to follow.

2
Trauma Care

Severely or multiply traumatized patients would be evaluated and managed in a systematic fashion, wth emphasis placed on establishing priorities of care based on the nature and severity of injury.

I. Airway Management

Airway management is of the highest priority. Patency of the upper airway should be ensured, with consideration given to the possibility of injury to the cervical part of the spine.

    A. In the unconscious patient, positioning maneuvers such as the chin lift and jaw thrust may produce airway patency. The neck should not be hyperextended in an effort to clear the airway.

    B. Suctioning of the airway may clear it of particulate matter.

    C. Insertion of a nasopharyngeal or oropharyngeal airway may maintain airway patency in an unconscious or stuporous patient.

II. Breathing and the Adequacy and Symmetry of Ventilatory Exchange

All trauma victims should have high-flow oxygen applied unless there is a specific contraindication to this treatment. Ventilatory support should be initiated if respiratory effort is inadequate.

III. Circulatory Evaluation

Initially circulatory evaluation consists of the control of external hemorrhage and the treatment of shock (see Chapter 1).

    A. Application of pressure to all visible external hemorrhage.

    B. Determination of the presence or potential for shock on the basis of an evaluation of vital signs, skin color and moisture, capillary refill, and mental status.

    C. Initiation of circulatory support should consist of the insertion of at least two large-gauge intravenous lines and the infusion of lactated Ringer's solution, the rate of infusion to depend on the patient's clinical status. Pneumatic antishock trousers may also be applied, as indicated.

IV. Resuscitation Monitoring

    A. Frequent evaluation of vital signs, including continuous monitoring of the cardiac rate and rhythm.

    B. Insertion of a Foley catheter and maintenance of a urinary output of at least 50 mL/hr in adults, 1 ml/kg/hr in children. A urinary catheter should not be inserted if there is suspicion of a urethral injury on the basis of blood at the urethral meatus, displacement of the prostate, or other findings. A retrograde urethrogram is indicated in this instance.

    C. Central venous pressure.—Serial assessment of central venous pressure may provide a guide to effectiveness of volume resuscitation in the patient without pre-existing cardiac or pulmonary disease. It may also indicate the presence of shock due to cardiac tamponade. A central venous pressure line should not, however, be inserted until large-gauge peripheral venous cannulation has been accomplished for purposes of volume infusion.

V. Clothing

The patient should be completely unclothed so that an evaluation of the entire body can be accomplished without impediment. At some point in the resuscitation, the patient's back (assuming an initially supine position) should be examined for evidence of injury.

VI. Intubation

Insertion of a nasogastric tube should be done by the orogastric route if there is midfacial injury that may produce a cribriform plate fracture. A nasogastric tube is useful for

    A. Relief of gastric distention.

    B. Removal of gastric contents.

    C. Diagnose the presence of gastrointestinal bleeding or diaphragmial herniation.

VII. Spinal Immobilization

Maintenance of the patient in spinal immobilization until radiographs can be performed is prudent if

    A. There is evidence of spinal bony injury or neurological deficit.

    B. The mechanism of injury strongly suggests the possibility of spinal injury.

VIII. Neurological Monitoring

Frequent reassessment of neurological status is mandatory in the patient with possible neural injury.

    A. In the patient with head trauma, emphasis should be placed on periodic re-evaluation of the level of consciousness.

B. The patient's responsiveness should be recorded through the use of a standardized system such as the Glasgow Coma Scale.
C. The rectal examination and evaluation of sacral sensory function should be a routine part of the examination of the patient with suspected spinal injury.
D. Hypoventilation may result from injury to the cervical spine. The patient's ventilatory status should be followed by assessment of arterial blood gases and measurement of vital capacity.

IX. Extremity Trauma

Generally, these are not life-threatening injuries and should be attended to only after more critical ones have been stabilized.

A. Assessment should include evaluation for swelling, deformity, ecchymosis, tenderness, and crepitation.
B. Evaluation and documentation of circulatory status is essential in all cases. This should include palpating distal pulses, evaluating capillary refill, and noting the color and warmth of the extremity distal to the injury.
   1. The Doppler stethoscope should be used if no pulse is palpable.
   2. Comparison should be made to the contralateral side.
C. Neurological deficit distal to the injury should be noted.
D. A fracture should be considered open if there is any disruption of the skin near a fracture site.
E. Management.
   1. Fractures and suspected fractures should be immobilized prior to radiographic evaluation, the nature of the immobilization depending on the injury.

2. Cooling and elevation should be instituted to reduce swelling.
3. Open wounds should be covered with dry, sterile dressings.
4. When an open fracture is present, broad-spectrum parenteral antibiotics should be instituted and tetanus prophylaxis administered (see Chapter 16).

3
Cardiac Emergencies

I. Acute Myocardial Infarction

A. Definition.— Acute myocardial infarction (AMI) occurs when myocardial necrosis results from an imbalance between the O_2 demands of the myocardium and its arterial blood supply. AMI is usually due to the occlusion of a coronary artery, but thrombosis or hemorrhage into an atheromatous plaque also causes AMI. It also may occur following arterial spasm or embolization of a blood clot or atheromatous material from a site proximal to the obstruction.

B. Incidence.—The disease must be suspected in all persons with chest pain, especially all men over 40 and all postmenopausal women. It also can occur in young men and in menstruating women. Knowing risk factors unless they are very significant is usually not very helpful in the emergency department. The significant risk factors include the following:

1. A history of death or AMI in family members at a relatively young age.
2. Specific disorders such as diabetes mellitus and lipoproteinemia type II.
3. Gross obesity.
4. Heavy smoking.

C. Diagnosis.—The classic uncomplicated AMI patient has a history of crushing substernal chest pain radiating into the left shoulder and arm, sweating, and nausea. The physical examination reveals an anxious patient in severe pain with no other abnormal physical signs. The early electrocardiograph (ECG) shows ST segment elevation and later Q waves corresponding to the site of the myocardial necrosis, and the blood creatine phosphokinase (CK) level is significantly elevated. Unfortunately many AMI patients do not follow this pattern. The threshold for suspecting that a patient has AMI must be relatively low in the emergency department to avoid discharging AMI patients erroneously.

1. Chest pain or discomfort may be relatively mild, may not radiate at all, or may radiate to any of the following: jaw, shoulder, left or right arm, wrist, back, epigastrium.

2. The ECG may be normal or nonspecifically abnormal or may have a pre-existing left bundle-branch block pattern which makes it impossible to rule out AMI by ECG.

3. The CK level may be normal in early stages of infarction but usually rises by 6 hours postinfarction.

4. History.—Stoic or frightened patients may minimize their symptoms; language and cultural barriers may lead to misinterpretation of the historical information.

5. Silent or missed AMI can cause or follow other clinical conditions, and the diagnosis may be very difficult. These conditions include the following:

a. Hypothermia from any cause.

b. Seizures that may be due to cardiac dysrhythmias or decreased cerebral perfusion.

c. Trauma occurring because of the loss of consciousness following an AMI that caused dysrhythmias or hypoperfusion of the brain.

        d. Unconsciousness and stroke.—AMI is not an uncommon cause here due to hypoperfusion or embolization from the damaged endocardium overlying the infarcted area in the heart.

        e. The elderly and diabetics often fail to manifest the usual signs and symptoms of AMI.

D. Evaluation and initial treatment.

    1. All suspected AMI patients must be taken immediately to the emergency department area equipped to deal with cardiac arrest. This must be done with a minimum of anxiety for the patient and with reassurance and confidence expressed by the physicians and nurses providing care.

    2. Begin immediate continuous cardiac rhythm monitoring and an intravenous (IV) line with 5% dextrose in water (D_5W) at a slow rate. Give oxygen by nasal cannula or mask at 8 to 10 L/min.

    3. There should be continuous nursing surveillance and immediate physician availability.

    4. Obtain 12-lead ECG.

    5. Consider ordering a complete blood cell count, serum enzyme determinations, especially cardiac CK, and blood electrolytes, and a urinalysis.

E. Nonspecific treatment.—If the diagnosis of uncomplicated AMI cannot be ruled out, arrange for prompt admission to the critical care unit and consider the following for treatment of pain.

    Nitroglycerine may be used as follows: sublingual (0.4 to 0.6 mg repeated every 10 minutes), in nitropaste form (1 to 2 in.), or IV (5–25 µg/min).

    Morphine sulfate may be administered IV in 2-mg increments to relieve pain and reduce anxiety. Drug-induced hypotension is treated with leg elevation and, if necessary, small increments of IV fluids: 200 cc over 5 to 10 minutes, paying careful attention to the neck veins, lung bases, and the appearance of an S_3 gallop for evidence of incipient cardiac failure. Rarely, morphine in these doses may cause altered levels of consciousness and respiratory depression and may require reversal with naloxone (Narcan), 0.8 mg by IV push.

Prophylactic lidocaine should be considered for all myocardial infarction patients, but definitely for any ventricular ectopy or anterior AMI. Give 1 mg/kg body weight by IV push slowly. A second bolus of 50% to 100% of the initial dose should be given within 10 minutes, and an IV infusion to provide 2 to 4 mg/min should be initiated immediately. Reduce the dose by up to 50% in patients 70 years or older and those with liver disease, cardiac failure, or hypotension.

F. Thrombolytic therapy.—Emergency department administration of IV streptokinase (STK) or tissue-type plasminogen activator (tPA) should be considered for patients who have pain of less than 6 hours' duration and significant ST changes on ECG.

1. Contraindications.—These drugs should be avoided in patients with a history of pathological bleeding (gastrointestinal [GI], central nervous system [CNS]), recent trauma, recent surgery, recent cardiopulmonary resuscitation (CPR), uncontrolled significant hypertension, other serious advanced disease, and receipt of STK within the past year.

2. Consultation.—These drugs should be administered with the cooperation of the cardiologist who will manage the patient's hospital stay.

3. Clotting studies.—In addition to routine AMI patient evaluation, patients need prompt evaluation of clotting studies. Premedication with phenylhydramine (Benadryl) (50 mg IV) and heparin (5,000 IU IV) is usually given.

G. AMI with complications.—The common emergency department complications are dysrhythmias producing hypotension, cardiac failure, cardiogenic shock, and cardiac arrest.

1. Cardiogenic shock.—This condition may occur within hours or several days of the onset of myocardial infarction and has a mortality of 80% or more. It can occur in any AMI patient but is more likely with very large infarcts, anterior infarcts, and combined anterior-inferior infarcts.

   a. Definition.—Cardiogenic shock is a syndrome caused by impaired circulation resulting primarily from poor cardiac pump activity. It usually has a relatively sudden onset, and its effect on vital organs is profound.

   b. Diagnosis.—In the emergency department, the diagnosis is made on the basis of

      (1) Diagnosis of AMI (see Section I, C).

      (2) Evidence of significantly diminished cardiac output, including hypotension, diaphoresis, clammy skin, and an altered level of consciousness.

      (3) Persistence of evidence of poor cardiac output after treating pain, anxiety, and dysrhythmias and a trial of volume expansion (see later).

   c. Treatment.—These patients should be transferred to a critical care unit as soon as possible where a catheter to measure pulmonary wedge pressure can be inserted. Emergency department management of cardiogenic shock patients should be limited to

      (1) Pain relief, reassurance, and continuous nursing surveillance pending transfer to a critical care unit.

      (2) Dysrhythmia prophylaxis and treatment.

      (3) Preload manipulation.

         a Leg elevation.

         b Fluid challenge of 200 cc D$_5$W over 10 minutes. Monitor neck veins and/or the central venous pressure (CVP) line, and remember that the CVP in this kind of patient may not accurately reflect left-sided pressures. Stop fluids if the CVP rises; continue fluid boluses if the CVP is unchanged and the clinical state is not deteriorating.

(4) Pharmacological augmentation.—Dopamine, 200 mg in 250 cc D$_5$W to provide 5 to 15 μg/hg/min. Remember that high doses of dopamine function as an adrenergic stimulant, therefore, start with 5 to 8 μg/kg/min. Dobutamine, 200 mg in 250cc D$_5$W is also useful with a starting dose of 2 to 10 μg/kg/min. Occasionally it is more effective when used with dopamine

(5) Note. Further preload and afterload (vasodilation) manipulation if necessary should be done in the intensive care setting with the appropriate hemodynamic monitoring information available.

2. Cardiogenic pulmonary edema.—This condition in its florid state is easily diagnosed. It is especially terrifying to patients who feel as if they are drowning in their own secretions. (The noncardiac causes of pulmonary edema are discussed in Chapter 5).

a. Definition.—Pulmonary edema results from the accumulation of liquid and solute in the extravascular tissues and spaces of the gas-exchanging areas of the lung. The cardiac causes include the following:

(1) AMI leading to
   a Mitral regurgitation.
   b Left ventricular failure.
   c Left ventricular aneurysm.
   d Ruptured ventricular septum.
(2) Systemic hypertension (severe).
(3) Acute valve damage, left ventricular outflow obstruction.

b. Diagnosis.—The common symptoms and signs are shortness of breath, orthopnea, and paroxysmal nocturnal dyspnea. Rales and, less commonly, bronchospasm may be audible on auscultation. The chest x-ray is extremely important, but x-ray findings may lag behind the clinical state. Early findings, if present, are redistribution of flow to the upper lobes. Later, evidence of increased interstitial fluid can be seen. Arterial blood gases will show hypoxemia and hypocarbia in the early stages. Hypercarbia may be present in later stages due to increased CO_2 retention and increased CO_2 production.

c. Treatment.—The following should be done rapidly:

   (1) Allow the patient to assume the most comfortable position, usually sitting up with legs over the side of the bed. Provide continual surveillance for dysrhythmias.

   (2) Administer high-flow oxygen by cannula or mask if the patient will tolerate it. Rarely, nasal or endotracheal intubation may be necessary.

   (3) In the absence of hypotension, give nitroglycerine, 0.4 mg (1/150 gm) sublingually, or 1 in. of nitroglycerine paste on the skin. For a rapid effect, IV nitroglycerine can be used, starting at 10 μg/min, increasing by 5 to 10 μg/min to a maximum of 250 to 500 μg/min.

   (4) Administer IV morphine sulfate in 2-mg increments to reduce anxiety and produce vasodilation.

   (5) Immediately evaluate a complete blood cell count, serum electrolytes, and arterial blood gases.

   (6) Administer diuretic therapy: furosemide, 20 to 40 mg IV, in a patient who is not currently taking this drug, otherwise dou-

ble the dose; double the dose if there is no response in 30 minutes.

(7) Dysrhythmia prophylaxis.—Reduce hypoxemia, correct the acid-base balance, consider an IV lidocaine bolus, 1 mg/kg body weight, and repeat 10 minutes later followed by IV infusion of 2 to 4 mg/min.

(8) Dysrhythmia treatment.—For pulmonary edema due to a dysrhythmia, speed of treatment is important. Consider cardioversion for fast atrial fibrillation, flutter, or other supraventricular rhythms. Less severe atrial tachyarrhythmias may improve promptly with drug treatment (see Section II, B). Bradyarrhythmias in this setting may require a pacemaker. If available, external pacemakers are very useful. If not, pharmacological pacemakers such as atropine, 0.5 to 1.0 mg IV slowly, should be used initially. Adrenergic drugs such as isoproterenol should be used only with great caution because they increase myocardial oxygen consumption.

(9) For significant bronchospasm, consider aminophylline, 5 mg/kg over 20 minutes, and a reduced maintenance dose of 0.4 mg/kg/hr.

(10) Phlebotomy removing 250 to 500 cc of blood may rapidly reduce the fluid overload. This is rarely needed.

II. Cardiac Dysrhythmias

A. General considerations.

1. Very often, cardiac dysrhythmias reflect an underlying pathological process that is not necessarily isolated to the heart. Patients with these dysrhythmias need careful assessment of their volume sta-

tus, a search for underlying disease, and evaluation of their electrolyte levels, acid-base balance, and medication intake.

2. Reassurance to reduce anxiety and therefore blood catecholamine levels is essential for these patients. Reassurance will not only revert some dysrhythmias to normal sinus rhythm but will also reduce the likelihood of benign dysrhythmias deteriorating into potentially more dangerous disturbances of cardiac rhythm.

3. When the effects of a cardiac dysrhythmia are assessed, particular attention should be paid to those patients who have diminished vascular supply to the brain, myocardium, and kidneys. Slight reductions in blood flow may severely damage these organs.

4. Pacemaker evaluation: with the widespread use of implantable pacemakers, emergency departments often receive patients complaining of "problems with their pacemaker" or who may be symptomatic from a malfunctioning pacemaker. The following approach is safe and useful:

   a. Reveiw the patient's cardiac history and try to identify pacemaker type. X-ray is helpful. Perform a full physical examination including a careful cardiac evaluation.

   b. Review a 12 lead ECG for pacemaker activity.

   c. If pacemaker activity is present, there should be appropriate capture, i.e., a pacemaker spike should be followed by a P wave or a QRS complex. Also, there should be appropriate sensing, i.e., a native P wave or a QRS complex should inhibit the pacemaker.

   d. If no pacemaker activity is present on the 12 lead EKG, there are three possibilities:

      (1) The patient's native rhythm is faster than the set rate of the pacemaker.

      (2) There is oversensing of the T wave or there is myopotential inhibition both of which inhibit the pacemaker activity.

          (3) There is complete battery failure with no output.

    e. Apply a magnet over the pacemaker for 20 seconds and observe the ECG tracing. If the pacemaker is functioning, it will fire at a fixed rate, often called the "magnet rate." If pacemaker activity is now present, the patient was either in a native rhythm faster than the set rate, or there was oversensing. If there is still no activity when the magnet is applied to the pacemaker, complete battery failure has occurred.

    f. Because magnet use carries a small risk of dangerous dysrhythmias, its application should be limited to a short period (20 seconds) for diagnosis only. Prompt communication with the physicians responsible for the insertion of the pacemaker and the management of the patient's care is most helpful in this setting.

B. Specific dysrhythmias.

    1. Sinus tachycardia.

        a. Diagnosis.

            (1) ECG rate.

                a Atrial, 100 to 160/min.

                b Ventricular, 100 to 160/min.

                c P waves normal.

                d PR interval normal.

                e QRS complex normal.

            (2) Causes.

                a Fever.

                b Hypotension.

                c Emotional factors.

                d Hypoxia from myocardial infarction, pulmonary embolism, heart failure.

                e Drugs including epinephrine derivatives, isoproterenol and its related compounds, atropine, caffeine, nicotine, and thyroid medication.

        b. Treatment.—Evaluate for the aforementioned causes and treat accordingly.

2. Paroxysmal supraventricular tachycardia (PSVT).
   a. Diagnosis.
      (1) ECG rate.
         a Atrial, 150 to 230/min (usually 160 to 190/min).
         b Ventricular, 150 to 230/min (usually 160 to 190/min).
         c P waves occasionally not seen.
         d PR interval normal or prolonged— >0.20/sec.
         e QRS segment normal or widened.
         f Carotid sinus massage (CSM) has no effect or terminates the episode.
      (2) Causes.
         a May occur in a "normal" person.
         b Precipitated by caffeine, alcohol, stress, exertion.
         c Wolff-Parkinson-White (WPW) syndrome, rheumatic heart disease, AMI.
   b. Treatment.
      (1) Reassurance and sedation often stop the "normal" types.
      (2) Vagal stimulation including CSM, gagging, face in ice water, Valsalva maneuver.
      (3) Pharmacological agents.
         a For patients who do not have serious evidence of WPW by history or ECG examination, treat as follows:
            (i) Verapamil is the treatment of choice; give 5 to 10 mg IV slowly over a period of 2 to 3 minutes. This may be repeated after 15 to 30 minutes. Contraindications to verapamil therapy include hypotension and congestive heart failure. When hypotension complicates the use of verapamil, it can be reversed with calcium chloride, 0.5 to 1.0 gm IV slowly. This

is more common in patients receiving chronic β-blocker therapy. Occasionally, IV fluids and vasopressors are needed.

(ii) If verapamil treatment is contraindicated or ineffective, alternate pharmacological agents are available and should be used with continuous close monitoring of the patient. These include edrophonium (5 to 10 mg. IV over a period of 1 minute given 5 minutes after administering a 1-mg IV test dose), neostigmine (0.5 to 2.0 mg intramuscularly [IM] or IV), phenylephrine (0.5 to 1.5 mg IV over a period of 30 seconds), metaraminol bitartrate (Aramine; 10 mg IV over a period of 5 minutes), propranolol (0.5 to 1.5 mg/min IV up to 5 mg), and digoxin (0.25 to 0.5 mg IV). Phenylephrine and Aramine should be used with great caution in hypertensive patients. Propranolol use is contraindicated in patients with congestive heart failure and asthma.

b Treatment for WPW patients with paroxysmal supraventricular tachycardia (SVT) or atrial fibrillation is as follows:

(i) Unless electrophysiological studies are available or known, initial therapy should be procainamide (100 mg IV slowly, repeated up to 1 gm) or lidocaine (1 mg/kg IV).

(ii) Atrial fibrillation can occur during treatment, and immediate cardioversion is indicated if the patient is hemodynamically unstable.

(iii) For the stable WPW patient with atrial fibrillation, drug treatment includes procainamide, quinidine, or disopyramide.

3. Paroxysmal atrial tachycardia (PAT) with block.
   a. Diagnosis.
      (1) ECG rate.
          a Atrial, 150 to 200/min.
          b Ventricular, 50 to 100/min—atrioventricular (AV) block, 2:1 or greater.
          c P waves regular and usually normal in shape.
          d PR interval normal in conducted beats.
          e QRS segment normal.
      (2) Causes.
          a Digitalis intoxication, hypokalemia, quinidine, isoproterenol.
          b Arteriosclerotic cardiovascular disease (ASCVD), AMI.
   b. Treatment.
      (1) Stop digitalis therapy.
      (2) Replace potassium, 20 to 40 mEq IV over a period of 2 to 4 hours.
      (3) Propranolol, 0.5 to 1.0 mg/min up to 5 mg unless there is bradycardia or a higher degree of block.
      (4) Phenytoin (Dilantin), 50 mg IV every 2 minutes up to 1,000 mg.

4. Multifocal atrial tachycardia (MAT).
   a. Diagnosis.
      (1) ECG rate.
          a Atrial, >100/min.
          b Ventricular, >100/min.
          c P waves have varying morphology from at least three different foci.
          d PR interval varies.
          e QRS complex is normal.
      (2) Causes.
          a Severe pulmonary disease.
          b Severe cardiac disease of any type.

        c Metabolic and electrolyte imbalances, infection.

        d Drugs: alcohol, bronchodilators.

    b. Treatment.

      (1) Evaluate for aforementioned causes and treat accordingly.

      (2) Occasionally lidocaine or procainamide may control the arrhythmia. However, dysrhythmia is a sign of serious underlying disease that must be treated.

5. Atrial flutter.

    a. Diagnosis.

      (1) ECG rate.

        a Atrial, 200 to 400/min.

        b Ventricular, 50 to 200/min, depending on AV block.

        c P waves are saw-toothed in leads II and V1.

        d QRS complex has normal shape and duration.

        e Relationship of P waves to QRS complex varies from 1:1 to 4:1.

        f CSM often transiently increases AV block for 2:1, 3:1, 4:1.

      (2) Causes.

        a Chronic heart disease.

        b Precipitated by hypoxia, stress, trauma, thyrotoxicosis, alcohol, pulmonary embolus.

        c Occasionally in patients who are receiving insufficient digitalis.

    b. Treatment.

      (1) Evaluate for aforementioned causes and treat accordingly.

      (2) Cardioversion, especially in hemodynamically compromised patient: use low energy, 25 to 50 W-seconds, and if initially unsuccessful, double the energy for the next shock. Digitalis intoxication is a relative contraindication, but cardioversion

may be necessary in the hemodynamically compromised patient. Start with very low energy, i.e., 5 to 10 W-seconds. Sedation using IV diazepam, 5 to 10 mg, or midazolam, 2 to 4 mg IV slowly, should be used to reduce patient discomfort.

(3) Verapamil, 5 mg IV, usually slows the ventricular rate even when conversion does not occur.

(4) Digoxin, by increasing the AV block, converts atrial flutter to atrial fibrillation with a slowed ventricular rate. The dose is 0.5 to 0.75 mg IV after checking the serum K^+ concentration. Following conversion, digitalize the patient fully.

(5) Propranolol, 0.5 to 1.0 mg/min IV up to 5 mg slowly, may be used in urgent situations. Contraindications are asthma, severe congestive heart failure, and AV block.

6. Atrial fibrillation.
   a. Diagnosis.
      (1) ECG rate.
         a Atrial, >400/min.
         b Ventricular, 100 to 200/min (irregular).
         c P waves not identifiable—wavy baseline.
         d QRS complex usually normal shape—irregularly spaced.
      (2) Causes.
         a Myocardial disease of any cause.
         b Precipitation by alcohol or stress.
         c Myocardial infarction.
         d Electrolyte imbalance, especially hypokalemia.
         e Mental stress, thyrotoxicosis, pulmonary embolism, WPW syndrome.
   b. Treatment.
      (1) Evaluate for underlying cause and treat accordingly.

(2) In hemodynamically stable patient, give digoxin IV or orally. The dose for IV use is 0.5 to 0.75 mg, followed by 0.25 mg every 1 to 4 hours for 1 to 3 doses. (The usual digitalizing dose is 1 to 1.5 mg.) When the rate is controlled, continue maintenance therapy of 0.125 to 0.25 mg daily.

(3) In a patient with WPW syndrome, use procainamide, quinidine, or disopyramide. Avoid digitalis. Drugs are much less effective when the shortest R–R interval is <0.25 sec. Cardioversion is a better alternative, especially in hemodynamically compromised patients.

(4) In hemodynamically compromised patients, synchronized cardioversion is indicated. Using IV sedation (diazepam, 5 to 10 mg, or midazolam, 2 to 4 mg IV slowly), starting with 50 W-seconds and increase by 50 W-seconds until successful.

(5) Verapamil can be useful in slowing the ventricular response to atrial flutter and atrial fibrillation. It acts by blocking calcium flow through the slow channels in the sinoatrial (SA) and AV nodes. The dosage is 0.075 to 0.15 mg/kg, 5 to 10 mg IV slowly. Side effects, which are uncommon, include bradycardia, hypotension, and AV block. Its use is hazardous in cardiogenic shock and severe sinus nodal disease, and it should be used with caution in patients taking β-blocking drugs or those with digitalis toxicity.

7. Sinus bradycardia.
  a. Diagnosis.
    (1) ECG rate.
      a Atrial, <60/min.
      b Ventricular, <60/min.

   c P wave normal.
   d PR interval normal.
   e QRS complex normal.
  (2) Causes.
   a Effect of vagal stimulation due to Valsalva maneuver, CSM, vomiting, raised intracranial pressure, anxiety.
   b Myocardial infarction, especially inferior.
   c Drugs: digoxin, morphine, propranolol, quinidine.
   d Sinus node disease, e.g., ASCVD, rheumatic fever.
   e Hypothyroidism, hypothermia, hypokalemia.
 b. Treatment.
  (1) In asymptomatic patients, no treatment except observation, e.g., in AMI.
  (2) In patients who show hemodynamic compromise
   a Atropine, 0.5 mg IV every 5 to 10 minutes up to 2 mg. If unsuccessful, see *b* or *c* below.
   b Isoproterenol, 1 to 2 mg in 500 cc at 1 to 4 µg/min, titrated to improve cardiac output and avoid ventricular dysrhythmias.
   c If available, an external pacemaker may be quite effective.
8. Atrioventricular block.
 a. Diagnosis.
  (1) First-degree AV block.—PR interval >0.20 seconds is of little clinical significance and needs no treatment.
  (2) Second-degree AV block.—ECG rate: atrial, 60 to 100/min, and ventricular, less than the atrial rate. There are two types:
   a Wenkebach (Mobitz I).—P waves are normal. The PR interval has progressive

prolongation and then one "dropped" beat. The R–R interval shortens with each beat. The QRS complex is normal.

   b Mobitz II.—P waves are normal. The PR interval is normal for a conducted beat or a dropped beat without progressive prolongation. The QRS complex is normal.

  (3) Third-degree AV block (complete heart block).

    a Rate.—Atrial is variable, and ventricular <50/min, but there may be a 60 to 100/min accelerated idioventricular rhythm.

    b ECG.—P waves can reflect normal or any supraventricular dysrhythmia. The QRS complex has a bizarre shape; the closer the focus to the AV node, the more normal the QRS shape.

    c Causes.

      (i) ASCVD, especially AMI.

      (ii) Drugs.—Digitalis, antihypertensives, propranolol.

      (iii) Myocarditis.

 b. Treatment.

  (1) Treat the patients with hemodynamic compromise, angina, or congestive heart failure.

  (2) Atropine, 0.5 to 1.0 mg IV every 5 to 10 minutes up to 2 mg, with larger rather than smaller doses because of the paradoxical vagotonia that may follow small doses.

  (3) Isoproterenol is occasionally successful at 1 to 2 mg in 500 cc, 1 to 10 μg/min IV, if atropine fails. Monitor for cardiac arrhythmias, especially premature ventricular contractions (PVCs), that are different from the idioventricular rhythm.

(4) Ventricular pacing is definitely indicated for third-degree AV block, Mobitz II, and a new bifascicular block associated with AMI. Pacemaker placement under fluoroscopy is preferred, but an external percutaneous pacemaker or blind transvenous placement of a floating pacemaker may temporize successfully in urgent situations.

9. PVCs.
   a. Diagnosis.
      (1) ECG rate.
         a Atrial, 60 to 100/min.
         b Ventricular, usually 60 to 100/min but irregular pulse.
         c P waves normal.
         d PR interval normal for basic rhythm, no P wave for PVC.
         e Normal QRS interspersed with bizarre-shaped QRS complexes, 0.12 seconds.
      (2) Potential for ventricular tachycardia (VT) and/or fibrillation (VF) especially in AMI if the following occur.
         a Unifocal PVCs more than six per minute.
         b Multifocal PVCs, i.e., different shaped QRS complex in same ECG lead.
         c Bigeminy or trigeminy, i.e., PVC coupled to normal QRS complex.
         d "Salvos of PVCs."
         e "R-on-T" phenomenon, i.e., PVC arises on T wave of preceding normal QRS segment (controversial).
         f VF or VT commonly occur without "warning" PVCs.
      (3) Causes.
         a Usually indicates significant heart disease.

    b Hypoxia from any cause.

    c Metabolic disturbances.

    d Electrolyte imbalance, especially hypokalemia.

    e Drugs.—Catecholamines, isoproterenol, tricyclic antidepressants, caffeine, alcohol, tobacco, digitalis, quinidine, procainamide.

    f Occasionally PVCs are benign.

  b. Treatment.

    (1) Evaluate for underlying cause and treat accordingly. Specifically, correct hypoxia and abnormal metabolic state and stop treatment with any precipitating drugs.

    (2) PVCs with sinus bradycardia may represent "escape beats." Atropine (0.5 to 1.0 mg IV) will increase the rate and abolish PVCs that occur in this setting.

    (3) Dangerous PVCs, i.e., salvos, multifocal, more than six per minute, and bigeminy need immediate treatment, especially in the setting of AMI.

      a Lidocaine (1 mg/kg), usually 100 mg by IV push, followed by a second bolus 10 minutes later of the same dose, followed by IV infusion of 2 gm in 500 cc at 2 to 4 mg/min. Reduce the bolus and maintenance dose by half in cardiac failure and liver disease patients. Use with caution in bradycardia.

      b Procainamide, 100 to 200 mg IV over 2 to 3 minutes, followed by 100 mg every 5 minutes until PVCs are suppressed. Do not exceed 1,000 mg. Follow with an IV infusion of 1 to 5 mg/min.

      c Other drugs, e.g., bretylium (5 to 10 mg/kg over a period of 10 minutes), propranolol (0.5 to 1.0 mg/min IV up to 5 mg, slowly), and phenytoin (50 mg

IV slowly every 2 minutes up to 1 gm), and override pacing may be indicated in selected cases.

10. Ventricular tachycardia.
    a. Diagnosis.
        (1) ECG rate.
            a Atrial variable.
            b Ventricular, 100 to 200/min.
            c P wave usually independent or retrograde.
            d QRS complex, bizarre shaped and widened, >0.12 seconds.
        (2) Causes are the same as for PVCs (see section 9,a,(3)).
    b. Treatment.—This is a very dangerous rhythm. The therapy depends on the impact of this rhythm on the patient's condition.
        (1) If patient is fully conscious and only mildly symptomatic, administer lidocaine, 1 mg/kg by IV bolus, repeat in 10 minutes, and initiate a lidocaine IV infusion to deliver 1 to 4 mg/min. If conversion does not occur, resort to following treatments.
        (2) If the patient is hypotensive or becomes confused, consider cardioversion immediately with low energy of 25 to 50 W-seconds and double the energy level with each unsuccessful attempt. If necessary, use IV sedation: Diazepam 5 to 10 mg IV, or Midazolam 2 to 4 mg IV, always given slowly. Administer lidocaine as in (1).
        (3) Correct hypoxia or abnormal metabolic state and stop treatment with any precipitating drugs.
        (4) Resistant or recurring VT may require the following:
            a Procainamide (Pronestyl), 100 mg/min IV for 2 minutes, then 200 mg over a

period of 5 minutes, repeated up to a loading dose of 1 gm. The maintenance dose is titrated at 1 to 5 mg/min.

b Bretylium, 5 to 10 mg/kg body weight IV, slowly over a span of 10 minutes. Profound hypotension is a well-documented side effect.

c Propranolol (Inderal), 1 mg/min up to 5 mg. Use cautiously in patients with bronchospasm, cardiac failure, and heart block.

d Search for rare causes of VT such as drug overdose, underestimated hypoxia, untreated acidosis, hypokalemia, sometimes with hypomagnesemia, and hypovolemia.

III. Torsade de Pointes

A. Diagnosis.
  1. ECG rate.
    a. Ventricular rate of 160 to 280 and long QT interval.
    b. Irregular ventricular rhythm with cycles of alternating electrical polarity and QRS peaks rotating around isoelectric line.
    c. Ventricular amplitude varies in sinusoidal pattern.
    d. Often occurs with bradyarrhythmias or ventricular bigeminy with long coupling interval; initiated by PVC on T wave.
  2. Causes.
    a. Antiarrhythmic agents (especially quinidine, procainamide, and disopyramide), phenothiazines and tricyclic antidepressants prolong the QT interval.
    b. Hypokalemia, hypomagnesemia, and hypocalcemia.

      c. Intracerebral hemorrhage, liquid protein diets, myocardial ischemia.

B. Treatment.

1. Patients are usually without major hemodynamic compromise, and withdrawl of offending agent or correction of electrolyte imbalance is sufficient.

2. When patient is hemodynamically compromised, lidocaine, phenytoin, or atrial or ventricular over-drive pacing are effective in reducing the QT interval. Bretylium may be useful. (For dosages see section II,9,b.)

3. Avoid quinidine, disopyramide, and procainamide.

IV. Cardiac Arrest

A. General considerations.

1. Cardiac arrest is the clinical state when cardiac output is effectively zero. Although it is usually due to VF, asystole, or electromechanical dissociation (EMD), it can be produced by other dysrhythmias that occasionally result in totally ineffective cardiac output. These include profound bradycardias and VT.

2. For most cardiac arrests, the evaluation and treatment plan should follow the principles and details described in this section. However, in special cases, specific drugs or surgical procedures are life-saving if administered or performed immediately. This means that every cardiac arrest must be evaluated for these relatively rare but therapeutically amenable causes. These include the following:

    a. Opiate or propoxyphene (Darvon) overdose requiring naloxone, 0.8 mg IV.

    b. Tricyclic antidepressant overdose appearing as a nonperfusing tachydysrhythmia requiring physostigmine, 2 mg IV.

    c. Massive pulmonary embolus requiring heparin, 5,000 units IV, immediately and consideration for subsequent embolectomy.

    d. Pericardial tamponade requiring needle or open pericardiotomy.

    e. Tension pneumothorax requiring immediate needle decompression and chest tube insertion.

    f. Hypothemia needing rewarming as described in Chapter 27.

3. Every cardiac arrest resuscitation team must have a single person identified as the leader. For the patient to have the best chance of success, this clinician should give all medication and procedure orders and receive all laboratory information for clinical decision making.

4. Every cardiac arrest resuscitation is a complex set of events, many of which must be done simultaneously. Throughout, every aspect must be scrutinized to be sure the resuscitation is being carried out as effectively as possible. Specifically, the following must be done:

    a. Frequent evaluation of mucous membranes and extremities, auscultation of the lungs, and rarely chest x-rays, when indicated, to check ventilation and oxygenation.

    b. Close attention to the technique of cardiac compression and to the presence of a palpable femoral pulse transmitted by cardiac compression.

    c. Measurement of arterial blood gases to identify hypoxemia, hypercarbia, and acidosis or alkalosis.

    d. Repeated evaluation of clinical history and physical findings to identify causes amenable to specific therapy.

5. Closed cardiac compression is effective in most situations. Ocasionally, due to specific causes or when the cardiopulmonary resuscitation tech-

nique is adequate but no femoral or carotid pulse is palpable, emergency thoracotomy and internal cardiac massage must be considered. This situation arises most commonly in the following cases:

a. Traumatic arrest secondary to
   (1) Penetrating heart wounds.
   (2) Cardiac tamponade that is unresponsive to pericardiocentesis.
   (3) Massive crush injuries to the chest.
   (4) Blunt chest injuries with suspected rupture of atria, ventricles, or aorta.

b. Severe hypothermia with ventricular fibrillation (pulses may be felt with CPR) and no availability of cardiopulmonary bypass, i.e., requiring direct rewarming of the heart.

c. Massive bleeding that is unresponsive to fluid and blood replacement, i.e., cross-clamping of the descending aorta.

d. Structural abnormalities precluding effective external chest massage.
   (1) Emphysematous patient with barrel-shaped chest.
   (2) Severe pectus carinatum.
   (3) Severe kyphoscoliosis.

e. Electric shock with refractory ventricular fibrillation. Pulses are often present with CPR.

6. The decision to terminate cardiac arrest resuscitation rests with the team leader and the patient's physician, if the latter is available. Although each decision is individual, the medical literature contains overwhelming evidence that under the following circumstances strong consideration should be given to halting resuscitation because the likelihood of a successful outcome is extremely small.

   a. Indications.
      (1) Pulselessness and apnea for more than 10 minutes prior to the initiation of CPR.
      (2) No clinical response after more than 30 minutes of advanced cardiac life support

(ACLS), including that given outside the hospital.

(3) No ventricular ECG activity, i.e., persistent asystole, after more than 10 minutes of ACLS.

(4) Pre-existing terminal illness such as terminal cancer and end-stage cardiac disease.

b. Exceptions.—Near drowning, hypothermia from any cause, and exsanguinating trauma, especially in young people. Under these circumstances, resuscitation efforts should be aggressively pursued, and the specific therapies listed earlier should be initiated promptly.

B. Evaluation and treatment.

1. Confirm unresponsiveness.—In trauma situations, minimize the risk of cervical spine injury. Call for help!

2. Establish an airway by using the head tilt–chin lift maneuver since cardiac arrest victims may fall and suffer neck injuries. If the head tilt–chin lift technique is unsuccessful, use the jaw thrust technique or the head tilt–neck lift maneuver to establish an adequate airway (Figs. 3–1 through 3–4). Inspect the mouth rapidly, clearing any food, vomitus, or dentures.

3. Attempt to give two quick breaths and confirm that the chest moves appropriately; if it does not, perform obstructed airway maneuvers.

   a. Again, check the mouth for foreign bodies or loose dentures by using a finger sweep.

   b. Direct examination of the pharynx and laryngeal area may reveal a foreign body accessible with McGill forceps.

   c. Administer four abdominal thrusts by kneeling next to the victim's hips or sitting astride him and pushing sharply into the epigastrium. For obese or pregnant victims, administer four chest thrusts by placing one palm on either

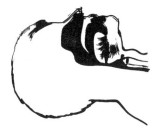 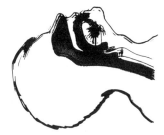

Closed Airway   **Open Airway**

FIG 3–1.

In the unconscious patient, inspiratory efforts may draw the tongue back into the throat. Tilting the head back usually causes the lower jaw to move forward and the airway to open.

side of the lower part of the chest anteriorly and thrusting posteriorly. Check the mouth and attempt ventilation for evidence of successful relief of airway obstruction. Repeat several times as needed. If absent, repeat the sequence until the obstruction is relieved.

d. If unsuccessful, do the following: roll the victim toward you and give four backslaps between the shoulder blades. Check the mouth with a finger sweep and attempt ventilation.

e. Finally, if all efforts fail, cricothyrotomy should be carried out. This procedure is much more effective and safer than tracheostomy is in this setting. The latter may be done later as an elective procedure if a more permanent tracheal opening is required.

f. Start CPR, and as team members arrive, delegate responsibility for airway management, ECG interpretation, and drug administration.

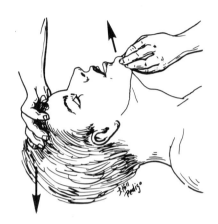

Head Tilt – Chin Lift

FIG 3–2.

For trauma patients and for patients in whom the tilt-neck lift does not provide an adequate airway, lifting the chin may be of value. Place the fingers under the bony part of the jaw near the chin and lift the jaw forward while supporting the jaw, i.e., the airway.

    g. Establish control of the airway as follows:
       (1) Continue mouth-to-mouth or mouth-to-mask ventilation until a bag-value mask is available.
       (2) Tracheal intubation is not necessary immediately since in most circumstances bag-valve mask ventilation is adequate to restore oxygenation. Tracheal intubation should be attempted only when a skilled person is present. Each attempt should be limited to 30 seconds, and failed efforts

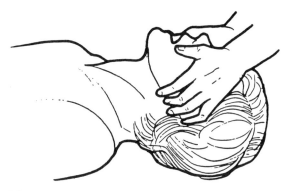

FIG 3–3.
Jaw-thrust method for opening airway. (From Rosen P, et al: *Emergency Medicine: Concepts and Clinical Practice.* St. Louis, CV Mosby Co, 1988, p 91. Used by permission.)

should be followed immediately by vigorous bag-valve mask ventilation to reduce hypoxia. Attention must be paid to the tube length to avoid right main-stem bronchus intubation. The endotracheal tube must be immobilized securely with adhesive tape.

(3) In trauma patients, care must be taken to minimize the risk of trauma to the cervical spine when intubation is attempted. In-line cervical traction is necessary.

h. Establish an IV line simultaneously with ECG interpretation since rapid defibrillation may be lifesaving (see later). A large-bore peripheral IV line should be established initially, and if possible, a long line should be passed into the central circulation. Extremity veins including the femoral veins should be tried. Subclavian

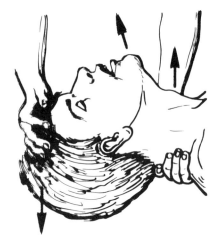

Head Tilt-Neck Lift

FIG 3–4.
With one hand on the patient's forehead and the other hand under the neck, tilt the head posteriorly, and lift the neck anteriorly. In trauma patients, this maneuver may increase the chance of cervical injury; it should, however, be done with the minimum amount of force necessary to open the airway. The head tilt-chin lift (see Fig 3–1) has less risk of causing cervical injury.

and internal or external jugular lines should be attempted after the airway is secure or if circulation has not been restored after initial drug administration via a peripheral vein. At this stage, a central line via one of these routes may also provide information that is useful for subsequent therapy. Intercardiac injections should be avoided because of the risk of coronary artery laceration and the likelihood of intractable dysrhythmias resulting from the inadvertent injection of drugs directly into the myocardium. Instillation of drugs into the trachea via the endotracheal tube is an effective alternative when it is not possible to establish an adequate IV line rapidly. Drugs should be in a volume of 5 to 10 mL, and initial doses of epinephrine, lidocaine, and atropine are similar to those for IV administration, but subsequent doses should be adjusted downward. These drugs should be injected into the endotracheal tube by using a CVP catheter or long needle, followed by vigorous bagging. Curently, no scientific evidence is available on the efficacy of other cardiac arrest drugs administered via the endotracheal route. The sublingual area, a very vascular tissue, should be considered for the administration of these drugs. IV doses should be used. Sodium bicarbonate administration should be considered only after initial specific drug therapy has been given without restoration of circulation. The initial dose is 1 mg/kg. Subsequent doses should be based on arterial blood gas results. When these are unavailable, sodium bicarbonate may be given every 10 to 15 minutes at half the initial dose.

i. Determine the ECG rhythm by using quick-look defibrillator paddles if available or standard ECG tracing. Treatment depends on the cardiac rhythm.

    (1) VF.

        a Administer 200 J of delivered energy immediately. If unsuccessful, administer a second shock of 200 to 300 J immediately and, if necessary, a third of up to 360 J. Give 0.5 to 1.0 mg of epinephrine

IV separately if defibrillation is unsuccessful. In an unwitnessed arrest consider sodium bicarbonate early. After epinephrine and bicarbonate administration, repeat defibrillation. Additional sodium bicarbonate administration should be based on arterial blood gas results. In out-of-hospital cardiac arrests, administer half the initial dose every 10 to 15 minutes. Epinephrine may be repeated every 5 minutes, or even more often.

b If VF is intractable, carefully re-evaluate the patient to rule out unrecognized hypoxia due to a pneumothorax, incorrect tracheal tube placement, or hypovolemia, and correct the acid-base imbalance. If unsuccessful, try these drugs and attempt defibrillation after each drug:

(i) Lidocaine, 1 mg/kg by IV bolus, and repeat defibrillation. If unsuccessful, repeat the bolus, and establish a maintenance infusion at 1 to 4 mg/min.

(ii) Bretylium, 5 mg/kg by IV bolus, and repeat defibrillation.

(iii) Procainamide, 100 mg by IV bolus over a period of 1 minute, 200 mg over 5 minutes, up to a loading dose of 1 gm, and repeat defibrillation.

(iv) Propranolol, 1 to 5 mg at 1 mg/min IV, and repeat defibrillation.

(v) Atropine, 1 mg IV, repeat defibrillation.

(2) Ventricular asystole (VA).

a Confirm in two ECG leads. If in doubt, treat as VF.

    b Administer epinephrine, 0.5 to 1.0 mg by IV bolus. If a peripheral IV line is not available, use a sublingual-route IV, or instill into the trachea and ventilate vigorously. If available, activate a percutaneous pacemaker. If ineffective, do the following:

    c Administer atropine, 1 to 2 mg, via IV bolus.

    d Consider administering sodium bicarbonate, 1 mEg/kg, especially if arrest is unwitnessed or there is prolonged downtime.

    e Very rarely, a transvenous pacemaker may restore an effective rhythm.

(3) EMD.

    a Characterized by a relatively organized ECG complex with no evidence of mechanical pumping action. Be sure to exclude pericardial tamponade, tension pneumothorax, hypovolemia, severe acidosis, and pulmonary embolism.

    b Administer epinephrine, O.5 to 1.0 mg IV.

    c Consider sodium bicarbonate, 1 mEq/kg.

    d If the ECG shows an idioventricular rhythm with no P waves and a wide, bizarre QRS, consider giving atropine, 1 mg IV.

4

Electrolyte and Acid-Base Disorders

I. Acid-Base Balance

A. General considerations.—Changes in the acid-base balance are identified by the evaluation of arterial blood gases. Nomograms or simple formulas (examples occur throughout the chapter) can be used to define acid-base abnormalities, which may be either acidosis or alkalosis. Both can be produced by respiratory or metabolic causes, and mixed abnormalities may coexist because one may compensate for the effect of the other. The four states are metabolic acidosis, metabolic alkalosis, respiratory acidosis, and respiratory alkalosis. Use the bicarbonate (HCO_3) value of the laboratory electrolyte results if there is a possibility of a complex abnormality. The HCO_3^- in blood gas evaluation is derived indirectly from pH and Pco_2 levels.

B. Respiratory acidosis.
   1. The mechanism of production is hypoventilation due to the following:
      a. Retention of CO_2 resulting from primary pulmonary disease e.g., chronic obstructive pulmonary disease (COPD) or asthma.
      b. Centrally acting drugs interfering with ventilation and producing CO_2 retention.

c. Neuromuscular diseases, thoracic or spinal trauma, massive obesity, and airway obstruction interfere with ventilation, which leads to CO_2 retention.

2. Clinical presentation.

a. The signs and symptoms of the condition that causes the hypoventilation.

b. Possible altered levels of consciousness due to cerebral edema following severe CO_2 retention.

c. Arterial blood gases.

   (1) $Paco_2$ elevated above the normal range of 38 to 42 mm Hg; calculate the expected pH for the patient's $Paco_2$. For every 10 mm Hg above a $Paco_2$ of 40, the pH usually falls 0.08. For example, for $Paco_2$ = 50, the calculated or expected pH = 7.32.

   (2) If the patient's pH is significantly below the calculated or expected pH, metabolic acidosis is present in addition to respiratory acidosis or alkalosis.

   (3) If the patient's pH is significantly above the expected value, metabolic alkalosis is present in addition to the respiratory abnormality.

   (4) The Po_2 value should be compared with the expected value for the patient's age:

   $$\text{Age-adjusted } Po_2 = 104 - 0.4 \times \text{Age}$$

   Because of the shape of the oxyhemoglobin dissociation curve, a Pao_2 above 60 mm Hg is acceptable because it represents 90% saturation. Even small decreases below 60 mm Hg represent significant falls in the saturation level, i.e., potential tissue hypoxia.

d. Serum electrolytes.—Serum bicarbonate levels will be normal in the acute setting and elevated in the chronic or compensated state due to reabsorption of bicarbonate by the kidney. Look for anion gap, and consider osmolal gap as well, if clinically appropriate (see Section C, 2, b, 3).

3. Treatment.
   a. Treat the underlying cause of the hypoventilation.
   b. Improve the ventilation by airway suction, bag-valve mask ventilation, and if necessary, nasal or endotracheal intubation.
   c. Rarely is $NaHCO_3$ administration indicated for pure respiratory acidosis. Correction of hypoventilation is the correct initial treatment. Recheck arterial blood gas concentrations as necessary to evaluate any improvement in the ventilation.

C. Metabolic acidosis.
   1. Mechanism of production.
      a. Diseases such as diabetic ketoacidosis, alcoholic ketoacidosis, and uremia result in an excess of acidic ions that cannot be excreted rapidly enough to prevent acidosis.
      b. Ingestion of acidic compounds such as methanol, aspirin, ethylene glycol, and paraldehyde produces severe metabolic acidosis.
      c. Anaerobic metabolism following cellular hypoxia produces lactic acidosis. This may occur in persons with sepsis, shock, convulsions, ketoacidosis, and uremia.
   2. Clinical presentations and diagnosis.
      a. The signs and symptoms of the underlying condition that causes the acidosis may be present.
      b. Arterial blood gases.
         (1) $Paco_2$ should be evaluated (see Section B, 2) for evidence of hypoventilation i.e., $Paco_2$ higher than 40 mmHg. The expected pH should be calculated.

(2) The patient's pH should be compared with the expected pH calculated from the $Paco_2$. If the patient's pH is less than the expected pH, metabolic acidosis is present. A pH below 7.1 can have serious effects on cardiac and neurological function.

(3) Check serum osmolality, electrolytes, and renal function tests.

    a Serum osmolality is calculated and compared with the measured level from the laboratory. A significant osmolal gap indicates the presence of additional solutes in the serum (see Chapter 29).

    b Electrolytes are evaluated to assess the anion gap.

$$Na - (Cl + HCO_3) = Anion\ gap$$

An anion gap greater than 15 indicates an excess of lactate or similar acidic ions producing metabolic acidosis.

    c An elevated blood urea nitrogen (BUN) level indicates renal failure or prerenal or postrenal azotemia.

(4) Toxicology screen.—If an overdose is suspected, a blood, urine, and gastric aspirate examination may identify the ingestion of drugs producing metabolic acidosis.

3. Treatment.

    a. Treat the underlying cause.

    b. $NaHCO_3$ administration should be considered if the pH is below 7.1 and HCO_3 is below 10.

$$Dosage = Desired\ HCO_3 - Observed\ HCO_3) \times (0.4) \times Weight\ in\ kg =$$
$$mEq\ HCO_3\ needed$$

But only one third to half of this dose should be administered before arterial blood gases and serum electrolytes are rechecked.
c. For patients with values for pH above 7.1 and $NaHCO_3$ above 10, only aggressive treatment of the underlying condition is indicated initially.

D. Respiratory alkalosis.
　1. Mechanism of production.
　　a. Hyperventilation due to psychogenic causes is the most common form of respiratory alkalosis seen in the emergency department. However, it should be diagnosed only after excluding the more dangerous causes.
　　b. Compensatory hyperventilation may follow metabolic acidosis due to stimulation of the medullary respiratory center by the acidic ions.
　　c. Hypoxia due to congestive heart failure and pulmonary disease such as pulmonary embolus produce hyperventilation.
　　d. The central action of certain drugs and brain stem diseases produce hyperventilation.
　2. Clinical presentation.
　　a. A common presentation of psychogenic hyperventilation is paresthesias of the extremities and the circumoral area, dizziness, chest discomfort, and rarely carpal pedal spasm.
　　b. Exclude potentially lethal conditions such as pulmonary embolism.
　　c. Arterial blood gases.
　　　The $Paco_2$ is decreased below normal, and the calculated or expected pH is elevated. If the patient's actual pH is significantly below the calculated or expected pH, metabolic acidosis is also present.
　3. Treatment.
　　a. If hypoxia is the cause, correct it immediately.

      b. Look for and treat any underlying cause, especially pulmonary embolism.

      c. For psychogenic hyperventilation only, use rebreathing CO_2 with a paper bag or administer a mild tranquilizer, diazepam, 5 to 10 mg orally or intravenously, as indicated.

E. Metabolic alkalosis.

  1. Mechanism of production.

      a. Loss of acid through vomiting or excessive gastric suction produces alkalosis.

      b. Chronic or excessive diuretic administration produces hyperchloremia leading to alkalosis.

      c. Severe pure K^+ depletion results in the movement of H^+ into the cells, thus producing alkalosis.

  2. Clinical presentation.

      a. Signs and symptoms of the underlying condition.

      b. Arterial blood gases.—Blood pH and HCO_3 level elevated above normal.

      c. Serum electrolytes.—Serum K^+ is decreased, Cl^- is decreased, and HCO_3 is increased.

  3. Treatment.

      a. Replace K^+ if needed as described in Section V, D, 3.

      b. Cl^- replacement is calculated by first determining the bicarbonate excess.

$$NaHCO_3 \text{ excess} = (\text{Desired } HCO_3 - \text{Observed } HCO_3) \times 0.4 \times (\text{Weight in kg})$$
$$= Cl^- \text{ deficiency}$$

      c. Replace the Cl^- lost when using NaCl and KCl, depending on the K^+ level (see Section V,D,3).

II. Hypernatremia

A. Mechanisms of production.
  1. Significant hypernatremia occurs only when thirst cannot compensate for the hypertonic state. This occurs most frequently with severe vomiting or diarrhea, obtundation, or environmental lack of water or in infants who are unable to make their needs known.
  2. Water loss in excess of sodium loss (both are lost).
     This is the most common mechanism of hypernatremia. Causes include gastroenteritis, sweating, and osmotic diuresis (due to hyperglycemia, iatrogenic mannitol, or the urea load of infant formulas).
  3. Pure water loss without sodium loss.
     This is much less common. Causes include diabetes insipidus (hypothalamic or nephrogenic) and excessive sweating from hypermetabolic states (hyperpyrexia or hyperthyroidism).
  4. Excess intake of sodium.
     This occurs mostly by accident. Among the causes are excessive administration of sodium bicarbonate during cardiac resuscitation, inadvertent use of intravenous hypertonic saline instead of dextrose solutions (e.g., 3% saline instead of 5% dextrose), accidental substitution of salt for sugar in the preparation of infant formulas, and drinking of seawater after shipwrecks.
B. Causes (*Note:* Table 4–1 compares the causes listed below with the mechanisms described above.)
  1. Gastrointestinal loss.
  2. Sweat loss.
  3. Osmotic diuresis.
  4. Diabetes insipidus.
  5. Hypermetabolic states.
  6. Accidental or iatrogenic.

TABLE 4-1.
Etiology of Hypernatremia

Etiology	H_2O Loss > Na Loss	Pure H_2O Loss	Increased NA Intake
Gastrointestinal loss	X		
Sweat loss	X	X	
Osmotic diuresis	X		
Diabetes insipidus		X	
Hypermetabolic states		X	
Accidental or iatrogenic	X		X

C. Clinical presentation.
   1. Nearly all the symptoms of hypernatremia are due to cellular dehydration caused by a fluid shift from the isotonic intracellular compartment to the hypertonic extracellular compartment. Sodium remains primarily in the extracellular space.
   2. If there is a net loss of total body sodium as well as water, then the volume of the extracellular (and therefore intravascular) compartment will decrease. This may lead to significant or even lethal hypotension.
   3. Neurological symptoms predominate in persons with hypernatremia: thirst, lethargy, coma, muscle irritability, and seizures. Severe cerebral dehydration may lead to hemorrhage as the brain shrinks away from its vascular attachments.
D. Treatment
   1. Replacement of water is central to correction of hypernatremia. Oral intake may suffice. Intravenous 5% dextrose in water may also be used.
   2. If a significant amount of sodium has been lost, intravenous normal saline will replace both water and sodium, and it is hypotonic relative to the patient's hypertonic serum.
   3. Rapid correction of hypernatremia may lead to significant rebound cerebral edema. Correction should therefore be limited to half the fluid loss over the first 24 hours.

Fluid loss = Normal total-body water −
$$\text{Current total-body water}$$
Normal total-body water (L) =
$$0.6 \times \text{Normal body weight (kg)}$$
Current total-body water =
$$\text{Normal total-body water} \times \frac{\text{Normal serum Na}^+}{\text{Current serum Na}^+}$$

III. Hyponatremia

A. Mechanisms of production.
1. Water retention greater than sodium retention (both are retained).
   a. The total-body water content is increased, total-body sodium content is increased, and urinary sodium levels are usually less than 10 mEq/L.
   b. The patient usually is clinically *edematous.*
   c. Disorders include congestive heart failure, nephrosis, and cirrhosis.
2. Sodium loss is greater than water loss (both are lost).
   a. The total-body water content is decreased, total-body sodium content is decreased, and urinary sodium levels are usually less than 10 mEq/L if sodium and water loss is nonrenal. Urinary sodium is usually more than 10 mEq/L if sodium and water loss is renal.
   b. The patient is in a net state of *dehydration.*
   c. Disorders include the following:
      (1) Nonrenal loss.—Vomiting, diarrhea, sweating, burns, pancreatitis, massive trauma.
      (2) Renal loss.—Diuretics, adrenal mineralocorticoid insufficiency, salt-wasting nephropathy, renal tubular acidosis.
3. Water retention without sodium retention (some sodium may be lost through compensatory mechanisms, but the principal abnormality is water retention rather than sodium loss).
   a. The total-body water content is increased, total-body sodium content may be somewhat decreased, and urinary sodium levels are usually more than 20 mEq/L.
   b. The patient does not frequently demonstrate edema or dehydration.
   c. Disorders include the syndrome of inappro-

priate secretion of antidiuretic hormone (SIADH), hypothyroidism, adrenocorticosteroid insufficiency, and water intoxication.

4. Additional osmotically active solutes in the serum. The elevated osmotic pressure of the serum attracts water into the intravascular space (from the intracellular compartment via the extracellular space; this additional water thus dilutes the serum sodium, which results in hyponatremia).

   a. The additional osmotic agents are most often glucose in hyperglycemia or mannitol added iatrogenically.

   b. Total-body water and sodium concentrations will usually be decreased due to osmotic diuresis.

   c. As hyperglycemia is corrected, the serum sodium level may rise approximately 2 mEq/L for each 100-mg/dL decrease in the serum glucose level.

B. Causes (*Note:* Table 4–2 compares the causes listed below with the mechanisms described above.)

1. Protein loss.—Nephrosis, cirrhosis.
2. Congestive heart failure.
3. Dehydration.—Vomiting, diarrhea, sweating, burns, pancreatitis, massive trauma.
4. Renal.—Nephrosis, salt-wasting nephritis, renal tubular acidosis.
5. Adrenal.—Mineralocorticoid insufficiency, corticosteroid insufficiency.
6. Diuretics.
7. SIADH.
8. Water intoxication.
9. Hypertonic states not due to sodium.—Hyperglycemia, excess mannitol administration.

C. Clinical presentation.

1. Symptoms and signs of the underlying process should be elicited.
2. Symptoms due to hyponatremia are largely rate

TABLE 4-2.
Etiology of Hyponatremia

	H_2O Retention > Na Retention	Na Loss > H_2O Loss	Pure H_2O Retention	Increased Osmoles
Protein loss (nephrosis, cirrhosis)	X			
Congestive heart failure	X			
Dehydration (vomiting, diarrhea, sweating, burns, pancreatitis, massive trauma)		X		
Renal				
Nephrosis	X			
Na-wasting nephritis		X		
Renal tubular acidosis		X		
Adrenal				
Mineralocorticoid insufficiency		X		
Corticosteroid insufficiency			X	
Diuretics		X		
SIADH			X	
H_2O intoxication			X	
Hypertonic states not due to Na (hyperglycemia, excess mannitol administration)				X

dependent. A sudden decrease in the serum sodium concentration from 140 to 130 mEq/L may cause severe symptoms, whereas a gradual decline to 120 mEq/L may be asymptomatic.

3. Symptoms generally occur at a serum sodium level below 120 mEq/L.

   a. Gastrointestinal.—Anorexia, nausea, vomiting.

   b. Neurological.—Lethargy, confusion, coma, seizures.

D. Treatment.

1. Water restriction is usually the principal treatment, particularly when water retention is the primary abnormality (see Sections III,A,1 and 3).

2. Administration of *isotonic* saline is often appropriate treatment for states in which sodium loss exceeds water loss (see Section III,A,2).

3. Correction of the underlying problem is, of course, important.

4. The antidiuretic hormone (ADH) inhibitor demeclocycline (300 to 600 mg given orally twice a day) may be useful for treating SIADH.

5. If potentially life-threatening symptoms occur (usually with a serum sodium level below 110 mEq/L), hypertonic saline may be indicated.

   a. Three percent saline is given intravenously in small quantities sufficient to correct the serum sodium level no more than halfway to normal over a period of 8 hours, (see Section II,D).

   $$Na^+ \text{ replacement (mEq)} = (\text{Desired serum } Na^+ - \text{Current serum } Na^+)$$
   $$\times \text{ Current total-body water}$$

   b. Hypertonic saline should be given only when *absolutely* necessary. This will usually be limited to states of acute water intoxication.

6. Another modality involves the use of a diuretic (furosemide or mannitol) to induce water diuresis and then replacement (if appropriate) of

sodium and potassium lost in the urine. This regimen is potentially quite *dangerous* if there is already a net total deficit of sodium or potassium. It should be used only for severe hyponatremia concurrently with treatment of the underlying abnormality. (Diuretics may, of course, be required for the treatment of specific disorders such as congestive heart failure.)

E. Falsely low serum sodium measurements—pseudohyponatremia.

1. The nonaqueous phase of serum is expanded in hyperlipidemias and hyperproteinemias such as macroglobulinemia and multiple myeloma.

2. Since sodium is confined to the aqueous phase but is measured per total volume of serum (aqueous plus nonaqueous), such states will lower the measured sodium concentration. The actual aqueous sodium concentration, however, is unchanged.

3. Because the symptoms of hyponatremia depend on the aqueous-phase sodium concentration, such states cause no symptoms and require no treatment.

IV. Hyperkalemia

A. Mechanisms of production.

1. Increase in potassium load.—This is an uncommon cause of hyperkalemia in the patient with normal renal function. However, the patient who receives medications containing potassium is at risk of hyperkalemia developing if renal function deteriorates. Potassium overload may also be the result of the release of potassium from injured tissue.

2. Alteration of the distribution of potassium in the body.—Since most of the body's potassium is intracellular, the redistribution of potassium to the

extracellular fluid may result in hyperkalemia. This is most commonly due to acidosis.

3. Decrease in the renal excretion of potassium.— This may be due to acute renal failure or the use of potassium-sparing diuretics. Patients with chronic renal failure usually maintain normal potassium excretion.

B. Causes.
   1. Acute renal failure.
   2. Acute acidosis.
   3. Adrenal insufficiency.
   4. Extensive transfusion with old banked blood.
   5. Cellular injury.
      a. Burns.
      b. Crushing injury.
      c. Rhabdomyolysis.
      d. Chemotherapy.
   6. Potassium-sparing diuretics (triamterene, spironolactone).

C. Clinical presentation.
   1. Neuromuscular.—Interference with resting neuromuscular membrane potential results in paresthesias, muscular cramping, weakness, or paralysis.
   2. Gastrointestinal.—Nausea, vomiting, anorexia, and abdominal pain.
   3. Cardiac.—Hyperkalemia affects the cardiac membrane potential, which results in conduction disturbances and dysrhythmias. Peaking of the T waves and shortening of the QT interval are early findings. These are followed by flattening or disappearance of the P wave and prolongation of the QRS complex. Ventricular fibrillation or asystole is the ultimate result of uncorrected hyperkalemia.

D. Treatment.
   1. The presence of neuromuscular symptoms, electrocardiographic abnormalities, and a serum po-

tassium level greater than 6.5 mEq/L are indications for treatment.

2. In the face of paralysis or severe cardiac conduction disturbance, the effects of hyperkalemia may be rapidly reversed by restoring normal membrane excitability. This is done by administering 10% calcium gluconate, 10 to 30 mL intravenously over a period of 3 to 4 minutes. The calcium has a transient effect, does not actually lower serum potassium levels, and should be followed by other treatment measures.

3. Promoting the movement of potassium into cells results in a lowering of the serum potassium level. The intravenous administration of 50 mL of 50% dextrose and 10 units of regular insulin may be expected to lower the serum potassium concentration by 1 to 2 mEq/L within 30 minutes. In the acidotic patient, the administration of intravenous sodium bicarbonate will accomplish the same purpose.

4. Removal of potassium from the body is a slower therapeutic process than the aforementioned. It may be accomplished by enhancing renal or gastrointestinal tract excretion. Diuresis with a thiazide diuretic or furosemide will increase urinary potassium excretion but is not appropriate for all clinical settings, e.g., hypovolemia or renal failure. Polystyrene sulfonate (Kayexalate) exchange resin causes potassium to transfer into the gastrointestinal tract by colonic cation exchange. The oral dose is 20 gm with 100 ml of 20% sorbitol solution. Retention enemas of 50 to 100 gm of Kayexalate with 50 to 100 mL of 70% sorbitol may be repeated every 4 hours as needed.

E. Falsely elevated serum potassium level measurements.

1. Hemolysis during sample collection results in falsely high levels.

2. Exercise of the extremity prior to sampling may result in muscular potassium being released into the serum.
3. Leukocytosis and thrombocytosis may also result in a falsely elevated potassium level.

V. Hypokalemia

A. Mechanisms of production.
 1. Inadequate potassium intake.—This is an unusual cause of hypokalemia except in persons with a remarkably deficient diet.
 2. Increased potassium excretion.—This is the most frequent cause of hypokalemia. Increased excretion may be renal or gastrointestinal.
 3. Alteration of the distribution of potassium in the body.—This is the mechanism of production of hypokalemia in alkalosis and other less common conditions.
B. Causes.
 1. Inadequate dietary intake.
   a. Starvation.
   b. Unusual diet.
   c. Alcoholism.
 2. Excessive potassium loss.
   a. Gastrointestinal.
     (1) Protracted vomiting.
     (2) Diarrhea, laxative abuse.
     (3) Nasogastric suction.
   b. Renal.
     (1) Diuretics.
     (2) Osmotic diuretics.
     (3) Aldosteronism.
     (4) Potassium-wasting nephritis.
 4. Hypokalemic periodic paralysis.
 5. Alkalosis.
 6. Cushing's syndrome.

C. Clinical presentation.
   1. Symptoms of hypokalemia tend to be vague and mild if the level of serum potassium is above 3.0 mEq/L. Severe complications usually occur at serum levels less than 2.0 mEq/L.
   2. Mental status.—Patients with hypokalemia may be depressed, confused, or agitated.
   3. Neuromuscular.—Fatigue, muscular weakness, or frank paralysis may develop. Interference with the neuromuscular transmembrane resting potential is the cause for muscular dysfunction. Apnea secondary to respiratory muscle failure may occur at serum potassium levels of 1.0 to 1.5 mEq/L.
   4. Cardiac.—Arrhythmias may be caused by hypokalemia. These include atrial, nodal, or ventricular premature beats or tachycardia. Hypokalemia is especially likely to lead to serious arrhythmia in patients taking digitalis. Electrocardiographic changes of hypokalemia include T wave flattening or inversion, QT interval prolongation, and prominent U waves. U waves are especially significant when they merge with the downstroke of the previous T wave.
D. Treatment.
   1. Whenever a condition is reversible, treatment should be directed toward this.
   2. If hypokalemia is minor, the dietary potassium intake may be supplemented by the addition of bananas or orange juice. Potassium chloride elixir, a 10% solution containing 20 mEq/15 mL, may be administered as a supplement. Forty to 60 mEq/day is adequate replacement therapy for most patients who have hypokalemia due to diuretic use.
   3. For severe hypokalemia—serum potassium level less than 2 mEq/L—intravenous replacement is necessary. The rate of infusion should depend

on the severity of symptoms. The administration of 5 to 20 mEq/hr is adequate for most cases. Potassium may be administered as rapidly as 50 mEq/hr in extreme emergencies. During intravenous potassium replacement, the electrocardiogram should be monitored for the reversion of inverted T waves to normal. Since hyperkalemia is generally far more hazardous than hypokalemia, all rapid potassium replacement should be watched with extreme caution.

VI. Hypocalcemia   (*Note:* Laboratory determinations of serum calcium levels measure total calcium, but clinical symptoms are based on only the ionized portion.)

A. Mechanisms of production.
   1. Hypoalbuminemia. Forty percent to 45% of the total serum calcium is protein bound. When the serum protein level decreases, homeostasis of the ionized portion of serum calcium is maintained, with an amount equivalent to that formerly bound to protein now absorbed into bone. Thus, the total serum calcium level falls in hypoalbuminemia, but the ionized portion remains normal, and there are no symptoms.
   2. Decreased mobilization of calcium from bone.—This involves the parathyroid hormone (PTH) system as well as magnesium interaction with this system.
   3. Decreased levels of vitamin D or its metabolites.—This may involve dietary insufficiency, malabsorption, metabolic abnormalities, or excessive excretion.
   4. Conversion of ionized to nonionized calcium.
B. Causes.
   1. Hypoalbuminemia.
   2. Disorders of the PTH system.
      a. Decreased PTH production.

  b. Decreased end-organ sensitivity to PTH (pseudohypoparathyroidism).

  c. Decreased level of serum magnesium.

 3. Disorders of vitamin D.

  a. Decreased dietary intake of vitamin D.

  b. Decreased gastrointestinal tract absorption of vitamin D.

  c. Decreased conversion of vitamin D to active metabolite.

  d. Increased conversion of vitamin D to inactive metabolite.

  e. Increased excretion of active metabolite.

 4. Precipitation of ionized calcium due to hyperphosphatemia or pancreatitis.

 5. Alkalosis.

 6. Increased incorporation of calcium into new bone formation due to osteoblastic metastases.

C. Clinical presentation.

 1. Neurological.—The initial symptoms are circumoral or peripheral paresthesias, muscle cramping, carpopedal spasm, and confusion. Symptoms may progress in severe hypocalcemia to frank tetany or convulsions. A significant decrease of the serum ionized calcium level is reflected by Chvostek's sign (facial muscle spasm induced by tapping over the facial nerve) and Trousseau's sign (carpal spasm induced by inflation of an arm tourniquet).

 2. Electrocardiographic.—Prolonged QT intervals may be seen.

D. Treatment.

 1. In persons with chronic hypocalcemia, the dietary intake of calcium and vitamin D is increased.

 2. Emergent treatment is necessary if the clinical signs of hypocalcemia are present. Unless these are due to a transient abnormality such as the respiratory alkalosis of hyperventilation, intravenous calcium should be given; 100 to 300 mg is

administered over a span of several minutes as 10 to 30 cc of a 10% solution of calcium gluconate. A slow intravenous infusion can be then titrated to serum levels.

3. If the level of serum magnesium is also low (less than 0.8 mEq/L), 1 to 2 gm of magnesium sulfate (8 to 10 mEq of elemental magnesium) is given intravenously as a 10% solution over a period of 15 minutes.

VII. Hypercalcemia

A. Mechanism of production.
   1. Increased gastrointestinal absorption, which may be due to the increased intake of dietary calcium, as in the milk-alkali syndrome, or to enhanced intestinal absorption.
   2. Mobilization of calcium from bone, which may be due to increased bone resorption or osteolysis.
   3. Reduced renal excretion of calcium.
B. Causes.
   1. Hyperparathyroidism.
   2. Malignant disease, most commonly cancer of the lung, breast, and kidney.
   3. Granulomatous illness.
      a. Sarcoidosis.
      b. Tuberculosis.
      c. Histoplasmosis.
      d. Coccidioidomycosis.
   4. Vitamin D intoxication.
   5. Immobilization.
   6. Milk-alkali syndrome.
   7. Hyperthyroidism.
   8. Addison's disease.
   9. Use of thiazide diuretics.
C. Clinical presentation.
   1. Gastrointestinal tract.—Anorexia, nausea, vomit-

ing, constipation, and abdominal pain are manifestations of hypercalcemia.

2. Urinary tract.—Hypercalcemia may cause polyuria, polydipsia, and stone formation in the urinary tract.

3. Neurological.—Fatigue, muscular weakness, and diminished deep-tendon reflexes are the result of hypercalcemia. Severe hypercalcemia is accompanied by alterations in mental status: apathy, depression, psychotic behavior, disorientation, stupor, or coma.

4. Electrocardiographic.—Hypercalcemia causes shortening of the QT interval.

D. Treatment.

1. Infusion of normal saline to overcome dehydration and lower the calcium concentration is the simplest measure available in the treatment of hypercalcemia. Urinary calcium excretion is enhanced by increased sodium excretion. The infusion of intravenous normal saline and the administration of 40 to 80 mg of intravenous furosemide may therefore be used to lower the serum calcium concentration. Care should be taken to prevent circulation overload. Thiazide diuretics, which may cause hypercalcemia, should be avoided.

2. Mithramycin lowers the calcium concentration by inhibiting bone resorption. A single dose of 25 µg/kg in 5% dextrose in water (D_5W) given in an intravenous infusion over a period of 3 to 4 hours results in a lowered calcium concentration in 12 to 24 hours. Repeated administration may result in thrombocytopenia and serious renal or hepatic toxicity.

3. Glucocorticoids reduce the level of serum calcium over the course of several days. Hydrocortisone, 250 mg intravenously every 6 hours, or the equivalent may be given.

4. Ethylenediamine tetraacetic acid (EDTA) increases the urinary excretion of calcium and forms complexes with calcium in the blood. It is the most effective way to reduce the calcium concentration. Fifteen to 50 mg/kg should be given over the course of 4 hours. Since there is a significant risk of acute renal failure with EDTA, its use should be restricted to life-threatening emergencies.

5. Administration of inorganic phosphate is also a rapid means of reducing the calcium concentration. Intravenous infusion of elemental phosphorus, 20 to 30 mg/kg over a period of 12 to 16 hours, will lower the calcium concentration rapidly. However, soft-tissue calcification, renal necrosis, and cardiac arrest may result from the use of elemental phosphate.

E. Falsely elevated serum calcium level measurements.

1. The level of serum calcium may be falsely elevated if there is venous stasis due to the prolonged application of a tourniquet.

2. Since almost half the serum calcium is protein-bound, a decrease in the levels of plasma albumin and globulin should result in a decrease in the upper limit for the normal calcium level. As a consequence, a patient with a low plasma protein level may display signs of hypercalcemia even though his measured serum calcium level is in the normal range. On the other hand, alkalosis results in increased binding of calcium to protein. The alkalotic patient may display signs of hypocalcemia even though the total serum calcium concentration is in the normal range.

5

Respiratory Emergencies

I. Pulmonary Embolus

A. Etiology
   1. The source of most pulmonary emboli is thrombosis of the deep venous systems of the pelvis and thighs.
   2. Venous stasis is the major predisposing factor to thrombosis. Patients who are subjected to prolonged bed rest or are immobilized are at the greatest risk.
   3. Other predispositions are malignancy, recent myocardial infarction, congestive heart failure, polycythemia vera, and sickle cell anemia. Persons who are obese, pregnant, postpartum, or taking oral contraceptive agents are also at risk.
B. Clinical diagnosis.
   1. Tachypnea is present in almost all cases. Dyspnea, pleuritic chest pain, hemoptysis, fever, or a pleural friction rub may be present.
   2. Arterial blood gas measurements usually indicate hypoxemia, but the Po_2 may be greater than 90 mm Hg. Therefore, a normal Po_2 does not rule out a pulmonary embolus.
   3. The electrocardiogram (ECG) is abnormal in most cases, but changes may be nonspecific. ST

segment changes and T-wave inversion are the most common findings. Other changes are the $S_1Q_3T_3$ pattern, right bundle-branch block, and left or right axis deviation. A change in the axis of more than 30 degrees from a previous tracing is significant, even if the axis is normal. Sinus tachycardia is usually present, and atrial premature beats, flutter, or fibrillation may appear.

4. Chest x-ray findings are normal in most cases. Elevation of a hemidiaphragm, infiltrate, pleural effusion, and platelike atelectasis are the most common abnormal findings. The loss of vascular markings in a portion of the lung (Westermark's sign) strongly suggests pulmonary embolism but is frequently difficult to distinguish.

C. Diagnosis (see also Chapter 3).

1. Perfusion scanning.

a. Other disease processes may mimic the appearance of pulmonary embolism, so abnormal scan findings may not be diagnostic.

b. A normal scan result, however, almost invariably excludes the diagnosis of pulmonary embolism. The false-negative rate is less than 1%.

2. Ventilation-perfusion (V-Q) scanning has a greater likelihood of providing a diagnosis, but only when there are segmental or lobar defects seen by perfusion scanning that are not matched by ventilation defects. In addition, either the chest x-ray must be normal, or any infiltrate present must be smaller than the corresponding perfusion scan defect.

3. Pulmonary arteriography.

a. This is the definitive diagnostic study.

b. Morbidity is 4% and mortality, 0.2%.

c. Indications.

(1) Clinical picture strongly suggestive of a

pulmonary embolus, but a nuclear scan is normal or not diagnostic.

    (2) Presence of congestive heart failure or parenchymal lung disease that interferes with perfusion scanning.

    (3) High risk in the use of anticoagulants.

    (4) Consideration for vena caval ligation.

D. Treatment.

  1. Heparin.

    a. This may be administered via continuous intravenous (IV) infusion (the preferred method) or a bolus every 4 hours. When the constant-infusion method is used, 5,000 to 10,000 units should be given as a primary dose and then 1,000 to 1,200 units each hour via infusion pump.

    b. The dose should be monitored by maintaining the partial thromboplastin time at 1½ to 2½ times normal.

  2. Coumadin.

    a. Administration should begin on the 3rd to the 5th day of anticoagulation.

    b. The dose should be monitored by maintaining the prothrombin time at twice normal. A daily dose of 10 mg should be given at the beginning.

    c. Oral anticoagulation therapy is continued for 3 to 6 months.

  3. Thrombolysis.—Thrombolytic therapy with streptokinase may be utilized in life-threatening massive pulmonary embolism, but most cases can be managed without such treatment.

  4. Surgery.—The indications for surgical embolectomy are controversial. Most authorities maintain that embolectomy should be performed on patients in shock who have had occlusion of more than 50% of the pulmonary vascular tree. Others hold to more liberal indications and maintain that embolectomy

should be done in patients in shock who are unresponsive to vasopressor therapy (see also Chapter 1), even if pulmonary artery obstruction is not 50%.

II. Pneumonia

A. Diagnostic workup.
   1. Chest x-ray.—Lung infiltrates in patients who are dehydrated may not become apparent on x-ray until the fluid balance is restored.
   2. Sputum sample for culture and Gram stain.— This may be coughed up by the patient, induced by ultrasonic nebulization, or even aspirated transtracheally.
   3. Blood culture.
   4. Arterial blood gases.
B. Pneumococcal infection.
   1. Clinical presentation.—The history may be several days of upper respiratory tract infection, or the disease may have an abrupt onset with fever and rigors. Cough and pleuritic chest pain are frequently present, and headache, nausea, vomiting, and abdominal pain may also appear. The patient displays tachypnea and tachycardia. Examination of the chest may reveal splinting, percussion dullness, increased tactile fremitus, bronchial breathing, rales, and whisper pectoriloquy. The white blood cell count is typically elevated with a shift to the left.
   2. Sputum.—The sputum is purulent or rust colored. Gram stain reveals gram-positive lancet-shaped cocci in pairs and short chains.
   3. Chest x-ray.—The typical radiographic appearance is that of a pleural-based lobar consolidation with air bronchograms. Multiple-lobe involvement is uncommon.
   4. Treatment.—Most pneumococci are sensitive to penicillin. IV crystalline penicillin, 2 to 10

million units/day, may be given. Alternatively, 600,000 units of procaine penicillin may be given twice daily as intramuscular injections or phenoxymethyl penicillin, 250 mg orally four times a day.

C. Staphylococcal infection.

  1. Clinical presentation.—The onset of illness is usually abrupt, with chills, fever, tachycardia, tachypnea, pleuritic chest pain, and sepsis. There may be physical findings of consolidation.

  2. Sputum.—The sputum is purulent and may be blood streaked. Staining reveals gram-positive cocci in clumps, and many may be within leukocytes.

  3. Chest x-ray.—Patchy bronchopneumonia is the most typical pattern, and rapid spread is the rule. Thin-walled, spherical cavitary lesions known as pneumatoceles are characteristic. Empyema is common.

  4. Treatment.—Nafcillin, 1 to 3 gm IV every 6 hours, is the treatment of choice. Therapy may need to be continued for 2 to 6 weeks until there is clinical resolution.

D. Streptococcal infection.

  1. Clinical presentation.—The typical findings of pneumonia are usually as outlined for pneumococcal and staphylococcal infections. In addition, most cases are accompanied by pharyngitis. Rheumatic fever and glomerulonephritis may be complications of streptococcal pneumonia.

  2. Sputum.—The sputum is purulent and displays gram-positive cocci in chains on staining.

  3. Chest x-ray.—Bronchopneumonic consolidation is typical, and pleural effusion may be seen. Empyema is a common complication.

  4. Treatment.—The drug of choice is penicillin in doses as for pneumococcal pneumonia (see Section II, B, 4).

E. *Haemophilus* infection.
   1. Clinical presentation.—Cough, dyspnea, fever, or pleuritic pain are the usual complaints. *Haemophilus* infection should be considered in alcoholic or debilitated patients and in those with chronic obstructive pulmonary disease. Physical findings of lobar consolidation are frequently absent.
   2. Sputum.—*Haemophilus influenzae* is a small gram-negative bacillus that may have the appearance of a coccobacillus.
   3. Chest x-ray.—Pleural effusion is present in about half the cases. Radiographic findings are otherwise similar to those of pneumococcal pneumonia.
   4. Treatment.—IV ampicillin, 50 mg/kg/day in divided doses, is the drug of choice. If there is a significant incidence of ampicillin-resistant *Haemophilus* infection in the community, IV chloramphenicol, 50 mg/kg/day, should be administered in addition to ampicillin until antibiotic sensitivities can be tested.

F. Gram-negative organisms.
   1. Clinical presentations.—Pneumonia due to gram-negative organisms is more common in middle-aged and elderly patients than in younger ones. Individuals with diabetes, malignancy, or alcoholism are particularly susceptible. The abrupt onset of cough, fever, chills, and pleuritic chest pain is the rule. Sepsis, endocarditis, gastroenteritis, or meningitis may be present.
   2. Sputum.—The sputum may be brick red due to the presence of blood and mucus. Gram-negative bacilli may be seen on staining.
   3. Chest x-ray.—*Klebsiella* is the most common organism to cause gram-negative pneumonia. Upper-lobe and multiple-lobe involvement is common. The classic appearance is that of an

infiltrate with bulging fissures. Abscesses may form.

4. Treatment.—Initial treatment should consist of cephalothin, 2 gm IV every 4 hours, and gentamicin, 3 to 5 mg/kg/day IV or intramuscularly. For *Pseudomonas* pneumonia, the drugs of choice are gentamicin and carbenicillin. 30 to 40 gm/day. Sputum and blood cultures should be checked and antibiotic regimens adjusted as sensitivities dictate.

G. Mycoplasma.

1. Clinical presentation.—*Mycoplasma* pneumonia is a disease primarily of children and young adults. Fever, dyspnea, tachypnea, headache, pharyngitis, and cough are usually present. Cervical adenopathy, skin rash, ear pain, and bullous myringitis are occasional features. Rales may be heard, but findings of lobar consolidation are usually absent.

2. Sputum.—Since *Mycoplasma pneumoniae* have no cell walls, they do not retain Gram stain. No organisms will, therefore, be seen on staining of the sputum, although neutrophils may be present.

3. Chest x-ray.—Segmental involvement of the lower lobes is typical. Patchy interstitial infiltrates are the rule, although lobar or segmental consolidation may be seen. Pleural effusion is not typical but does occur. Radiographic findings are often more impressive than are findings from a physical examination.

4. Treatment.—The drug of choice is erythromycin, 250 to 500 mg four times a day. Alternatively, tetracycline may be given in a similar dosage. Therapy should be continued for 2 to 3 weeks, although clinical improvement usually occurs in 2 to 3 days.

H. Legionnaire's disease.

1. Clinical presentation.—Symptoms may be mild

or extremely severe. Fever, chills, myalgias, and headache may be present. Nausea, vomiting, and watery diarrhea may also occur. Hemoptysis and pleuritic chest pain are seen in some patients. Fine rales are typically heard early in the course of the disease, but findings of consolidation may become evident as the disease progresses.

2. Sputum.—Gram staining typically reveals neutrophils but no predominant bacterial organism. *Legionella pneumophilia* is a gram-negative bacillus.

3. Chest x-ray.—Bronchopneumonia involving multiple lobes is typical. There may be small pleural effusions. As the disease progresses, lobar consolidation may appear.

4. Treatment.—Erythromycin is the drug of choice. The dosage should be 500 mg every 6 hours, and treatment should be continued for 3 weeks because a relapse may occur if it is discontinued prior to this course. Hospitalization is usually indicated.

I. Viral pneumonia.

1. Clinical presentation.—Several viruses may produce pneumonia. The clinical picture varies with the various organisms. Fever, chills, pharyngitis, cough, myalgias, and malaise may precede the appearance of dyspnea and tachypnea. Cyanosis may be present. Fine rales may be noticed on auscultation.

2. Sputum.—The cough is typically nonproductive or produces nonproductive sputum. No predominant bacterial organism is seen in the sputum.

3. Chest x-ray.—Infiltrates are usually patchy and may involve multiple lobes. The development of diffuse alveolar infiltration or consolidation may indicate the development of adult respiratory distress syndrome.

4. Treatment.—Treatment is largely supportive. The previously healthy patient who does not appear severely ill may be treated on an outpatient basis. However, viral pneumonia may progress to adult respiratory distress syndrome, respiratory failure, and death within hours, so good follow-up must be maintained. Young children, the elderly, those with chronic illness, and pregnant women are particularly susceptible. These individuals as well as those in severe respiratory distress should be admitted to the hospital. If the pneumonia is thought on epidemiological grounds to be due to influenza A virus, amantadine may be given, 100 mg twice a day.

J. Immunodeficiency.—Respiratory symptoms in the immunocompromised patients should bring to mind the possibility of *Pneumocystis carinii* pneumonia. Characteristic symptoms include nonproductive cough and exertional dyspnea.

III. Acute Respiratory Failure

A. Definition.
   1. This disease is acute, life-threatening deterioration of respiratory function associated with hypoxemia (Po_2 less than 50mm Hg) and hypercarbia (Pco_2 greater than 50mm Hg) or hypoxemia alone.
   2. The preceding figures may not apply to patients with chronic lung disease in whom long-standing hypoxemia or CO_2 retention may be present. Baseline blood gas values must be known for these individuals.

B. Etiology.
   1. Central nervous system (CNS) dysfunction.— Central hypoventilation, drug overdose, trauma, cerebral vascular accident, poliomyelitis, Guillain-Barré syndrome.

2. Neuromuscular dysfunction.—Muscular dystrophy, myasthenia gravis.
3. Mechanical factors.—Abdominal distention, flail chest, tension pneumothorax, obesity, pleural effusion.
4. Upper-airway obstruction.
5. Pulmonary embolus.
6. Obstructive disease.—Emphysema, chronic bronchitis, asthma.
   a. The most common precipitant of respiratory failure in chronic obstructive pulmonary disease is infection.
   b. Other precipitating causes are pneumothorax, congestive heart failure, bronchospasm, and oxygen- or drug-induced respiratory depression.
7. Pneumonitis.
8. Adult respiratory distress syndrome.—Shock lung, fat embolism, toxic inhalation, drug overdose–induced pulmonary edema.

C. Physical examination.
   1. Signs of pulmonary parenchymal or extrapulmonary disease.
   2. Signs and symptoms of hypoxemia.—Confusion, restlessness, irritability, impaired mental status, cyanosis, diaphoresis, tachycardia.
   3. Signs and symptoms of hypercarbia.—Headache, drowsiness, sedation, cutaneous and scleral vasodilation.
   4. Tachypnea, dyspnea, cough. Use of accessory muscles of respiration.

D. Diagnostic tests likely to be useful.
   1. Chest x-ray.
   2. Complete blood cell count.
   3. Electrolytes.
   4. Total eosinophil count.
   5. Smear and culture of sputum.
   6. ECG.
   7. Arterial blood gases.

E. Arterial blood gas formulas.
1. Age-correction formula.—Expected Po_2 = 103 − (0.4 × Age).
2. Correlation.
    a. Acute.—For each 10–mm Hg deviation from normal in Pco_2, there is an expected inverse change of 0.07 in pH.
    b. Chronic.—For each 10–mm Hg deviation from normal in Pco_2, there is an expected inverse change of 0.03 in pH.
3. Respiratory compensation of acute metabolic acidosis.—For every fall in serum bicarbonate concentration of 1 mEq/L, there is an expected 1–mm Hg fall in Pco_2.
4. Calculation of alveolar-arterial Po_2 gradient.
    a. Calculated alveolar Po_2 = 150 − (Pc_{O_2} × 1.2).
    b. Gradient = Calculated Pa_{O_2} − Po_2 (measured).
    c. Normally, the gradient is less than 15 mm Hg.
    d. Hypoxemia may occur in all the following: hypoventilation, V-Q mismatch, shunting, and diffusion impairment. There is an increased alveolar-arterial Po_2 gradient in persons with all these abnormalities *except* hypoventilation. The application of high-flow oxygen can significantly correct hypoxia in all persons *except* those with arteriovenous shunting. This must be done with care in the patient in whom the hypoxia may be due to chronic obstructive pulmonary disease.
F. Treatment.
1. Oxygenation.
    a. For the patient without CO_2 retention, oxygen should be administered so that the Po_2 is maintained at 60 to 70 mm Hg. This may be done by nasal prong or mask application,

but the recognition that prongs usually cannot deliver more than 40% oxygen at even high flow rates. A nonrebreathing mask is necessary for delivery of more than 60% oxygen.

b. For the patient with CO_2 retention, oxygen should be administered with care, beginning with a 24% Venturi mask or nasal prongs at a 0.5- 2.0-L/min flow. The Po_2 should be maintained at 50 to 60 mm Hg.

c. Oxygen therapy should be continuous, because intermittent oxygenation may result in precipitously low Po_2 levels and CO_2 retention.

2. Bronchodilation is indicated if bronchospasm is present (see Chapter 25).

3. Chest physiotherapy.

4. Tracheobronchial hydration.

5. Antibiotics for infection.

6. Endotracheal intubation and mechanical ventilation.

a. This should be avoided in patients with chronic obstructive pulmonary disease because there is high morbidity and mortality associated with prolonged intubation and mechanical ventilation in these patients.

b. Indications for intubation should be altered to suit each individual. Some recommendations follow:

(1) Cardiorespiratory arrest.

(2) Coma with respiratory depression.

(3) Inability to maintain a Po_2 within a range of 50 to 60 mm Hg despite high-flow O_2.

(4) Progressive hypercarbia accompanied by the deterioration of mental status, muscular fatigue, or respiratory acidosis with a pH less than 7.20.

(5) Inability to clear airway secretions with chest physiotherapy and suctioning.

IV. Noncardiogenic Pulmonary Edema

A. Definition.—Increased alveolar and interstitial fluid accumulation unassociated with left ventricular failure.

B. Etiology.
   1. High altitude.
   2. Drugs.
      a. Narcotics.
      b. Salicylates.
      c. Pentazocine.
      d. Propoxyphene.
   3. Neurogenic.
      a. Head and spinal cord injury.
      b. Cerebral vascular accident.
      c. CNS infection.
      d. Postconvulsion.
   4. Organophosphate insecticides.
   5. Near drowning.
      a. Occurs in both saltwater and freshwater near drowning.
      b. Evidence for pulmonary edema may be delayed for as long as 48 hours following near drowning.
   6. Toxic inhalation.
   7. Airway obstruction.
   8. Sepsis.
      a. Miliary tuberculosis.
      b. Viral pneumonia.
      c. Gonococcal sepsis.
   9. Fat embolism.
   10. Gastric contents aspiration.
   11. Posttraumatic.

C. Pathophysiology.
   1. Although the common feature of noncardiogenic pulmonary edema is damage to the pulmonary alveolar-capillary membrane and

resultant exudation of fluid into the interstitial and alveolar spaces, the precise mechanism is unknown.

2. Hypoxia undoubtedly plays a role in some forms of the syndrome. However, hypoxia alone has not been shown to disrupt the capillary-alveolar membrane.

3. Membrane disruption by toxic materials is a possibility.

4. Pulmonary release of vasoactive substances may be involved.

D. Clinical presentation.

1. Patients display a variable degree of respiratory distress with chest pain, cough, tachypnea, dyspnea, and cyanosis.

2. Rales, rhonchi, or wheezing may be diffuse or localized or absent altogether.

3. Cardiomegaly and jugular venous distension are not present.

4. Arterial blood gas measurements typically reveal hypoxemia and respiratory alkalosis.

5. The chest x-ray pattern is usually one of bilateral pulmonary vascular congestion and infiltrates with a normal cardiac silhouette. However, asymmetrical and unilateral patterns may be seen.

E. Treatment.

1. Treatment of the underlying cause, if apparent, is most important.

2. The mainstay of treatment is oxygen administration and mechanical ventilation when necessary. The addition of positive end-expiratory pressure should be considered if the Po_2 cannot be maintained in the desired range despite mechanical ventilation and high inspired oxygen levels.

3. Near-drowning victims who do not have noncardiogenic pulmonary edema should nevertheless be admitted to the hospital for obser-

vation of this complication. The treatments for cardiogenic pulmonary edema—morphine, diuretics, rotating tourniquets—are of no benefit to persons with pulmonary edema due to near drowning.

V. Pulmonary Aspiration

A. Occurrence.—Aspiration of gastric contents occurs with the greatest frequency in persons who have reduced levels of consciousness or mechanical abnormalities of gastrointestinal tract and airway function. The latter group includes those patients with gastric dilation, achalasia, hiatus hernia, and medical devices such as esophageal obturator airways or Blakemore-Sengstaken tubes.

B. Pathophysiology.—Aspiration of acidic gastric contents results in atelectasis, bronchial mucosa injury, alveolar destruction, and increased capillary permeability. Fluid and blood fill the alveoli which results in noncardiogenic pulmonary edema.

C. Clinical presentation.—The severity of findings depends on the extent of lung involvement and the time from aspiration. Respiratory distress of variable degree develops 1 to 2 hours following aspiration. Dyspnea, cough, frothy sputum production, cyanosis, fever, tachycardia, and hypotension may be present. Auscultation may reveal rales, rhonchi, or wheezes. Arterial blood gas measurements typically reveal hypoxemia with a normal or low Pco_2. Central venous pressure is low.

D. Chest x-ray.—The areas of lung involvement depend on the patient's position at the time of aspiration. Central, mottled, or streaky infiltrates develop in the right upper lobe of the supine patient or in the right middle or lower lobe of the sitting or semirecumbent patient. Abnormal x-ray findings do not appear for several hours following aspiration, and they may develop during the next 36 hours.

E. Treatment.

1. Position.—If the aspiration is witnessed, the patient should be placed in the head-down, prone or lateral decubitus position and the pharynx suctioned of any remaining vomitus.

2. Oxygenation.—High-flow oxygen should be applied and the respiratory status observed carefully. The development of tachypnea or falling Po_2 is an indication for endotracheal intubation and positive-pressure ventilation. Positive end-expiratory pressure has been shown to enhance oxygenation and should be used in treating patients receiving positive-pressure ventilation.

3. Fluid replacement.—This may be necessary in the unusual circumstance of a large amount of fluid having been extravasated into the lungs.

4. Bronchoscopy.—This is indicated for the relief of segmental or lobar obstruction by large particles. Fiberoptic bronchoscopy may also be useful to confirm the extent of injury.

5. Antibiotics.—Although antibiotics are frequently used to treat aspiration pneumonia, their efficacy is in question. Penicillin or methicillin and gentamicin (see the dosages described in Section II, B to F) are the drugs of choice when antibiotics are indicated.

6. Corticosteroids.—The use of corticosteroids in aspiration is controversial. The benefits of steroid administration have been difficult to demonstrate, and serious gram-negative infection may complicate the illness of the patient who is receiving corticosteroids. If steroids are to be used, they must be administered at the time of aspiration or within 5 minutes. A dose of 30 mg/kg methylprednisolone is recommended.

VI. Smoke Inhalation

A. Carbon monoxide (CO) poisoning.
   1. CO results from the incomplete combustion of organic material. Fires and automobile exhaust are common sources.
   2. The general effects of CO on the body are caused by the inhibition of oxygen transport, delivery, and utilization.
   3. The clinical manifestations of CO poisoning include cardiac ischemia and arrhythmias in susceptible individuals, visual and auditory impairment, and diminished cognitive and psychomotor performance. Late CNS effects include parkinsonism, mental retardation, disorientation, and psychosis.
   4. Signs and symptoms can be correlated with levels of carboxyhemoglobin (COHg) on a rough basis.
      a. COHg less than 10%, usually no symptoms.
      b. COHg 10% to 20%, frontal and temporal bandlike headache.
      c. COHg 30% to 40%, headache, weakness, visual impairment, nausea, vomiting.
      d. COHg 40% to 50%, impaired consciousness.
      e. COHg 50% to 60%, coma, convulsions.
      f. COHg greater than 60%, cardiorespiratory depression, death.
   5. The aforementioned should be used only as a guide because significant clinical findings may occur at levels lower than these. Cherry red coloration of the skin and mucous membranes is not a sensitive index of poisoning.
   6. Treatment outline.
      a. Determine the COHg level. Arterial Po_2 levels may be normal in persons with CO poisoning. They are not a valid reflection of exposure.
      b. Apply high-flow oxygen to the patient while

awaiting the COHg reading. Oxygen displaces CO from hemoglobin and hastens its elimination from the body.

c. Oxygen via mask at 100% should be administered to all symptomatic patients with a COHg level greater than 10%.

d. Patients with significant mental impairment or COHg greater than 40% should be treated in a hyperbaric chamber if one is available.

e. Patients with cardiac dysfunction, those who were rendered unconscious, and those with COHg levels higher than 25% should be admitted to the hospital for cardiac monitoring and oxygen administration.

B. Other toxic inhalation.

1. Fires and industrial exposure may result in the inhalation of other toxic gases, including sulfur oxide, nitrogen oxide, hydrogen chloride, phosgene, and chlorine.

2. Prolonged inhalation, especially in an enclosed area, is particularly likely to result in injury.

3. The major result of such injury is chemical pneumonitis, with loss of surfactant, atelectasis, leakage of fluid across damaged pulmonary capillary membranes, and noncardiogenic pulmonary edema.

4. The onset of respiratory symptoms and chest x-ray abnormalities may be delayed for 24 hours.

5. Diagnostic evaluation of arterial blood gases, chest x-ray, and COHg level.—The patient should be admitted to the hospital if he meets the admission criteria in section VI,A,6,d and e or VI,C,2 or displays significant respiratory distress, blood gas abnormalities, or x-ray evidence of pulmonary edema.

6. Treatment.—Adequate oxygen levels (Po_2 higher than 60 mm Hg) should be maintained by the application of oxygen via mask. Progres-

sive hypoxemia should be treated with endotracheal intubation and positive-pressure ventilation. Positive end-expiratory pressure may be added if hypoxemia persists or pulmonary edema develops. Efforts should be made to prevent overhydration, which exacerbates pulmonary fluid accumulation.

C. Respiratory "burn."

1. Damage to the respiratory tract due to thermal exposure is most frequently the result of toxic inhalation rather than heat injury per se. The exception is exposure to steam, which has been demonstrated to cause epithelial necrosis and edema in the tracheobronchial tree.

2. Burns on the face and nasal hairs, hoarseness, and carbon particles in the sputum indicate that respiratory injury may have taken place. However, significant injury may occur even in the absence of any of these signs. If there is a strong suspicion of exposure on the basis of history, physical findings, or signs of respiratory distress, the patient should be admitted to the hospital for observation and treatment.

3. Treatment should proceed as outlined in Section VI,B,6. Early endotracheal intubation should be considered for patients with extensive facial or mucous membrane burns because the development of edema will render the procedure more difficult subsequently.

VII. Differential Diagnosis Listing for Hemoptysis

A. Aortic aneurysm.
B. Aspergillosis.
C. Bacterial pneumonia, especially gram-negative.
D. Bronchiectasis.
E. Bronchitis.

F. Broncholithiasis.
G. Coagulopathy.
H. Congenital heart disease.
I. Cystic fibrosis.
J. Foreign body aspiration.
K. Goodpasture's syndrome.
L. Idiopathic.
M. Mitral stenosis.
N. Neoplasm, especially bronchogenic carcinoma and bronchial adenoma.
O. Parasitic infection.
P. Polyarteritis nodosa.
Q. Pulmonary arteriovenous fistula.
R. Pulmonary hypertension.
S. Pulmonary infarction.
T. Systemic lupus erythematosus.
U. Tracheoesophageal fistula.
V. Trauma.
W. Tuberculosis.

VIII. Differential Diagnosis Listing for Pleural Fluid Accumulation—Effusion, Empyema, Hemothorax

A. Bacterial infection.
B. Cirrhosis.
C. Coagulopathy.
D. Congestive heart failure.
E. Hypoproteinemia.
F. Meigs' syndrome.
G. Neoplasm.
    1. Bronchogenic carcinoma.
    2. Lymphoma.
    3. Metastatic disease.
H. Nephrosis.

    I. Pancreatitis.

    J. Post-thoracic surgery.

    K. Pulmonary embolus.

    L. Pulmonary fibrosis.

    M. Rheumatoid disease.

    N. Spontaneous pneumothorax.

    O. Subdiaphragmatic abscess.

    P. Systemic lupus erythematosus.

    Q. Trauma.

    R. Tuberculosis.

IX. Asthma   (see Chapter 25).

6
Thoracic Injuries

I. General Considerations

A. Patients with injuries to the chest are frequently in critical condition and require rapid diagnosis and adequate treatment. Emergency thoracotomy is needed in only about 10% of the cases of major thoracic trauma. The other 90% need resuscitation procedures that are available in a well-equipped emergency department (ED) followed by appropriate inpatient care.

B. The ABCs should be evaluated immediately after the patient arrives in the ED: *Airway, breathing,* and *circulation* must be secured.

C. Airway.

1. If the airway is not patent, it must be made so immediately. The obstruction is often caused by the patient's tongue, and a jaw thrust extending the mandible forward often is sufficient to clear the airway. Adjuncts such as an oral or a nasal airway may also help. Foreign bodies, including displaced dentures, must be removed.

2. Endotracheal (ET) intubation may be required if the airway cannot be secured by the aforementioned measures or if the patient is not ventilating adequately.

   a. Orotracheal intubation can be undertaken if

cervical spine trauma is ruled out clinically or radiographically.

b. Blind nasotracheal intubation is preferable if an impaired airway necessitates immediate intubation before cervical spine injury is ruled out. The head must be maintained in a neutral position by an assistant. (Orotracheal intubation and nasotracheal intubation under direct visualization are less optimal because the use of a laryngoscope may result in unintentional motion of the cervical spine.)

3. Cricothyrotomy may be necessary if intubation is unsuccessful, if there is a strong possibility of cervical spine injury, or in cases of massive facial trauma.

a. Cricothyrotomy is preferred over formal tracheostomy in the emergency department because there is less danger of major bleeding and because the trachea lies closer to the skin at the cricothyroid membrane.

b. Cricothyrotomy is performed in the following manner:

(1) The cricothyroid membrane is located at the tranverse slit lying caudal to the thyroid cartilage and cephalad to the cricoid cartilage.

(2) The thyroid cartilage is stabilized with one hand while a 1- to 2-cm transverse incision is made with the other hand. The scalpel penetrates in one stroke through both skin and cricothyroid membrane.

(3) The incision is then spread and a tube inserted. Either a tracheostomy device or a small ET tube (e.g., no. 4 ET tube cut short) can be used.

(4) If a surgical airway must be maintained beyond several days, a formal tracheostomy should be performed in the operating room.

(5) A large-bore needle or commercially available cricothyrotomy device may be inserted temporarily as an easier and more rapid alternative to a formal surgical cricothyrotomy. However, such smaller airways should be replaced as soon as possible with a larger tube inserted through an incision.

D. Breathing.—Even if the airway is clear, the patient's breathing may still not be adequate. Observe the chest and auscultate the lungs. If needed, assist ventilation with a bag-valve device connected to a mask or ET tube.

E. Circulation.—Perfusion must be maintained by control of bleeding, infusion of fluid and blood through large-bore-intravenous (IV) lines as indicated, decompression of tension pneumothorax or pericardial tamponade, or open thoracotomy with aortic compression and internal cardiac massage (see the following items).

F. The initial evaluation may reveal underlying serious pathology such as the following:

1. Pneumothorax.—Dyspnea with decreased breath sounds and tympany on one side, perhaps with subcutaneous emphysema.

2. Tension pneumothorax.—The aforementioned signs plus the eventual development of tracheal deviation to the opposite side, distended neck veins, cyanosis, shock, and perhaps cardiac displacement as determined by percussion and auscultation.

3. Open pneumothorax (sucking chest wound).—An obvious penetrating wound with air flow through the chest wall defect.

4. Flail chest.—A segment of the chest wall moving paradoxically, i.e., inward during inspiration and outward during expiration.

5. Pericardial tamponade.—Hypotension with distended neck veins but symmetrical breath sounds.

II. Diagnosis and Treatment of Thoracic Trauma

Trauma to the chest can be either blunt or penetrating, and may result in injuries that range from trivial to lethal.

    A. Rib fracture.

        1. General.

            a. A simple rib fracture is painful but rarely serious. However pain may curtail respiration and prevent adequate coughing, particularly in the elderly, thereby leading to atelectasis and pneumonia.

            b. Multiple rib fractures may cause a flail chest (see Section II,B).

            c. Fractures of the first or second rib are associated with a significant incidence of major vessel injury. Strong consideration should be given to aortography.

            d. Fractures of the lower ribs may be associated with splenic or hepatic injury.

        2. Diagnosis.

            a. The patient with a simple rib fracture has tenderness on palpation and complains of pain aggravated by coughing, deep breathing, or motion.

            b. A chest x-ray, including rib detail, confirms the diagnosis and helps rule out the presence of underlying pneumothorax or hemothorax.

            c. Much of the anterior chest wall consists of noncalcified cartilage, which is not radio-opaque. A fractured rib cartilage thus does not appear on radiography but clinically resembles a rib fracture.

        3. Treatment.

            a. Pain is usually relieved with oral analgesic such as 60 mg codeine with 600 mg aspirin every 4 hours.

    b. Intercostal block can be used to manage severe pain from rib fracture.

      (1) Bupivacaine (Marcaine), 0.5%, is infiltrated around the intercostal nerve of the fractured rib as well as the ribs one space (and if possible two spaces) above and below.

      (2) The site of injection is beneath the lower edge of the rib, between the fracture and the spinous process. Care must be taken to avoid the intercostal vessels and the lung parenchyma.

    c. Tight binding is not recommended because it may restrict breathing. An easily removable rib belt fastened with Velcro can provide comfort, but the patient must be reminded of the importance of periodic sighing or deep breathing to prevent hypoaeration, retention of secretions, and pneumonia.

    d. Factors that might warrant hospital admission are age, underlying cardiorespiratory disease, significant associated injuries, multiple fractures, abnormal blood gas values, or complications such as pneumothorax.

B. Flail chest.

  1. General.

    a. When several ribs and/or the sternum are fractured on both sides of the point of impact, an unstable or flail chest may result (Fig 6–1).

    b. The unsupported chest wall segment moves in a paradoxical manner, moving inward with negative intrathoracic pressure during inspiration and moving outward during expiration.

    c. This paradoxical motion results in decreased tidal volume, which leads to a functional right-to-left shunt and hypoxia.

  2. Diagnosis.—The paradoxical motion of the flail segment can be discerned by direct observation or palpation.

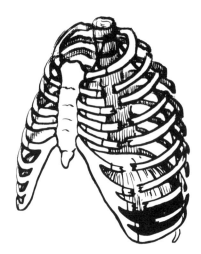

FIG 6–1.
Flail chest.

3. Treatment.
   a. The flail segment must be stabilized. The position of the segment is not important so long as there is no paradoxical motion.
   b. In the field, paramedics may place the patient in a supine or decubitus position so that the flail segment lies against the gurney.
   c. In the ED, internal stabilization is the best approach for significant cases of flail chest, especially if blood gas analysis reveals inadequate ventilation and/or oxygenation. Internal stabilization consists of ET intubation and positive-pressure ventilation.
   d. Associated injuries such as pneumothorax and hemothorax are treated with tube thoracostomy.

Because positive-pressure ventilation can induce pneumothorax in an injured lung, prophylactic chest tubes are often inserted (see Section C).

e. Pulmonary contusion is not uncommonly associated with flail chest (see Section E).

f. Intercostal blockade is particularly helpful for severe pain.

C. Pneumothorax.

1. General.

a. Traumatic pneumothorax may follow blunt or penetrating injuries and can be associated with hemothorax. Air may enter the pleural space from either the trachea, bronchi, or lungs, if these are damaged, and/or from the surrounding atmosphere if the chest wall is penetrated.

b. It is important to ascertain the relative amount of air in the pleural space and to determine whether it is under tension.

c. It is also important to determine whether so much air is moving through a chest wall defect that little air is entering the mouth and nose.

d. Pneumothoraces may be classified as *simple, tension,* or *open.* The last two categories in particular may be rapidly fatal.

2. Simple pneumothorax.

a. The parietal and visceral pleura are normally held in contact by the combined actions of negative intrapleaural pressure and the capillary attraction provided by a small amount of pleural fluid.

b. When air enters the pleural space, both of these factors are negated.

c. The lung on the affected side begins to collapse, and oxygenation becomes impaired (Fig 6–2).

3. Tension pneumothorax.

a. If more air enters the pleural space during inspiration than escapes during expiration, a ball-valve effect is created.

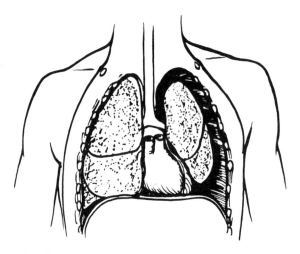

FIG 6–2.
Simple pneumothorax.

b. Intrapleural pressure increases even after the lung completely collapses.

c. Eventually this pressure becomes so high that the mediastinum is pushed to the opposite side, thus leading to compression of the opposite lung as well (Fig 6–3).

d. Extreme hypoxia can result.

e. As intrapleural pressure increases and both lungs are compressed, venous return to the heart declines significantly, thereby resulting in arterial hypotension and shock.

f. Tension pneumothorax is an extreme emergency. It can be lethal within minutes if not immediately corrected (see Section C,6,e).

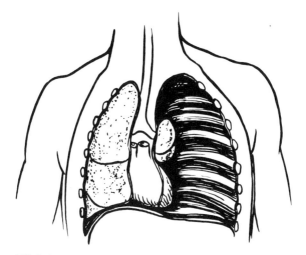

FIG 6–3.
Tension pneumothorax.

4. Open pneumothorax (sucking chest wound).
   a. Even with penetrating trauma to the chest wall, most air enters the pleural space from the damaged lung rather than through the chest wall defect.
   b. If the chest wall defect is sufficiently large, however, air may enter and leave the pleural space with each breath, thus leading to paradoxical collapse of the underlying lung during inspiration and expansion during expiration.
   c. A large defect may also offer less resistance to air flow than do the mouth and nose, thereby leading to preferential ventilation of the pleural space through the chest wall rather than venti-

lation of the lungs through the upper portion of the airway. A chest wall defect two thirds the diameter of the trachea may preclude effective pulmonary ventilation.

    d. An open pneumothorax can be rapidly fatal unless corrected immediately (see Section C,6,f).

5. Diagnosis.

    a. Symptoms.—Dyspnea and pleuritic chest pain.

    b. Physical examination.

        (1) Simple pneumothorax.

           a Diminished breath sounds are auscultated over the affected side of the chest.

           b Tympany to percussion may be elicited.

           c Subcutaneous emphysema may or may not be present.

           d These signs may not be apparent if the pneumothorax is small. As the amount of pleural air increases, breath sounds may disappear entirely.

        (2) Tension pneumothorax.

           a Neck vein distension—*unless there is significant blood loss.*

           b Tracheal deviation to the opposite side as detected by palpation of the neck.

           c Cardiac displacement to the opposite side as detected by percussion and auscultation of the chest.

           d Shock.—*Shock with distended neck veins strongly suggests tension pneumothorax if breath sounds are diminished or asymmetrical, or pericardial tamponade if breath sounds are normal (see Section J). Shock due to blood loss should cause collapse of the neck veins.*

        (3) Open pneumothorax.

           a Air bubbles may be seen to move through blood overlying the wound.

           b A characteristic hissing sound may be

heard as air traverses the chest wall defect.

c. X-ray.

(1) Separation of the visceral from the parietal pleural surface is the hallmark of pneumothorax.

    a A distinct lung margin is seen medial to the parietal pleura.

    b Pulmonary vascular markings are absent in the region between the two pleural surfaces.

(2) An expiratory view may help reveal a subtle pneumothorax because the lung is smaller with more concentrated markings on expiration, while the amount of pleural air remains constant.

(3) An upright film is strongly recommended if the spine is stable and the patient not significantly hypotensive. Small- and moderate-sized pneumothoraces may not be readily apparent on supine films because the air is layered above the entire lung surface in the supine position.

(4) The following clues to pneumothorax may be detected on a supine film:

    a Lucency of one lung field compared with the other.

    b Pneumomediastinum.

    c Pneumopericardium.

    d Subcutaneous emphysema.

6. Treatment.

a. Observation may be sufficient treatment for small (<10%) spontaneous pneumothoraces with no significant symptoms.

b. Insertion of a unidirectional valve device through the chest wall may be used to drain small pneumothoraces.

c. Tube thoracostomy with continuous suction is

advisable for all but the most minor traumatic pneumothoraces as well as for spontaneous pneumothoraces of moderate to large size.

d. Technique of tube thoracostomy:

(1) The second intercostal space, midclavicular line, can be used in a spontaneous pneumothorax.

(2) The 4th to 6th intercostal spaces, midaxillary line, should be used in trauma for better drainage of a possible hemothorax. The location will leave a less obvious scar and may therefore be advisable for a spontaneous pneumothorax in young women.

(3) Percuss during full expiration to be sure the site does not overlie the liver or spleen.

(4) The midaxillary line at the level of the tip of the scapula is often a good site.

(5) After preparing the skin, infiltrate thoroughly with lidocaine (Xylocaine) down to the periosteum and the pleural surface.

(6) Make a small incision down to the rib.

(7) Using a small hemostat, dissect bluntly up over the superior margin of the rib, thereby avoiding the neurovascular bundle running along the bottom rib margin.

(8) Enter the pleural spread the hemostat to enlarge the pleural opening.

(9) Insert a gloved finger into the pleural space to make sure that the pleural space has been entered and that no adhesions will interfere with placement of the tube.

(10) Attach a clamp to the tube and insert. Direct posteriorly if there is any possibility of hemothorax.

(11) Be sure that all side holes in the tube are inside the pleural space.

(12) The tube is then connected to a water seal and continuous suction at -20 cm water.

    (13) The tube is secured to the chest wall with a horizontal mattress suture and an airtight petrolatum dressing.

    (14) Use of a trochar is controversial but is definitely dangerous if the pneumothorax is small.

    (15) For patients with trauma, use a large-bore tube (36 French). A spontaneous pneumothorax can be treated with a smaller tube (10 to 12 French).

e. Tension pneumothorax.

    (1) Air under tension must be removed rapidly!

    (2) A large-bore needle (preferably mounted on a saline-filled syringe) should be used to relieve the tension.

    (3) This is performed safely through the second intercostal space in the midclavicular line.

    (4) A chest tube is then inserted with water seal and suction.

f. Open pneumothorax.

    (1) The sucking wound must be closed immediately by any means available.

    (2) The examiner's gloved hand can be used initially, with a petrolatum gauze dressing applied as soon as possible.

    (3) Tube drainage of the thorax should begin as soon as possible through a separate incision.

    (4) The patient is then taken to the operating room, if necessary, for definitive repair of the chest wall.

    (5) If occlusion of the sucking wound is not followed immediately by tube thoracostomy—especially if intubation and assisted ventilation are required—a tension pneumothorax may sometimes develop. If this occurs, remove the occlusive dressing to allow the air to decompress through the chest wall defect.

D. Hemothorax.
1. General.
   a. Hemothorax is an accumulation of blood in the pleural cavity. It occurs frequently in the setting of major chest trauma and is often—but not always—accompanied by a pneumothorax.
   b. Hemothorax may be caused by injury to the chest wall vasculature, the great vessels, or the intrathoracic organs such as the lung, heart, or esophagus.
   c. Large hemothoraces may lead to
      (1) Hypovolemic shock.
      (2) Hypoxia due to interference with lung expansion.
2. Diagnosis.
   a. Symptoms.
      (1) Pleuritic chest pain.
      (2) Dyspnea.
   b. Physical examination.
      (1) Diminished breath sounds.
      (2) Dullness to percussion unless there is a significant accompanying pneumothorax.
   c. Chest x-ray.
      (1) Fluid is apparent below the base of the lung on an upright film.
      (2) Hemothorax may be subtle on a supine film and cause only a hazy dullness on the affected side.
3. Treatment.
   a. A very small hemothorax can be managed by observation.
   b. Any significant hemothorax is drained with a tube thoracostomy and connected to a water seal and constant suction (− 20 cm of water).
   c. The blood is removed and the lung *must* be re-expanded.
   d. Drainage through the chest tube should reflect the rate of hemorrhage.

    e. Restoration of blood volume with IV fluid or blood should begin immediately.

    f. Thoracotomy in the operating room should be strongly considered if the patient fails to respond to the aforementioned measures.

E. Contusion of the lung. (See Chapter 5 "Respiratory Emergencies.")

    1. Lung contusion may develop within the first 72 hours and is characterized by dyspnea, decreasing arterial Po_2, rales, and infiltrates seen on x-ray.

    2. Severe lung contusion is associated with voluminous tracheobronchial secretions, hemoptysis, and pulmonary edema.

    3. The treatment of a significant contusion is ET intubation to permit suctioning and to apply mechanical ventilation with continuous positive end-expiratory pressure (PEEP).

    4. Lung contusion may lead to adult respiratory distress syndrome (ARDS).

F. Tracheal or bronchial rupture.

    1. Pneumomediastinum or pneumothorax usually occurs.

    2. Tension pneumothorax may develop.

    3. If the patient requires a ventilator, tension pneumomediastinum may arise and cause tracheal compression.

    4. Rupture of the airway can result in inadequate air delivery to the lungs.

    5. Subcutaneous emphysema, especially in the neck, may indicate a serious airway injury.

    6. Bronchoscopy will establish a diagnosis.

    7. Tracheostomy may be used to control respiration, to remove secretions, and to prevent further leakage of air from the high intratracheal pressures that occur with coughing or the Valsalva maneuver.

    8. One or more chest tubes should be inserted if a pneumothorax is present.

    9. Operative repair of the tracheal or bronchial lac-

eration is indicated as soon as possible after the patient's condition is stable.

G. Diaphragmatic rupture.

1. Rupture of the diaphragm is often seen after blunt trauma to either the chest or the abdomen. Evidence of rupture may be present immediately or may be delayed many months.

2. If the defect is large, the abdominal contents will herniate into the chest. The tear is usually on the left.

3. Changes in respiratory physiology are much like those seen with a pneumothorax.

4. With acute herniation, the first complaints are dyspnea and left-sided chest pain, which may be referred to the shoulder.

5. The diagnosis is made with a chest x-ray, which may reveal loops of bowel in the thorax. Do not confuse herniated bowel with intrapleural fluid!

6. Treatment.—Operative reduction of the herniation and repair of the ruptured diaphragm are performed as soon as possible.

H. Injuries to the aorta and great vessels.

1. Penetrating injuries to the aorta may result in cardiac tamponade or hemothorax, depending on whether the site of the vessel injury is intrapericardial or extrapericardial.

2. In nonpenetrating injuries, the most common site of rupture is near the aortic isthmus just below the origin of the subclavian artery.

3. Such injuries are usually fatal immediately, but a small number of victims may survive long enough to reach the hospital.

4. Fluid resuscitation and medical antishock trousers (MAST suit) are used to maintain blood pressure.

5. Aortography is performed immediately if x-rays reveal a widened mediastinum or a fracture of the first (or second) rib or if there is a strong clinical suspicion of major-vessel injury.

6. If an aortic tear is documented, the aorta is re-

paired, or a graft is inserted. Facilities for cardio-pulmonary bypass should be available.

I. Myocardial contusion.

1. Blunt trauma to the chest may cause contusion of the myocardium.

2. The resulting injury resembles myocardial infarction, although the damage may heal completely and the clinical course is usually more benign.

3. Enzyme changes and electrocardiographic (ECG) abnormalities may occur over the same time course as in nontraumatic infarction. Thus, a contusion may not be apparent for a day or two.

4. ECG changes may include sinus tachycardia, right bundle-branch block, various conduction disturbances, and other dysrhythmias.

5. The clinical course has a risk of serious dysrhythmias and other complications. The patient must be monitored in a critical care unit.

J. Cardiac tamponade.

1. Cardiac tamponade occurs from an accumulation of blood in the pericardial sac due to either blunt or penetrating trauma.

2. Diastolic filling and stroke volume decline.

3. In persons with thoracic trauma, falling blood pressure and distended neck veins (in the absence of other signs of tension pneumothorax) strongly indicate acute pericardial tamponade.

4. Severe shock out of proportion to the severity of the chest wound and to the amount of blood lost strongly suggests tamponade.

5. Other findings in tamponade may include narrowed pulse pressure, muffled heart sounds, and pulsus paradoxus (blood pressure fall of more than 10 mm Hg during inspiration). However, these signs may not be present, and their absence does not rule out acute pericardial tamponade.

6. Treatment.

a. If a pulse is palpable, needle aspiration is the initial treatment and often is lifesaving (Fig 6–

4). (If there is no pulse, see Section K on emergency thoracotomy.)

(1) Aspiration is performed with a 16- or 18-gauge, short-bevel spinal needle attached to a three-way stopcock and a 50-mL syringe.

(2) The needle is inserted slightly to the left of the xyphoid and is directed cephalad and to the left until blood can be aspirated. The depth of insertion usually is 3 to 4 cm. Unless there is great urgency, this should be

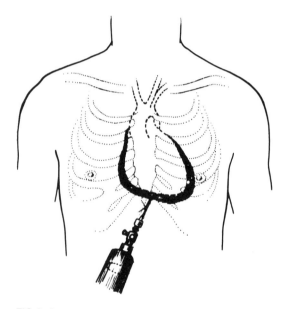

FIG 6–4.
Needle aspiration of pericardial fluid.

done with ECG monitoring. An alligator clamp is used as an ECG lead and attached to the needle, which is then advanced until a current of injury appears on the monitor. The needle, which is now touching the epicardial surface, is then slightly withdrawn back into the pericardial space, and fluid is aspirated.

(3) A central venous catheter can be threaded through the needle and left in place to allow periodic aspiration to prevent the reaccumulation of fluid.

b. Needle aspiration of an acute traumatic pericardial tamponade may be difficult and is often only a temporizing procedure. Traumatic pericardial fluid is primarily blood (hemopericardium), and clots are not easily aspirated through a needle. Immediate thoracotomy in the ED is sometimes necessary to sustain life until definitive surgery can be done in the operating room (see Section K).

c. Thoracotomy in the operating room is the definitive treatment for all patients with penetrating wounds of the heart and acute hemopericardium and tamponade.

(1) All blood and clots must be evacuated.

(2) The wounds of the heart should be closed.

(3) A wide aperture is made in the pericardium to provide for drainage.

K. Open thoracotomy in the ED.

1. Indications.

a. Trauma.

(1) Hemorrhage from any source with unobtainable carotid and femoral pulse.

(2) Chest injury with an unobtainable pulse.

b. Refractory ventricular fibrillation with a basically healthy heart.

(1) Electrocution.

(2) Hypothermia.

2. Procedure.
    a. An incision is made in the left fourth intercostal space from a point 2 to 3 cm lateral to the sternum (to avoid the internal thoracic vessels) to the midaxillary line.
    b. Rib-spreading retractors are used if available. If not, the incision can be extended to the sternum and one or both adjacent costosternal cartilages cut with a scalpel.
    c. For exsanguinating hemorrhage, the aorta is compressed just above the diaphragm with a vascular clamp or the physician's finger. Blood is thus shunted to the vital organs.
    d. If there is any possibility of hemopericardium, the pericardium is opened.
        (1) The phrenic nerve is first identified.
        (2) A longitudinal incision is made parallel to the phrenic nerve.
        (3) The pericardial sac is evacuated of clots, and the heart is delivered outside the pericardium.
        (4) Most cardiac lacerations involve the right ventricle and can be controlled with finger pressure, and only a minority require suturing in the ED.
    e. In persons with refractory ventricular fibrillation, internal paddles are used to apply direct defibrillation. Moist saline gauze pads should be used to separate the paddles from the pericardial surface. Thirty to 50 W-seconds may be used.
        (1) In electrocution, this may be sufficient.
        (2) In hypothermia, warming the heart in warm saline may allow successful defibrillation.
    f. Throughout the procedure, internal cardiac massage is performed as needed.
    g. The patient is taken to the operating room as soon as possible for definitive treatment.

7

Neurological Emergencies: Altered Level of Consciousness

I. General Considerations

A. Patients with altered levels of consciousness cover a spectrum from mild confusion and disorientation to profound coma.

B. Every arousable patient needs a mental status examination (Table 7–1). Frequent repeated evaluations by the same observer are needed to document changes in the level of consciousness over time.

C. For stupor and coma patients, a standard format such as the Glasgow Coma Scale should be used for optimal continual evaluation (Fig 7–1).

D. All these patients should receive 50 cc of 50% glucose and 0.8 mg of naloxone (Narcan) intravenously (IV) early in the evaluation. Attention to airway management is essential. If the patient cannot protect the airway adequately, the patient should be placed on his side with the head positioned to allow adequate ventilation and drainage of secretions as well as to mini-

TABLE 7-1.
Mini-Mental State*

Maximum Score	Score	
		Orientation
5	( )	What is the (year) (season) (date) (day) (month)?
5	( )	Where are we: (state) (country) (town) (hospital) (floor).
		Registration
3	( )	Name 3 objects: 1 second to say each. Then ask the patient all 3 after you have said them. Give 1 point for each correct answer. Then repeat them until he learns all 3. Count trials and record.
		Attention and Calculation
5	( )	Serial 7s. 1 point for each correct. Stop after 5 answers. Alternatively spell "world" backwards.
		Recall
3	( )	Ask for the 3 objects repeated above. Give 1 point for each correct.

9 ( )   Language

Name a pencil, and watch (2 points)

Repeat the following "No ifs, ands or buts." (1 point)

Follow a 3-stage command: "Take a paper in your right hand, fold it in half, and put it on the floor." (3 points)

Read and obey the following: "Close Your Eyes." (1 point)

Write a sentence. (1 point)

Copy design. (1 point)

Total score

ASSESS level of consciousness along a continuum

            Alert Drowsy Stupor Coma

Score Interpretation

>26 = normal

20-26 = usually normal

<20 = always abnormal

*From Folstein MF, Folstein SE, McHugh PR: "Mini-mental state." A practical method for grading the cognitive state of patients for the clinician. *J Psychiat Res* 1975; 12:189-198. Used by permission.

Glasgow Coma Scale

Eyes	Open	Spontaneously	**4**
		To verbal command	**3**
		To pain	**2**
	No response		**1**
Best motor response	To verbal command	Obeys	**6**
	To painful stimulus*	Localizes pain	**5**
		Flexion – withdrawal	**4**
		Flexion – abnormal (decorticate rigidity)	**3**
		Extension (decerebrate rigidity)	**2**
		No response	**1**
Best verbal response**		Oriented and converses	**5**
		Disoriented and converses	**4**
		Inappropriate words	**3**
		Incomprehensible sounds	**2**
		No response	**1**
Total			**3-15**

The Glasgow Coma Scale, based upon eye opening, verbal, and motor responses, is a practical means of monitoring changes in level of consciousness. If response on the scale is given a number, the responsiveness of the patient can be expressed by summation of the figures. *Lowest* score is 3; *highest* is 15.

*Apply knuckles to sternum; observe arms.
**Arouse patient with painful stimulus if necessary.

FIG 7–1.
Glasgow Coma Scale.

mize the risk of aspiration. However, in trauma patients, cervical spine precautions including the use of a rigid immobilizing collar should be instituted. If ventilation is inadequate, very careful endotracheal or nasal intubation may be necessary. If alcohol abuse is suspected, give thiamine, 10 mg IV and 100 mg intramuscularly (IM) initially, with the glucose.

E. Causes.
  1. Drugs or poisons.
  2. Head trauma.
  3. Alcohol abuse.
  4. Hyperglycemia with and without ketosis.
  5. Hypoglycemia.
  6. Uremia.
  7. Hepatic failure.
  8. Central nervous system (CNS) infection.
  9. Adrenal crisis, myxedema, and thyroid storm.
  10. Hypertensive encephalopathy.
  11. Cerebrovascular accidents and mass effects.
  12. Catatonia and hysteria.

F. Three important cerebral herniation syndromes are shown in Table 7–2. Herniation of the brain is commonly caused by one of the following: brain metastasis, intracerebral hemorrhage, subdural hematoma, brain abscess, acute hydrocephalus, radiation necrosis. These patients present with symptoms and signs of raised intracranial pressure and focal neurologic findings.

G. Evaluation.—Immediate treatment to ensure an adequate airway and ventilation and maintain a blood pressure sufficient to perfuse vital organs must precede the comprehensive evaluation. A rapid assessment using the following five clinical signs is extremely helpful in deciding whether the cause is structural (i.e., hemorrhage or thrombosis either causing increased intracranial pressure [ICP] or disrupting CNS tracts), or metabolic and/or drug related.
  1. Level of consciousness.—Deep coma is rarely caused by lesions in the cerebral cortex. Excep-

TABLE 7–2.
Cerebral Herniation Syndromes*

I. Transtenorial Herniation
   A. Uncal Herniation
        Headache
        Vomiting
        Unilateral pupillary dilatation
        Rapid progression to stupor and
        coma
        Decorticate and decerebrate
        posturing
   B. Central Herniation
        Headache
        Progressive drowsiness
        Small reactive pupils
        Periodic respirations (Cheyne-Stokes)
        Paucity of focal motor signs
        Bilateral extensor plantar responses
II. Tonsillar (Foramen Magnum) Herniation
        Headache
        Vomiting
        Hiccoughs
        Stiff neck
        Rapid progression to stupor and
        coma
        Skew deviation of the eyes
        Irregular respirations
        Hypertension

*From Cairncross JG, Posner JB: Neurological complication of systemic cancer, in Yarbro JW, Bornstein RS: *Oncologic Emergencies*. New York, Grune & Stratton, p 76. Used by permission.

tions are massive intracerebral hemorrhages, mass effects of an intracerebral lesion, and profound prolonged hypoxia. Thalamic lesions usually produce stupor. Deep coma is usually due to brainstem hemorrhage or thrombosis or to metabolic causes and drug ingestion.

2. Pupils.—Metabolic factors or drug ingestion rarely completely destroys the pupillary response to light. Exceptions are overdoses of glutethimide (Doriden), anticholinergics such as atropine, and lysergic acid diethylamide (LSD). "Apparently" nonreacting pupils should be rechecked by using a magnifying glass or the positive lens of an ophthalmoscope. Small reactive pupils occur with thalamic lesions. Midposition-fixed pupils indicate structural damage in the midbrain or medulla. Pinpoint-fixed pupils indicate pontine lesions. A single dilated pupil indicates third nerve pressure that is usually due to uncal herniation of the same side or ocular trauma.

3. Doll's eyes (use the terms *present* or *absent* rather than *positive* or *negative*).—The normal response, i.e., doll's eyes present, occurs in the supine patient when the head is turned to the side and both eyes turn together to the ceiling. Very limited or absent movement is reported as "doll's eyes absent" and indicates a structural lesion below the upper pons. Note: in the patient with suspected head trauma, until radiology and the clinical examination show no neck fracture, this test cannot be done.

4. Tone position and abnormal reflexes.—Increased muscle tone is found with midbrain lesions, less so with pontine lesions, and tone is often flaccid with medullary lesions. Decorticate positioning occurs with thalamic lesions, and decerebrate positioning occurs with midbrain and upper pontine lesions. Abnormal reflexes, especially Babinski's sign, are more likely to be present the farther

down the brain stem the structural lesion has occurred.

5. Respiration.—Careful observation of the respiratory rate and rhythm is necessary. Cheyne-Stokes breathing occurs with metabolic causes, hyperventilation in midbrain and upper pontine lesions, and apneustic or ataxic breathing with lesions of the pons and medulla.

H. Laboratory and radiological investigations.

1. Complete blood cell count (CBC), urinalysis for glucose and acetone, and microscopy.

2. Serum electrolytes, and serum glucose drawn prior to the administration of glucose. Calculate the serum osmolality (see page 128), and check for anion gap (see Chapter 2).

3. Calcium and blood urea nitrogen (BUN).

4. Arterial blood gases.

5. Toxicology screen of blood urine and gastric aspirate if drug ingestion cannot be ruled out. Consider the carbon monoxide level and the measured serum osmolality.

6. Computed axial tomography scan (CAT scan) to exclude structural lesions.

7. Cervical x-rays if trauma may have occurred.

8. Chest x-rays.

I. Treatment.

1. Airway management with 100% oxygen initially. If trauma is suspected as the cause of coma, protect the cervical spine when securing the airway (see Chapter 2).

2. Glucose, 50 cc of 50% dextrose in water, and naloxone (Narcan), 0.8 mg by IV push. If an IV line is not possible, immediately give glucagon, 1 cc IM, instead of IV glucose, and give naloxone sublingually.

3. Through a large IV line, restore the volume if necessary by using a normal saline or lactated Ringer's solution until electrolyte, BUN, and arterial blood gas results are available. Then replace fluids and electrolytes as indicated. The military antishock

trousers (MAST) suit and Trendelenburg position may be indicated.

4. Correct the acid-base balance.

5. If alcohol abuse is suspected, administer thiamine, 10 mg IV and 100 mg IM, with or before the glucose.

6. Monitor fluid intake and output by using a Foley catheter as indicated.

II. Treatment of Specific Types of Stupor or Coma

A. Drug-induced or poison-induced (see Chapter 29).

B. Head trauma (see Chapter 12).

C. Alcohol abuse.

1. All these patients should be evaluated for other causes of stupor and coma in addition to the effects of alcohol.

2. A blood alcohol level should be obtained.

3. All these patients should receive thiamine, 100 mg IM and 10 mg IV, with 50 cc 50% dextrose in water IV.

4. Alcohol is associated with an altered level of consciousness in the following clinical states:

a. Acute intoxication.

   (1) Diagnosis.

   a History of heavy or "binge" drinking.

   b Clinical state varies from "drunk" to coma.

   c Blood alcohol level.

   (2) Treatment.

   a Observation.

   b Airway management.

   c Coma nursing care.

b. Early withdrawal.

   (1) Diagnosis.

   a History of cessation of drinking 12 hours to 2 days before.

   b Clinical state of mild confusion; mild tremor, hyperreflexia, seizures, and occasional hallucinations.

   c Blood alcohol level usually in lower levels of intoxication. However, it is the fall in level that is important, not the absolute level.

  (2) Treatment.

   a Sedation with benzodiazepine, e.g., chlordiazepoxide (Librium), 50 to 100 mg orally every 4 to 6 hours, or paraldehyde, 5 to 10 mL orally every 2 to 4 hours. May require admission for observation.

   b Seizures should be treated with phenobarbital, 100 to 150 mg IM, or IV diazepam (Valium) in 5-mg increments.

 c. Delirium tremens.

  (1) Diagnosis.

   a History of cessation of drinking for several days.

   b Clinical state of confusion, severe memory loss, severe tremor, hyperreflexia, and auditory or visual hallucinations. Seizures are less common; the full-blown picture develops over several days. The autonomic nervous system is very overactive.

   c Blood alcohol levels may be low. Liver enzymes and bilirubin levels may be elevated.

  (2) Treatment.

   a Needs admission for close monitoring and IV hydration. This condition has a 5% mortality rate.

   b To reduce autonomic overactivity symptoms sedate with chlordiazepoxide, 100 mg every 1 to 2 hours, or any other benzodiazepine. It may require very large doses to control the symptoms.

    d. Wernicke's encephalopathy.
- (1) Diagnosis.
  - *a* History of chronic alcoholism and malnutrition.
  - *b* Clinical state of confusion, amnesia, confabulation, ataxia, nystagmus, ophthalmoplegia, usually unilateral bilateral sixth or third nerve palsies.
  - *c* The blood alcohol level may be low; occasional evidence of hepatic dysfunction.
- (2) Treatment.
  - *a* Thiamine hydrochloride, 50 to 100 mg IM or IV.
  - *b* Long-term dietary supplementation with thiamine and vitamins.

    e. Hepatic encephalopathy.
- (1) Diagnosis.
  - *a* History of chronic alcoholism; precipitation of coma by abuse of drugs, gastrointestinal tract bleeding, infection.
  - *b* Clinical state of progressive confusion, agitation, and asterixis; evidence of liver failure on physical examination.
  - *c* Abnormal liver function test results.
- (2) Treatment.
  - *a* Treat the precipitating cause.
  - *b* Reduce protein intake.
  - *c* Sterilize the gastrointestinal tract with neomycin, 4 to 6 mg/day orally, and by an enema.
  - *d* Avoid tranquillizing and sedating drugs, and use caution with drugs that require hepatic detoxification.

D. Hyperglycemia with and without ketoacidosis.
1. Diagnosis.
   a. History of diabetes mellitus, brittle or under poor control, or recent infection, myocardial infarction, emotional episode, or trauma.

  b. Clinical state of confusion through coma, hyper-ventilation, or signs of dehydration.

  c. Elevated blood sugar level, glucosuria and keto-nuria, metabolic acidosis.

2. Treatment.—The amount of ketoacidosis is more important than is the blood sugar level when therapy is initiated. For unconscious patients, treatment should begin before laboratory studies are available and should be based on a urine estimation of the degree of glucosuria and ketonuria and serum dilution gauged by acetone tablets for the degree of ketonemia. Note that acetone tablets may underestimate the degree if the ketone is predominantly β-hydroxybutyric acid.

  a. IV fluids.—Use normal saline (rapidly, 1 Liter per hour, if dehydration is present) until serum electrolyte and BUN levels are available. Monitor for evidence of fluid overload. Serum osmolality may be estimated by using the formula

$$2(Na + K) + \frac{Blood\ sugar}{18} = \frac{Serum}{osmolality}$$

Hyperosmolar, nonketotic patients may require large amounts of IV fluid to restore homeostasis. Careful close monitoring is essential.

  b. Potassium replacement should be based on blood levels. Until they are available, use the electrocardiograph (ECG) to rule out severe hyperkalemia or hypokalemia.

  c. Insulin.—When ketosis is absent, give insulin only if the blood sugar is above 600 mg/dL. Two methods are available: regular insulin, 50 to 100 units by IV push or regular insulin by continuous infusion, 6 to 10 units/hr. Add 100 units to a mixture of 1 gm of human serum albumin and 100 mL of normal saline. Administer 6 to 10 cc/hr by using a Harvard or IVAC pump.

  d. Acid-base balance.—Correct metabolic acidosis by the administration of $NaHCO_3$ only if there is shock or hyperkalemia or the serum pH is below 7.1. Avoid bolus therapy except in resuscitation. Add $NaHCO_3$ to IV fluids, 2 ampules to 1 L 0.45 normal saline. Carefully monitor the electrolytes, especially potassium, because of hypokalemia, which may follow the correction of severe acidosis. When the level falls to 4.5 mEq or less, begin replacement.

    e. Search for the precipitating cause. Provide coma patient care including a nasogastric tube, corneal protection, and a bladder catheter.

E. Hypoglycemia.

  1. Diagnosis.

    a. Almost always occurs in a diabetic patient with inadequate intake following insulin administration or excessive exercise.

    b. Can occur in alcoholic patients and may appear as persistent seizures.

    c. Rapid onset, bizarre behavior, confusion, occasional seizures, obvious overactivity of autonomic nervous system.

  2. Treatment.

    a. A semiquantitative (Dextrostix) blood sugar estimation should be performed if possible; draw a clot for immediate laboratory estimation.

    b. IV glucose, 50 cc of 50% dextrose in water.

    c. If an IV is impossible, use glucagon, 1 cc IM.

    d. Naloxone (Narcan), 0.8 mg IV, if drug abuse cannot be ruled out.

F. Uremia.

  1. Diagnosis.

    a. Slow onset of coma, usually with a history of the cause.

    b. Elevated BUN and creatinine levels.

  2. Treatment.

    a. Rule out dangerous hyperkalemia. If present, treat as in Chapter 4, Section IV.

    b. Coma management.

    c. Medical consultation.

G. Hepatic failure.
1. Diagnosis.
   a. Progressive deterioration of mental state and history of liver disease.
   b. Jaundice, flapping tremor, fetor hepaticus, spider nevi, liver palms.
2. Treatment.
   a. Coma management.
   b. Medical consultation.
H. CNS infection.—In the emergency department, meningitis and encephalitis are the most common urgent problems in this category.
1. Clinical presentation and diagnosis.
   a. Patients usually have fever and headache.
   b. Elicit a careful history for symptoms that suggest a stiff neck, photophobia, altered mentation, and neurological deficit. Be more cautious with immunosuppressed or malnourished patients. (See Chapter 23, Section II, B, 4.)
   c. Carefully examine for the source of infection, papilledema, a stiff neck or other meningeal irritation signs, neurological deficit or abnormal reflexes, and skin rash, especially petechiae.
   d. Perform a white blood cell count, urinalysis, and a spinal tap before or after a CAT scan, depending on the rate of deterioration of CNS function, the presence or absence of localizing signs, and the age of patient. Unless the CAT scan will delay urgently needed antibiotic treatment, the scan should precede the spinal tap. Consider a space-occupying lesion with rapid onset in an older patient, especially with focal findings (see Table 7–3 for cerebrospinal fluid findings).
2. Treatment.
   a. Antibiotic treatment should begin in the emergency department on the basis of clinical information and cerebrospinal fluid examination. In

TABLE 7–3.
Common Cerebrospinal Fluid Findings in Meningitis

	Opening Pressure (mm CSF*)	Cells (per mL)	Protein (mg/100 mL)	Glucose (mg/100 mL)
Normal values	<150	≤5 monocytes	15–45	40–80 (draw blood for glucose simultaneously)
Acute bacterial meningitis	Usually elevated	>300, may be few but predominantly PMNs	40–100	Low, <50% of simultaneous blood glucose
Tuberculous meningitis	Usually elevated	50–300	60–500	Low, <30% of blood glucose
Fungal meningitis	Rarely elevated	<300, usually lymphocytes	100–500	Low, <50% of blood glucose
Viral meningitis	Usually elevated	<300, usually lymphocytes, occasionally PMNs early	40–80	Normal to low

*Abbreviations: CSF = cerebrospinal fluid; PMN = polymorphonuclear leukocytes.

urgent cases empirical treatment without spinal tap results is indicated.

b. For neonatal and pediatric information, see Chapter 24.

c. For meningitis of unknown cause, in an immunocompetent adolescent or adult initiate treatment with penicillin G, 2 to 3 million units IV every 4 hours, and chloramphenicol, 1 gm every 6 hours. (See Chapter 23, Section II, B, 4.)

d. For elderly or debilitated patients, give penicillin G, 2 to 3 million units IV every 4 hours, plus cefotaxime, 2 gm IV every 4 hours.

e. For known organisms: meningococcus, penicillin G, 2 to 3 million units IV every 4 hours; *Streptococcus pneumoniae (Pneumococcus),* penicillin G, 2 to 3 million units every 4 hours; *Hemophilus influenzae,* cefotaxime, 2 gm IV every 4 hours is more effective than chloramphenicol, 1 gm IV every 6 hours, and penicillin G, 2 to 3 million units IV every 6 hours; gram-negative bacteria (e.g., *Escherichia coli*), cefotaxime, 2 gm IV every 4 hours.

f. Meningococcal prophylaxis is usually only necessary for intimate contact such as household contact; give rifampin, 600 mg/day orally for 2 to 3 days. It is unnecessary for emergency department staff.

I. Endocrine conditions.—These endocrine entities—adrenal crisis, myxedema coma, and thyroid storm—while relatively uncommon, do appear in the emergency department. They require rapid assessment and therapy.

1. Adrenal crisis.

a. Diagnosis.

(1) Usually in the steroid-dependent patient who suddenly stops taking steroid drugs or has infection and/or stress.

(2) Can occur in patients with carcinoma or tuberculosis spreading to the adrenal gland.

        (3) Presents with hypotension, confusion, and a cushingoid appearance if the patient is taking steroid drugs.

        (4) Hyponatremia, hyperkalemia, and acidosis.

    b. Treatment.

        (1) Rapid volume replacement using normal saline.

        (2) Rapid corticosteroid replacement using IV hydrocortisone, 100 mg immediately and 100 mg 4 to 6 hours later.

2. Myxedema coma.

    a. Diagnosis.

        (1) Stupor followed by coma may occur suddenly if precipitated by drug ingestion, infection, cold, or trauma.

        (2) May be a history of insidious onset of clinical signs and symptoms of myxedema.

        (3) Clinical examination characterized by hypothermia, hyperventilation, pericardial and pleural effusion, ascites, and myxedema of the facies and skin.

    b. Treatment.

        (1) Adequate ventilation and careful IV fluid administration.

        (2) Hydrocortisone, 100 to 200 mg IV immediately.

        (3) Thyroid hormone IV as L-thyroxine, 0.3 to 0.5 mg, under cardiac surveillance.

        (4) Reversal of hypothermia that ranges from passive surface rewarming to active core rewarming in severe hypothermia (temperature lower than 29.7°C, or 85°F).

3. Thyroid storm.

    a. Diagnosis.

        (1) Thyroid storm usually occurs in a known case of hyperthyroidism at the beginning of treatment or precipitated by infection, metabolic disorders, severe illness, or abrupt withdrawal from drugs.

> (2) Signs and symptoms of hyperthyroidism are exaggerated.
> (3) Persons with severe cases may have high output failure, confusion, or coma and may die suddenly.
> b. Treatment.
> > (1) Treat hypotension with fluids and vasopressors.
> > (2) Hydrocortisone, 100 mg IV immediately.
> > (3) Propranolol, 0.5 to 1.0 mg/min IV up to 2 to 10 mg every 2 to 4 hours. (Reserpine may be a useful substitute for patients with CNS agitation.)
> > (4) Treat the underlying cause.
> > (5) Treat hyperthyroidism with propylthiouracil, 300 to 400 mg orally every 8 hours. Start sodium iodine, 1 to 2 gm IV every 24 hours, 2 to 3 hours after thiourea.

J. Hypertensive encephalopathy. (For a discussion of hypertensive conditions, see specific diseases in the index.)

1. Diagnosis.
   a. Sudden severe elevation of blood pressure with development of confusion and stupor. It may progress to coma. Seizures may occur.
   b. History of preexisting hypertension or associated acute glomerulonephritis, preeclampsia, or rarely pheochromocytoma.
   c. Clinical findings of papilledema and focal neurological signs.

2. Treatment.
   a. Obvious CNS signs indicate the need for rapid evaluation and initiation of therapy. Order an ECG, chest x-ray, CBC, BUN, and urinalysis.
   b. Drug therapy.—Either of the following is considered the drug of choice.
      (1) Nitroprusside is suitable for virtually all conditions. Administration requires con-

stant nursing surveillance and usually an arterial line to monitor its immediate and often profound effect. The dose is 50 mg in 500 cc 5% dextrose in water, with the bottle covered with aluminum foil to limit the drug's exposure to light. The infusion rate should start at 0.5 μg/kg/min and be increased based on the response. The average required rate is 3 μg/kg/min.

(2) Nifedipine, sublingual, acts in 30 minutes and is given by piercing the capsule. The dose is 10 or 20 mg, and the duration of action is 4 to 5 hours.

(3) Labetalol, 20 mg IV bolus and then 20 to 80 mg every 10 minutes to achieve rapid control; an effect occurs within 5 minutes. It can be given as a continuous IV infusion, 2 mg/min.

(4) Diazoxide is useful for refractory hypertension requiring urgent, aggressive treatment. It is not indicated for patients with myocardial infarction, aortic dissection, or intracerebral hemorrhage. Diazoxide should be given as a combined, slow continuous (15 mg/min) and small-dose intermittent (1 to 2 mg/kg every 10 minutes) infusion. A response should occur within 20 minutes. Furosemide (Lasix), 40 mg, is usually given simultaneously to counteract the sodium retention of diazoxide.

(5) Hydralazine may be useful in milder cases. It is given IM or IV, 10 to 20 mg, for an effect in 20 minutes and can be repeated every 30 minutes until a response is achieved.

(6) A hypertension control program using oral drugs should be started soon. A good combination is a thiazide diuretic plus propranolol or methyldopa.

K. Cerebrovascular accident (CVA) and mass effects (see Section I, F).
   1. Diagnosis.
      a. CVAs that affect the cortex or the internal capsule rarely alter the level of consciousness. Exceptions are massive intracerebral bleeds, profound prolonged hypoxia, or the mass effect of an intracerebral lesion.
      b. Thalamic lesions usually produce stupor, and brain stem lesions produce coma.
      c. Special consideration should be given to the diagnosis of a transient ischemic attack because this condition may require immediate invasive evaluation and therapy. Similarly, if a CVA is of relatively sudden onset with the maximal neurological deficit evident from the start, the diagnosis of cerebral embolism should be carefully considered. Sources of emboli include plaques in the carotid vessels and cardiac emboli secondary to a silent myocardial infarction or a cardiac dysrhythmia, especially atrial fibrillation.
      d. Lumbar puncture is rarely indicated, and computed tomography scanning should be used as soon as possible to delineate the pathological process.
   2. Treatment.
      a. Airway management and coma care including IV glucose (50% dextrose in water) and IV naloxone, 0.8 mg.
      b. Neurological consultation for the consideration of invasive evaluation and subsequent therapy. Only very high levels of blood pressure should be treated urgently in the emergency department, and then only over several hours.
L. Catatonia and hysteria (see Chapter 30 "Psychiatric Emergencies").

8
Syncope

I. Definition

A sudden, transient loss of consciousness, with or without prodromal symptoms, followed within seconds to minutes by regaining of consciousness to the level of pre-event mental status. Confusion may persist for a short time, especially if the causative factor is still present.

II. Evaluation

A. It is essential to take an accurate history of events preceding the syncope and to obtain a complete drug history.

B. The physical examination focus is on cardiac and neurological systems and to exclude concealed hemorrhage (gastrointestinal [GI] bleed, ectopic).

C. The blood pressure and pulse should be measured with the patient lying and after standing for several minutes.

D. A complete blood count (CBC), electrocardiogram (ECG), and chest x-ray are usually part of the workup, with additional tests as needed.

E. Unfortunately, the cause is often not found in the emergency department, and close follow-up is essential. Admission to the hospital may be necessary in those patients where life-threatening cardiac or vascular causes are likely.

III. Causes

A. Cardiac
   1. Dysrhythmias.—All fast or very slow rhythm disturbances can produce decreased cerebral perfusion. Episodes of light-headedness often precede actual syncope.
   2. Myocardial infarction.—Conduction abnormalities, poor cerebral perfusion, and peripheral vasodilation produce syncope in these patients, as does pain and stress.
   3. Valvular.
      a. Aortic and mitral valve disease are common causes.
      b. Anxiety and exercise may precipitate syncope through ischemia or a sudden onset of arrhythmia.
      c. Mitral myxomas and left atrial thrombi cause syncope through the ball-valve effect or embolization.
      d. Congenital heart disease may cause syncope in children due to valve or shunt abnormalities.
      e. Hypertrophic aortic stenosis occurs in young people, and syncope is often precipitated by exercise in these patients.

B. Neurological.
   1. Carotid sinus syndrome.—A very sensitive carotid sinus responds to head and neck movement, coughing, and sneezing and leads to bradycardia. Some drugs (digitalis and propranolol) may act directly on the sinus. Other drugs cause hypotension through volume depletion or decreased peripheral resistance.
   2. Micturition syncope.—The idiopathic form occurs in young men. In older men syncope occurs when, during micturition and defecation, vagal stimulation produces bradycardia and consequent decreased cerebral perfusion.

C. Vascular.
   1. Vasovagal syncope.—This is the most common cause of syncope and results from anxiety and major stress. Syncope is usually preceded by tachycardia and hypertension. The syncope reverses promptly unless underlying cerebral cardiovascular disease results in the persistence of an altered level of consciousness.
   2. Orthostatic hypotension.—Certain drugs and numerous conditions cause a loss of vasoconstriction when the upright position is assumed. These include antihypertensive drugs, Parkinson's disease, diabetic and alcoholic neuropathies, syphilis, Guillain-Barré and Shy-Drager syndromes, and syringomyelia.
   3. Arterial diseases.—Rarely, diseases of the major arterial vessels produce pure syncope. Concealed bleeding may present as syncope. Takayasu's disease specifically produces syncope when the disease causes cerebral ischemia.
D. Miscellaneous.
   1. Endocrine.—Hypothyroidism, Addison's disease, pheochromocytoma, and hypoglycemia can cause syncope.
   2. Anemia and toxic exposure by inhalation or a direct effect may cause weakness and syncope.
   3. Hysterical.—This is a most difficult group to identify. A useful test is the cold water caloric test, which produces horizontal nystagmus away from the ear being irrigated in the normal hysterical patient. Deviation toward the cold occurs in the pathological situation.
   4. Hyperventilation and breath holding in children may produce syncope.

9
Headache

I. Causes

    A. Primary.—Most patients with headache in the emergency department have primary headaches, i.e., not due to structural lesions or identifiable systemic illnesses.

    B. Secondary.—A significant number have secondary headaches due to intracranial causes (tumors, bleeds, infections), extracranial causes (sinusitis, neuritis, temporal arteritis), and systemic causes (infection, fever, hypertension, anemia, vasoactive drugs, and carbon monoxide).

II. Evaluation

It is most important to rule out the presence of secondary headache, especially to exclude those conditions with high morbidity when the diagnosis is delayed or missed. The history is most important.

    A. Previous history.—A history of prior similar headaches suggests the primary syndrome. Migranes almost always start before the age of 30. Vascular headaches begin in childhood.

    B. Provocation.—Recurring similar headaches provoked by agents such as stress, lack of sleep, fatigue, exertion, and specific foods (cheese, alcohol, chocolate, monosodium glutamate [MSG], nitrites) are suggestive of the primary headache syndrome.

C. Time.

1. Daily headaches starting late and waxing and waning suggest tension as a cause.

2. Daily headaches starting early morning are more suggestive of migraine. These do not occur every day, and the asymptomatic periods may be long.

3. Cluster headaches start abruptly, last several hours, recur daily for days to weeks, and return after months or years.

D. Severity.—"The worst headache in my life" should be carefully evaluated for a secondary cause (subarachnoid hemorrhage), as should the patient who complains that this particular headache is worse than or different from all the previous ones. Tumors sometimes cause less severe, fluctuating pain with gradual onset that is occasionally affected by position.

E. Pain site and quality.

1. Migraine is usually pulsatile, unilateral, and temporal.

2. A tension headache is usually bandlike and at the temples, vertex, or neck.

3. Cluster headaches are severe, constant, unilateral, and often retro-orbital.

F. Prodrome.

1. Classic migraine is defined as having prodromal symptoms or signs. These can include nausea and vomiting, diarrhea, photophobia, scotomas, visual hallucinations, unilateral paresthesia, hemiparesis, vertigo, and blindness. Neurological signs may appear before the migraine and resolve during it. Aggressive evaluation is indicated when neurological signs appear after the headache starts or persist when the headache ceases.

2. Cluster headaches often have ipsilateral lacrimation, a red eye, and nasal congestion.

III. Physical examination

This should include pupil size, fundi, cranial nerves, gross motor and sensory testing, tendon reflexes, and exclusion of abnormal reflexes. In primary syndromes, findings should be limited to physiological effects as described earlier and should be normal when the patient is asymptomatic. Any neurological finding of significance warrants consultation promptly.

IV. Laboratory studies

When the evaluation suggests a secondary syndrome, a computed tomography (CT) scan followed by a spinal tap in appropriate cases is indicated. Primary headache patients seldom need laboratory evaluation.

V. Treatment

A. Ergotamine.—For vascular headaches give 2 to 3 mg, repeated every 30 to 60 minutes, to a total dose of 8 to 10 mg. The patient should be encouraged to take the drug during the prodrome. Caffeine is a useful addition as in Cafergot. If the patient is vomiting, the rectal (2 mg), intramuscular (IM) (0.3 to 0.5 mL), or aerosolized (two puffs) route is helpful.

B. Opiates.—These are effective for vascular or tension headaches, especially those resistant to other drugs. Use either codeine (30 to 60 mg orally [PO] or IM) or meperidine (75 to 125 mg with 25 to 50 mg hydroxyzine). There is a problem of the risk of dependency, especially in the chronic patient, or patient with a propensity for substance abuse.

C. Recently, intravenous (IV) prochlorperazine (Compazine) has been found useful.

D. Prophylaxis should be encouraged. Possible drugs to use include amitriptyline, propranolol, low-dose ergot, indomethacin, and methysergide or IV dihydroergotamine with metoclopramide. Avoidance of precipitating factors is also important.

10
Dizziness and Vertigo

I. Definition

The term *dizziness* is very nonspecific and is used by different people to mean different things.

    A. Vertigo.—Patients have the feeling that they or the surroundings are rotating. This is usually due to a peripheral or central cause of vestibular function disturbance.

    B. Faintness.—A feeling of weakness and impending loss of consciousness that often precedes syncope can occur.

    C. Dysequilibrium.—This is a loss of balance without the strange sensations in the head that are usually caused by problems with sensations of touch, vision, proprioception, and occasionally vestibular function.

    D. Psychogenic vertigo.—Hyperventilation due to anxiety can cause light-headedness or faintness.

II. Causes

    A. Peripheral.—About 80% of patients with dizziness have labyrinthine dysfunction.

        1. Meniere's disease.—Usually occurs in the middle-aged and presents with tinnitus, hearing loss, and

145

vertigo, with pallor, nausea, and vomiting. Attacks last minutes to 1 hour, and usually terminate abruptly. It is often bilateral, with persistence of some symptoms for many years.

2. Vestibular neuronitis.—Occurs in the younger and middle-age group and is usually unilateral with sudden severe attacks of vertigo, nausea, and vomiting. Vertigo usually resolves spontaneously over days to weeks and is often associated with a recent viral infection.

3. Benign positional vertigo.—Lasts for less than a minute and is precipitated by certain movement and position. It usually occurs in young people and is often associated with an upper respiratory tract infection.

4. Other causes.—Drugs, allergy, congenital syphilis, and bacterial and viral infections.

B. Central.—The dizziness in these situations is much less rotational and not intermittent. Nausea and vomiting are usually absent.

1. Posterior fossa tumors.—The most common are acoustic neuromas.

2. Vertebrobasilar artery insufficiency.—Atherosclerotic disease causes ischemia and, consequently, the symptoms. The attacks are short, usually relating to sudden changes in head position.

3. Post-traumatic dizziness.—This is very common following head injury and is often associated with headaches. The mechanism is not fully understood.

C. Evaluation.—Physical examination includes provocative tests to bring out the symptomatology.

1. Valsalva maneuver.

2. Carotid sinus stimulation.

3. Hyperventilation.

4. Postural vital signs.

5. Nylen-Barany test.

   a. The patient is abruptly brought from a sitting to a lying position, with the head extended to 45 degrees and held over the edge of the table.

    b. When the head is moved from the right to the left with a pause of several minutes between, the patient is observed for nystagmus and vertigo at each position.

    c. When nystagmus occurs spontaneously in acute peripheral conditions, the slow component is directed toward the involved ear.

D. Treatment.

  1. Symptomatic treatment is often helpful, and most of these diseases are self-limiting and benign. However, for those patients with unexplained neurological signs or where the cause is potentially more serious and possibly treatable, management should be aggressive, and appropriate consultation should be obtained promptly.

  2. Antihistamines.

    a. Diphenhydramine or dimenhydrinate, 50 mg orally (PO) every 4 to 6 hours; meclizine, 25 to 50 mg PO every 12 hours; or cyclizine, 50 mg intramuscularly (IM) every 4 to 6 hours.

    b. Promethazine, 25 to 50 mg can be given po, IM, or by rectal suppositories every 4 to 6 hours.

  3. Scopolamine.—A dosage of 0.06 mg PO or IM every 6 hours is often effective in severe cases, but patients occasionally have hallucinations and delirium.

11
Convulsive Disorders

I. General Considerations

A. Determine the status of the patient presenting in the emergency department (ED) with convulsive disorders.
   1. Posticteral state after having a single seizure or several seizures.
   2. In the process of having a seizure or a series of seizures (status epilepticus).
B. Distinguish *generalized status epilepticus,* which requires prompt emergency therapy, from *nonconvulsive status* (petit mal) and *partial status* (focal motor or the rare case of psychomotor status), which may be treated with less urgency and often with oral or intramuscular anticonvulsants.
C. Single seizures often do not require emergency therapy.
D. History of seizures.
   1. Determine anticonvulsant drug levels, particularly if the patient's seizures had been controlled for a long time.
   2. Augment doses of drugs found to be in a subtherapeutic range before the patient is discharged from the ED.

3. Determine the increase in the dose on the basis of the serum level of the drug and the drug's half-life.

4. If the patient is an epileptic with poorly controlled seizures, administer adequate antiseizure medication prior to discharge from the ED. The patient should also be referred back to his physician for further manipulation of the chronic anticonvulsant medication.

E. No history of seizures.

1. Conduct a more complete diagnostic evaluation.

2. If the patient is comatose and a neurological examination shows no focal neurological dysfunction, perform a computed tomography (CT) scan and, if necessary, a lumbar puncture.

3. If focal neurological abnormalities and/or papilledema are present or if the history suggests a progressive neurological process, a CT scan should be obtained immediately.

4. Avoid a lumbar puncture unless the patient is febrile or the history or physical examination suggests an acute subarachnoid hemorrhage or meningitis with no evidence of raised intracranial pressure.

II. Diagnostic Examinations

A. Status epilepticus patient.

1. Levels of serum glucose, calcium, and electrolytes and a complete blood count (CBC) should be determined.

2. Serum anticonvulsant levels should be determined if the patient is an epileptic. A serum sample may be stored for further analysis if there is no history of chronic epilepsy.

3. Serum and urine samples and a gastric aspirate should be analyzed for illicit drugs if the patient is not a known epileptic. (Phencyclidine [PCP] toxicity and barbiturate withdrawal are common

causes of status, particularly in adolescents and young adults.)

4. Prolonged seizures rarely produce lactic acidosis and myoglobinuria. Check arterial blood gases and serum creatine phosphokinase (CK) levels. The urine may need to be examined for myoglobin content.

B. Fully conscious patient with a first-time seizure without neurological deficit or evidence of infection.

1. CBC and a determination of the levels of serum electrolytes, calcium, magnesium, and glucose.

2. CT scan.

3. Consideration of phenytoin (Dilantin) loading (500 to 1,000 mg intravenously (IV) slowly), and ongoing treatment, 300 mg/day for adults.

4. Recommendations about automobile driving and operation of heavy machinery.

C. Patients with chronic seizures.

1. If the patient's baseline state is well known to the ED staff, the workup should be very limited. Uncessary CT scans and blood tests can be avoided.

2. If the patient's baseline status is unknown or if one cannot reasonably rule out the possibility of infection, intracranial bleeding, or metabolic abnormalities, a careful evaluation should be done, including a CT scan, lumbar puncture, and blood tests as needed.

III. Treatment of Status Epilepticus

A. Diazepam is used to stop the seizures and is an effective drug when administered IV, but its effectiveness is often short-lived. Respiratory arrest is an occasional complication, especially when the drug is given immediately before or after parenteral phenobarbital. The IV dose is 10 to 50 mg (not faster than 10 mg/5 min). It is often effective in the treatment of minor absence status.

B. Phenobarbital, also used to stop seizures, especially

in children, is given slowly IV or by intramuscular injection (adults, 200 to 300 mg; children, 5 to 10 mg/kg). In less urgent cases, phenobarbital may be given as an oral loading dose (5 mg/kg). The parenteral dose may be repeated in 30 to 60 minutes if seizures persist.

C. Phenytoin is used to prevent further seizures, and 15 mg/kg of body weight should be administered slowly IV (not faster than 50 mg/min) with continuous electrocardiographic (ECG) monitoring. This drug is particularly effective in treating idiopathic status epilepticus in known epileptics, but it is less effective for patients who have seizures secondary to infections or intracerebral hemorrhage. Phenytoin should *never* be given intramuscularly because of the unpredictability of its absorption. An oral loading dose of 500 to 1,000 mg may be given in less urgent cases such as brief focal motor seizures or other partial seizures. Maintenance phenytoin (5 mg/kg) should be given during the first 12 hours by the oral or IV route. The serum phenytoin level should be determined in 24 hours if the patient is kept in the ED for observation.

D. Paraldehyde should be administered if phenytoin and phenobarbital are ineffective. It may be given rectally (5 to 15 mL), IV with a glass syringe (3 to 5 mL), by slow IV infusion (up to 2.5 mL/kg of a 5% solution with saline), or by deep intramuscular injection (10 to 12 mL) and repeated if necessary (5 mL every 30 minutes). Frequent intramuscular injections should be avoided because of the risk of a sterile abscess.

E. Lidocaine is a potent anticonvulsant but has a narrow safety margin. Large doses may exacerbate or precipitate seizures. An initial bolus of 1 mg/kg may be followed in 5 minutes by a second injection of 0.5 mg/kg if the initial dose is ineffective. If seizures stop, an infusion of 30 µg/kg/min should be started. Phenobarbital may augment the anticonvulsant effect of lidocaine and suppress its neurotoxicity. Phenobarbital (100 mg) may be given intravenously with the initial bolus of lidocaine.

F. Other drugs used infrequently in the treatment of status epilepticus are chloral hydrate, 4 gm by rectal infusion, and sodium amytal (sodium amobarbital), by slow intravenous infusion (500 mg in a 10-ml solution at a rate of 1 ml or 50 mg/minute).

G. In rare instances if seizures persist, it may be necessary to proceed to general anesthesia, intubation, and neuromuscular paralysis. In such cases continuous or intermittent EEG monitoring may be necessary because the neuromuscular paralysis will block the peripheral manifestations of seizures.

12
Neurological Trauma

I. Head Injuries

A. Be sure the airway is clear, and ensure that ventilation is adequate. If intubation is needed use the orotracheal route with manual in-line traction or the nasotracheal route. If facial injuries make intubation hazardous, consider immediate cricothyroidotomy.

B. Stop active bleeding with pressure unless a spurting vessel can be seen and clamped.

C. Investigate other parts of the body for life-threatening injuries (e.g., sucking sound in the chest).

D. Keep the neck immobilized until cervical injury is ruled out on clinical grounds or, when indicated, radiological grounds.

E. Do a brief but thorough neurological examination, and record the results as soon as possible (see Chapter 7, Section I).

   1. Evaluate the state of consciousness. Changes in this state are more important than all other examination findings in raising the suspicion of intracranial hemorrhage.

      a. Is the patient awake?

      b. Does he answer questions and obey commands?

      c. If drowsy, can he be readily awakened?

    d. Is he oriented for time, place, and person?

    e. If unresponsive verbally, does he respond to painful stimuli such as pressure between the mastoid and the mandible or on supraorbital nerves or squeezing the Achilles tendon?

    f. If he moves, is the movement purposeful (i.e., can he respond to directions)?

    g. Do all four extremities move?

    h. Is the movement restricted to flexion or extension of arms and legs (decerebrate response)?

2. Examine the eyes for pupillary size and reaction to light.

    a. Unilateral enlargement of a pupil may indicate increasing intracranial pressure, especially when the patient is unresponsive.

    b. Fixed midsize or small pupils may indicate a midbrain or pontine lesion.

    c. Whenever pupillary inequality is visible in the initial examination, it should be carefully evaluated. Even in the alert patient, it may indicate early herniation.

    d. The finding of normal fundi does not preclude intracranial trauma. The examination should be deferred, especially if the patient is restless or uncooperative.

3. Eye movement.

    a. If the eyelids are not too swollen to prevent the examiner from seeing eye movement, the simple turning of the eyes in response to a command gives a baseline for recording.

    b. If the patient is unconscious and cervical injury has been ruled out, gently rotating the head to one side permits one to see whether the eyeballs stay with the head (doll's eyes absent) or move to the opposite side (doll's eyes present); movement indicates preservation of the oculocephalic (proprioceptive head turning) reflex. If cervical injury has not been ruled out, keep the neck immobilized. Consider caloric testing if it is important to rule out brain stem injury and computed tomographic (CT) scan is not available.

4. Assessments of the motor functions of jaws, face, palate, and neck are readily done in conscious patients.

5. Palpation of the neck posteriorly for tenderness may permit recognition of dislocation or fracture and must precede any attempt to turn the patient to examine the spine.

6. Deep-tendon reflexes.

    a. Deep-tendon reflexes should be elicited. Abdominal and cremasteric reflexes are not of immediate vital importance.

    b. Babinski and similar abnormal reflexes indicate impairment of central nervous system pathways and should be elicited.

7. Bleeding from the ear and nose.

    a. Investigate to see whether the blood is from an adjacent laceration.

    b. Admixture with cerebrospinal fluid or leakage of clear fluid alone indicates a basal skull fracture regardless of skull radiographs.

    c. Hospitalization for observation is indicated.

    d. If blood is present in the ear canal or nose, do not insert instruments, and do not try to dam it up with cotton or gauze. For cleanliness, gauze can be taped against the external ear to still allow otorrhea.

    e. Obvious blood arising in the ear (e.g., bulging or discolored eardrum) indicates a basal skull fracture. The patient should be hospitalized.

8. Nystagmus may be noted in the examination of eye movements and may mean cerebellar or vestibular disturbance or recent indulgence in alcohol or other drugs such as phencyclidine (PCP).

F. Closed head injuries.

1. Blood pressure, pulse, and respiration recordings are made at admission and at 30- to 60-minute

intervals at first and then at 1- to 4-hour intervals if the patient remains comatose or the state of consciousness deteriorates. Early CT scanning is very important.

2. Pupillary changes and responsiveness are also charted. Increased pupil size, expecially if unilateral, and decreased alertness indicate the need for prompt neurosurgical attention.

3. Sedation will interfere with these criteria and should be minimized. Acetaminophen or acetylsalicylic acid (aspirin) is useful for analgesia and may help restlessness; if there is pain from an additional serious injury, narcotics may be necessary.

4. If a convulsion occurs, anticonvulsants may be administered. For persistent seizures i.e., status epilepticus, Diazepam (Valium), 10-15 mg· given intravenously, 5 mg/min, has the advantage of minimizing sedation. To prevent additional seizures in the immediate future, phenytoin loading should be initiated. Alternative drugs are available (see Chapter 7).

5. X-ray films of the head are not the first priority for patients with severe, closed head injuries; repeated clinical observations are more important. With missile injuries and compound fractures, determining the location of bone and foreign objects becomes important, and films may be used when CT scanning is not available. Skull x-rays are more useful clinically in children, often identifying unsuspected fractures. These x-rays are also of value in awake adult patients who have received a direct temporal-area blow or injury. When the patient is alert and there is no serious neurological problem, skull radiographs may be used as part of the basis for deciding about the release of the patient from the emergency department. A fracture usually indicates the severity of the head trauma and ordinarily indicates hospitalization for observation. In a patient with altered mental sta-

tus, a negative skull x-ray finding does not rule out significant head injury.

6. Cervical spine x-rays should be considered in any patient with a head injury or injury above the clavicle accompanied by unconsciousness. Care must be taken to consider injuries to the spine before twisting or turning the patient's neck; when there is doubt, it is best to take just anteroposterior and across-the-table lateral views without turning the head. For every patient, the C7 and T1 bodies must be visualized on the x-ray. Downward traction on the arms by an adequately protected individual and/or swimmer's views may be required.

7. CT scanning should be considered for head injury patients who do not improve promptly and for all patients who show signs of neurological deterioration.

8. Hyperventilation to a Pa_{CO_2} of 25 to 30 mm Hg is indicated if cerebral edema is suspected.

9. In the rapidly deteriorating patient, mannitol 1 to 1.5 gm/kg, should be given intravenously, once only. Place a Foley catheter in the unconscious patient.

10. The use of steroids to reduce cerebral edema resulting from trauma is no longer supported scientifically. If used, dexamethasone (Decadron), 20 mg, should be administered intravenously, immediately followed by 10 mg every 4 hours for 24 hours.

G. Penetrating head injuries.

1. All penetrating wounds of the cranial cavity require debridement and closure. If the dura has been breached, a neurosurgeon and operating room facilities will be required. If a knife or foreign object protrudes from the head, it should be removed in the operating room.

2. The patient's condition should be evaluated regularly, as in closed head injuries (see Section F).

3. If there is active scalp bleeding, figure-of-eight or vertical mattress sutures are better than applying hemostats to vessels that are smaller than superficial temporal, frontal, or occipital arteries.
4. Before closure, the wound can be probed gently with sterile forceps or a sterile gloved finger to see whether there is a fracture. If unsure, obtain skull x-rays.

II. Spine Injuries

A. Any patient who has fallen or has been involved in an accident including drowning may have an injury to the spine and its contents. Consequently, a high degree of suspicion is warranted for any unconscious patient who is brought into the emergency department, and movements should be gentle and guarded. A rigid cervical collar should be applied to prevent neck movement, and the patient should be on a spine board.

B. Examination.
1. In the examination of the unconscious patient, the spine should be palpated from head to sacrum for obvious protrusions, malalignments, and areas of reflex pain withdrawal responses.
2. If the patient needs to be turned, the head and body should be moved en bloc to avoid twisting the neck and spine until the examiner is sure there is no injury.
3. Determination of the presence of knee and ankle stretch reflexes and withdrawal responses to pinprick or other painful stimuli will aid even the unconscious patient. The absence of such reflexes and responses may indicate trauma to the spinal cord. It is important to check for priapism and to assess rectal sphincter tone and reflex.
4. If the patient is conscious, neurological examination can rapidly detect spinal cord damage.
   a. Voluntary movement of various parts of the extremities is requested.

b. Reflexes are elicited, including plantar, abdominal, and cremasteric responses in men and biceps, triceps, knee, and ankle stretch reflexes. Responses to a pinprick also are elicited. Rectal sphincter tone must be assessed. Priapism suggests cord injury.

5. The level of spinal cord injury can be determined by the neurological findings with reasonable accuracy in most cases (Tables 12–1 and 12–2).

a. The thoracic levels of most injuries cannot be determined by muscular movements except that forceful ventral flexion of the neck normally produces contraction of the recti abdomini mus-

TABLE 12–1.
Motor Levels

Action	Muscles	Spinal Cord Levels
Shrugging shoulders	Trapezius	Accessory nerve, C2, C3
Flexion of forearm at elbow	Biceps	C5, C6
Extension of arm at elbow	Triceps	C6, C7
Abduction and adduction of fingers	Interosseous and lumbricals	C8, T1
Flexion of thigh on abdomen	Iliopsoas	L1, L2, L3
Extension of lower leg at knee	Quadriceps	L2, L3, L4
Dorsiflexion of foot and great toe	Anterior tibial and peroneal muscles	L4, L5
Plantar flexion of foot	Gastrocnemius	L5, S1

TABLE 12–2.
Sensory Levels

Areas of Body	Spinal Cord Levels	Vertebral Body Levels
Neck to clavicle	C2–4	C2–4
Outer deltoid	C5	C5
Thumb	C6	C6
Index finger	C7	C7
Little finger	C8	T1
Nipple	T3	T2
Umbilicus	T10	T8
Inguinal area (groin)	L1	T10
Thigh above knee	L3	T11
Lateral part of calf	L4	T11–12
Foot dorsum	L5	T12
Lateral part of foot and small toe	S1	L1
Buttock	S3–5	L1–2

cle (T8–T12). If the umbilicus moves upward (Beevor's sign), the upper recti (T8–T10) are active, and the lower ones (T11–T12) are not.

b. In the cervical area, the vertebral bodies correspond to the spinal cord segments; in the thoracic region, the bodies are 1 to 2 segments higher than the cord levels; the lumbar and sacral areas of the cord are compressed from the level of T10 to the interspace between L1 and L2, where the cord normally ends. Pinprick sensation should be checked on both sides of the body and also on the back and front for discrepancies and better localization.

c. Retention of superficial and deep pain discrimination indicates an incomplete lesion, and lateral-column preservation. Sacral sparing, (retained anal sensation and voluntary contraction) also indicates an incomplete lesion and is often a good prognostic sign.

6. The most common serious injuries to the spine that are compatible with life are those at C5–6 and those at T12–L1.

   a. Lesions at or above C4 usually involve phrenic centers and apnea. Those at C5–6 cause sensory loss below the clavicles and on the tricipital and ulnar areas of the arm and hand.

   b. Lesions at L1 involve the conus medullaris and produce saddle anesthesia and sphincter tone loss.

   c. Once the presumed locus of the neurological lesion is determined, radiographs of the spine corresponding to this area should be done. Movement of the patient with a suspected spine lesion should be minimized; hence, a complete x-ray examination may not be warranted.

   d. The area at C6–T1, especially in large men, may be difficult to visualize unless the arms are pulled down while the film is taken. Swimmer's views may be required. Oblique views, again without moving the patient, may be needed.

   e. CT scanning of the spine may be very helpful.

C. Treatment.

1. Ensure that the airway is patent and ventilation is adequate. High cord lesions sometimes produce apnea. If tracheal intubation is needed, use the oro-tracheal route with manual in-line traction or the nasotracheal route.

2. If x-rays show a fracture and/or dislocation in the cervical spine, spine immobilization if not already in place should be immediately instituted wherever the patient is—in the x-ray department, the emergency department, or the operating room.

3. Whenever possible, the Regional Spinal Cord Center physicians should be involved in the care of these patients as early as possible. Patients with un-stable fractures, fracture-dislocations, or a neuro-

logical deficit should be considered for transfer to the regional center as soon as clinically stable (see Table 12–3). Early telephone consultation should address spinal cord aspects of patient management, including the value of Gardner-Wells tongs, the

TABLE 12–3.
Classification of Spinal Injuries

Mechanisms of Spinal Injury	Stability
Flexion	
Wedge fracture	Stable
Clay shoveler's fracture	Stable
Subluxation	Potentially unstable
Bilateral facet dislocation	Always unstable
Flexion teardrop fracture	Extremely unstable
Atlanto-occipital dislocation	Unstable
Anterior atlantoaxial dislocation with or without fracture	Unstable
Odontoid fracture with lateral displacement fracture	Unstable
Fracture of transverse process	Stable
Rotation	
Unilateral facet dislocation	Stable
Rotary atlantoaxial dislocation	Unstable
Extension	
Posterior neural arch fracture (C1)	Unstable
Hangman's fracture (C2)	Unstable
Extension teardrop fracture	Usually stable in flexion; unstable in extension
Posterior atlantoaxial dislocation with or without fracture	Unstable
Vertical compression	
Bursting fracture of vertebral body	Stable
Jefferson fracture (C1)	Extremely unstable
Isolated fractures of articular pillar and vertebral body	Stable

composition of the clinical team for transfer, and selection of transfer vehicle type. In the absence of a specific recommendation to use Gardner-Wells tongs, it is acceptable to transfer these patients in strict immobilization by using a semirigid collar and spine board plus sandbags and tape as needed to ensure a minimum of mobility. It may be necessary for a physician and/or nurse to accompany the patient during transfer.

4. For any patient with a stable spine fracture without a neurological deficit, prompt neurosurgical and/or orthopedic consultation is recommended.

13

Acute Abdominal Emergencies

I. Intestinal Obstruction

A. Mechanical obstruction of the bowel is a common cause of acute abdominal pain. From almost every clinical standpoint, obstructions of the small and large bowel are two different diseases.

B. The diagnosis of obstruction cannot be made on the basis of any single group of symptoms.

1. Nearly all patients at some time during the course of obstruction have pain, vomiting, distension, obstipation, and abnormal x-ray findings.

2. Distension and obstipation occur most consistently, yet neither is diagnostic.

3. Pain and vomiting are more prominent with small-bowel obstructions and may be absent with obstructions of the large bowel.

4. Obstructive pain is typically cramping, starts without warning, is frequently followed by vomiting, tends to build to a peak of severity, and then suddenly subsides. The next episode follows in 5 to 15 minutes. Such rhythmic periodicity is characteristic of obstructive pain and differentiates it from the cramping of minor intestinal disturbances.

 5. The vomiting varies somewhat with the level of the obstruction. It is frequent and abundant with high obstructions and occasionally absent with colon obstructions.

 6. Although the absence of bowel movement is a natural sequence to a mechanical block, a preliminary period of diarrhea may occur as the obstruction becomes complete.

 7. Stool may be passed for as long as 24 hours after the onset while the colon distal to the obstruction is being evacuated.

C. Distension is invariably present unless the obstruction is quite high. Ordinarily, the distension begins in the lower abdomen and progresses upward as more and more loops become distended.

D. A characteristic finding in intestinal obstruction is the presence of high-pitched, rushing bowel sounds, which result when intestinal contents are squirted through a narrow lumen. The sounds may be followed by relief from pain, thus identifying that pain as an obstructive paroxysm.

E. The plain x-ray film of the abdomen supplies important information for the diagnosis of obstruction and especially for the differentiation between that of the small bowel and the large bowel.

 1. Films should be made with the patient both supine and upright and should include the diaphragm and the lowest part of the pelvis.

 2. Gas in the intestinal tract produces typical patterns that identify the bowel as either small intestine or colon.

 3. Gas patterns are not always seen if only a supine film is made because the dammed-up fluid proximal to the obstruction obliterates the gas pattern.

 4. The upright film will show multiple horizontal fluid levels, which indicate the existence of stasis.

F. It is most important to differentiate mechanical obstruction from adynamic ileus.

1. Adynamic ileus follows a variety of processes such as peritonitis, excessive trauma during surgery, injury to intra-abdominal organs, hypokalemia, and other diseases.
2. Pain is often absent, except in persons with post-operative ileus.
3. Bowel sounds are characteristically absent.
4. The plain x-ray film of the abdomen shows distended loops of both large *and* small bowel with multiple fluid levels.
5. In mechanical obstruction, either the small or the large bowel is predominantly involved, depending on the level of the obstruction.

G. The differentiation between large- and small-bowel obstruction usually is not difficult.

1. Typical small-bowel obstruction is seen in young or middle-aged patients.
2. The patient usually has had previous abdominal surgery or a hernia.
3. The symptoms are sudden in onset and consist of severe pain and persistent vomiting.

H. Large-bowel obstructions, because they are usually caused by carcinoma, are seen mostly in older persons. The history is one of chronic constipation slowly progressing to obstipation, with episodes of pain and bloating and frequently the passage of blood. Vomiting is often minimal or absent. X-ray interpretation of plain films of the abdomen is a most valuable diagnostic procedure. Mechanical obstruction primarily involves either the small intestine or the colon; gas appears in one or the other but rarely in both. An exception is large-bowel obstruction with an incompetent ileocecal valve. The characteristic small-bowel pattern is that of a distended bowel marked by thin feathery lines, the valvulae conniventes (Fig 13–1). The pattern of colon obstruction outlines the haustra of the colon as large segmented collections of gas (Fig 13–2).

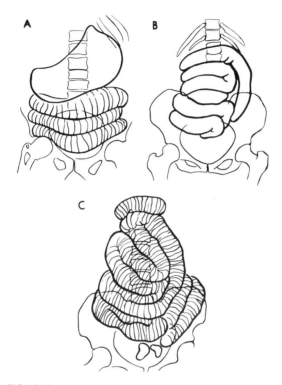

FIG 13–1.
Mechanical small-bowel obstruction. **A,** bowel caught in an implant of carcinoma. Valvulae conniventes indentify the pattern as being of the small bowel. Gastric distension is present. **B,** valvulae conniventes is not seen, but the "ladder formation" indentifies the gas pattern as small-bowel obstruction (due to postoperative adhesion). **C,** advanced obstruction indicated by the oblique position of the loops in an obstruction secondary to adhesion. The almost complete absence of air in the large bowel is characteristic of complete small-bowel obstruction.

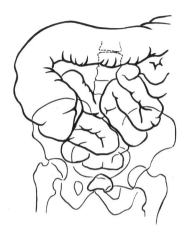

FIG 13–2.
Large-bowel obstruction: diagram from a plain x-ray film of the abdomen that shows a distended cecum and transverse colon. The distended small bowel indicates incompetence of the ileocecal valve and advanced obstruction.

I. Recognition of strangulation.
 1. Strangulation rarely occurs with a large-bowel obstruction except in volvulus.
 2. Strangulation is a constant hazard with all small-bowel obstructions.
 3. The most significant clinical finding is abdominal tenderness of varying intensity, usually associated with rebound tenderness. Fever and leukocytosis develop.
 4. The obstructive pain, which at first is periodic, tends to become constant and very severe.
J. Sigmoid volvulus.
 1. Cramping abdominal pain, abdominal distension,

nausea and vomiting, and obstipation are the clinical findings.

2. An abdominal x-ray displays a distended loop of the large bowel on the left side, with the curve in the upper portion of the abdomen and the "beak" in the pelvis.

3. Treatment consists of derotation by passage of a rectal tube through a sigmoidoscope. Dramatic decompression is the rule.

4. The patient should then be admitted to the hospital and observed for signs of a gangrenous bowel.

K. Cecal volvulus.

1. Findings are the sudden onset of colicky midabdominal pain, nausea, vomiting, and moderate abdominal distension. The abdomen may be diffusely tender and tympanitic, or the tenderness may be localized to the right lower quadrant.

2. An abdominal x-ray reveals a distended, oval, or kidney-shaped loop of bowel in the midabdomen or left upper quadrant. There may be distended loops of small bowel and no colonic gas.

3. Immediate surgery is the treatment of choice.

II. Acute Inflammatory Disease

A. The pain of inflammatory disease frequently begins slowly, away from the involved organ, and later tends to shift and localize over the organ.

1. The pain is often described as cramping, but it does not have a definite periodic seizure like the seizures of obstruction.

2. Some pain persists at all times, even between the periods of intense pain. The pain of intestinal obstruction on the other hand, is intermittent rather than remittent, i.e., between episodes, the patient is free from pain.

    3. A particular feature of an acute inflammatory process is pain when the patient walks, coughs, moves about, or is jarred.

B. Appendicitis.

    1. Pathognomonic of acute appendicitis is generalized abdominal pain that later localizes to the right lower quadrant.

    2. Vomiting may be absent, but anorexia is nearly always present. Hunger in a patient with abdominal pain is strong evidence against the diagnosis of appendicitis.

    3. A low-lying appendix produces lower abdominal pain and tenderness that do not localize well, but it usually can be diagnosed by tenderness on the right on rectal examination.

    4. If the diagnosis is uncertain, any patient who has abdominal pain with localized tenderness in the right lower quadrant usually requires observation and consideration for laparotomy.

C. Pelvic inflammatory disease.

    1. Pain begins in the lower abdomen, is quite persistent, and may be severe. Its onset frequently coincides with the menses.

    2. Because the gastrointestinal tract is not involved, it is not unusual for the patient to eat regularly.

    3. Tenderness is usually bilateral, although it may be localized in the right lower quadrant.

    4. Adnexal tenderness and, most important, excruciating pain on movement of the cervix are of considerable diagnostic significance.

    5. Fever, leukocytosis, and elevation of the erythrocyte sedimentation rate may be present.

    6. For treatment, see Chapter 15.

D. Acute diverticulitis produces symptoms similar to those of appendicitis except that the findings are localized to the left side of the abdomen. They are more often seen in older patients and there may be a prior history of diverticulosis.

E. Cholecystitis.
  1. Gallbladder pain characteristically is in the right upper quadrant or the epigastrium, with radiation through to the interscapular region and shoulder. Pain in other parts of the abdomen lasting more than a few hours usually does not arise from the biliary tract.
  2. Tenderness over the gallbladder is frequent, and occasionally there is a significant rise in the quantitative serum bilirubin level, even though there is no stone in the common bile duct.
  3. An ultrasound of the gallbladder is indicated if cholecystitis is considered: biliary stones are consistently visualized, and other signs of gallbladder inflammation may be seen.

F. Perforated peptic ulcer.
  1. The sudden outpouring of gastroduodenal contents into the abdominal cavity produces a dramatic clinical picture.
  2. The pain is sudden, reaches maximum intensity immediately, and usually remains constant and unremitting. It may, however, subside for a period following perforation as a result of the transudation of fluid into the peritoneal space. This fluid dilutes gastric contents.
  3. The patient has an anxious, pale appearance, the skin is diaphoretic, and the abdomen is held rigid. The patient does not move in bed at all.
  4. The rigidity is absolutely unyielding and results in the term *boardlike*.
  5. Peristaltic sounds are usually absent, and tenderness is most marked in the upper portion of the abdomen.
  6. The most reliable diagnostic procedure is x-ray demonstration of free intraperitoneal air. The best view for visualizing the presence of free air in the abdomen is the upright chest or lateral decubitus.

G. Acute pancreatitis is predominantly a disease of heavy drinkers. It may also be seen in the patient with gallbladder disease.

1. It is characterized by a sudden onset of severe pain, following a large meal.

2. The pain is quite severe, is constant, and radiates through the back.

3. The patient is acutely ill; the abdomen may be soft, but tenderness and rebound tenderness are usually present.

4. Proper management of acute pancreatitis is rarely operative.

5. The level of serum amylase is almost always elevated at some time during an episode of acute pancreatitis, especially in the early hours of the disease. The rise is frequently transitory, and there may be no abnormal result; nevertheless, the diagnosis cannot often be established with certainty unless the serum or urine amylase value is known to be abnormal.

6. In acute pancreatitis, the renal clearance of amylase exceeds that of creatinine. The amylase/creatinine ratio is calculated with the following formula:

$$\frac{\text{Urine amylase}}{\text{Serum amylase}} \times \frac{\text{Serum creatinine}}{\text{Urine creatinine}} \times 100$$

In acute pancreatitis this is elevated above a normal of 5%.

III. Constipation and Diarrhea

A. Constipation has a variety of causes including fecal impaction, dehydration, intestinal obstruction, hypercalcemia, and the use of medications that reduce intestinal motility.

1. The history and physical examination should

stress the aforementioned areas. The abdominal and rectal examinations are particularly important.

2. Abdominal x-rays should be obtained if intestinal obstruction is considered.

B. Diarrhea may be the result of several mechanisms. Disorders of gastrointestinal motility in chronic illnesses such as diabetes may produce diarrhea.

1. Acute diarrhea frequently has an infectious etiology. The organism responsible may be viral, bacterial, or protozoal.

2. The history should stress that of foreign travel, involvement of other family members, and the presence of mucous or blood in the stool.

3. Rectal examination should be done and the stool tested for blood and fecal leukocytes.

   a. Blood in diarrheal stool is commonly seen in *Shigella* enteritis infection, amebiasis, *Campylobacter* infection, and ulcerative colitis.

   b. Fecal leukocytes are present in infection with *Salmonella, Shigella,* amebas, and *Yersinia.*

4. Stool bacterial culture or a search for ova and parasites should be performed as clinically indicated.

5. Symptomatic treatment with bismuth subsalicylate is recommended. Opiates should be avoided, as they may prolong the duration of a bacterial infection.

IV. Traumatic Wounds of the Abdomen

A. Nonpenetrating or blunt injury to the abdomen may rupture a hollow viscus and cause peritonitis or may rupture a solid viscus and cause internal hemorrhage.

1. Many abdominal contusions occur without serious visceral damage, but the possibility of such injury must be kept in mind constantly and the

patient examined at frequent intervals until a decision can be made regarding surgery.

2. A very trivial injury may rupture the bowel or spleen. Serious injuries may occur without a visible mark or contusion on the abdominal wall.

3. Difficulties in diagnosis arise because clinical evidence of injury may not appear until several hours after the injury.

4. It is mandatory that the same physician examine the patient at frequent intervals.

5. An intravenous line, nasogastric tube, and Foley catheter are installed. As soon as the patient's condition permits, plain x-ray films of the abdomen and chest are made and examined for pneumoperitoneum or for a characteristic intestinal gas pattern. The absence of free intraperitoneal air does not rule out rupture of a hollow viscus.

6. The correct diagnosis depends to a great extent on the frequency and character of the clinical examinations.

7. Absolute indications for a laparotomy are the following:
   a. The evisceration of abdominal contents.
   b. The presence of free intraperitoneal air.
   c. Abdominal lavage that yields blood.
   d. Persistent shock in the absence of thoracic, spinal, or significant extremity injury.

B. Solid-organ injury.
   1. Visceral injury occurs most often to the spleen or liver.
   2. Plain films of the abdomen are occasionally of considerable help in diagnosing a splenic rupture.
   3. Even small tears of the spleen may continue to bleed, so once the diagnosis is made, a decision regarding operative intervention is indicated.
   4. The typical picture of traumatic rupture of the spleen consists of the following:
      a. Abdominal pain.

  b. Tenderness.
  c. Evidence of internal hemorrhage.
  d. Pain in the left shoulder.
5. Signs of hypovolemia may be present at the time of the initial examination or be delayed by hours or days.

C. The bladder is the hollow viscus most frequently damaged. Injury is suspected in any patient who has a pelvic fracture or in whom only a few drops of bloody urine are obtained by catheterization.
  1. Diagnosis is made by extravasation of contrast material on retrograde cystourethrography.
  2. If blood is present at the urethral meatus, urinary catheterization should not be done until this study is performed.

D. Peritoneal lavage is performed by inserting a renal dialysis catheter below the umbilicus. A liter of saline is run in and then aspirated to determine whether free blood exists in the peritoneal cavity. An abnormal tap is helpful, but a normal tap does not rule out intra-abdominal injury.

E. Computed tomographic (CT) body scanning has been used in abdominal trauma patients who are hemodynamically stable. CT is especially useful for delineating hepatic, splenic, and renal injury. Because CT visualizes the retroperitoneal space, it is useful for identifying injuries in this area.

F. Penetrating wounds.
  1. A problem in such wounds is to determine whether the abdominal cavity has been penetrated and, if so, what intra-abdominal structure has been injured.
  2. An intravenous line should be started and hemoglobin, hematocrit, and urine examinations performed.
  3. A nasogastric tube, a bladder catheter, and a rectal examination are indicated.
  4. Abdominal and chest x-ray films are made to examine for pneumoperitoneum and for localization of the missile if the wound is from a bullet.

5. Presumptive evidence of penetration of a viscus is based on the following:
   a. Abdominal tenderness and rebound tenderness.
   b. Increasing pulse rate and decreasing blood pressure.
   c. Pneumoperitoneum.
   d. Discharge of intestinal contents or bile from the wound.
   e. Blood emanating from catheters in the stomach or bladder.
6. Gunshot wounds.
   a. Unlike knife wounds in which viscera may slip away from the path of the knife, a bullet rips through the abdomen and damages structures in its path and even some distance away.
   b. Massive peritoneal contamination or serious hemorrhage frequently results.
   c. The mortality from gunshot wounds of the abdomen is high and can be decreased by shortening the interval between injury and operation.
   d. Laparotomy is mandatory because of the serious nature of these wounds.
   e. Antibiotic therapy should be instituted early and should cover both aerobic and anaerobic bowel flora. Tetanus prophylaxis should be administered. Give gentamicin, 60 to 80 mg intramuscularly or intravenously and then 3 to 5 mg/kg/day, and intravenous cefoxitin, 1 gm every 4 hours, or intravenous clindamycin, 600 mg every 6 hours.

V. Massive Gastrointestinal Hemorrhage

A. Patients with massive gastrointestinal tract hemorrhage present a most urgent problem and require immediate treatment. The majority of these patients have peptic ulcer disease, gastroesophagitis, or gastroesophageal varices.

1. A smaller proportion of persons with gastrointestinal tract hemorrhage have erosive gastritis, gastric carcinoma, or polyps as a cause of bleeding.
2. Severe bleeding from the lower part of the gastrointestinal tract may be due to ulcerative colitis, bleeding diverticulosis, adenocarcinoma, or large hemorrhoidal veins.

B. A rapid history is taken, and inquiry should be made as to the use of steroids, salicylates, and anticoagulants as well as to hypertension.

C. Evaluation of the patient.

1. Blood is taken for a complete blood cell count, typing, and crossmatching, and an intravenous catheter is inserted. Oxygen is given, and intravenous fluids are infused as indicated. A nasogastric tube is inserted, and blood is evacuated from the stomach.
2. A search is made for signs of cirrhosis such as enlargement of the liver, spider nevi, palmar erythema, and dilated superficial veins around the umbilicus.
3. An abdominal mass, enlarged supraclavicular lymph nodes, a rectal shelf, or an enlarged liver may indicate a gastric carcinoma.
4. All patients with massive hemorrhage should be admitted to the hospital promptly. Endoscopy may be very helpful in localizing the site of bleeding.
   a. If the bleeding is due to esophageal varices, it may be necessary to use a Sengstaken-Blakemore tube.
   b. After inflation of the balloons, traction must be maintained to hold the gastric balloon in place and to keep pressure on the bleeding point.
   c. Continuous-infusion intravenous vasopressin, 0.3 to 0.9 units/min, may be useful to control variceal bleeding. However, it has not been shown to affect eventual mortality.

d. If the bleeding arises from an ulcer, blood is replaced as indicated, and the patient is observed for evidence of persistent or continued bleeding.

VI. Anorectal Conditions

A. Fecal impactions.
  1. History.
     a. Change in bowel habits.
     b. Feeling of constant rectal pressure.
     c. As a rule, the patient has been taking antidiarrheal medication.
     d. The condition is generally found in elderly or debilitated patients.
  2. Objective findings.
     a. Rectal examination will reveal a large, rocklike fecal bolus with soft stool oozing around the mass.
     b. If no mass is palpable, have the patient strain as if defecating, and the mass will be palpable to the index finger.
     c. In rare cases, a large mass will be revealed in the sigmoid on sigmoidoscopy.
  3. Treatment.
     a. Two oil-retention enemas are given and retained as long as possible.
     b. If the mass is not passed, digital manipulation will aid in breaking it up for evacuation.
     c. Follow-up treatment:
        (1) Instruct the patient to drink more fluids.
        (2) Have the patient increase the bulk of the stool with more vegetables, bran cereal, and fruit.
        (3) Prescribe a bulk laxative.
B. Perirectal abscess.
  1. History.
     a. This abscess can occur in persons of any age but is rare in children.

       b. The patient complains of rectal pain, pressure, inability to sit, and chills and fever for 24 to 48 hours.

   2. Objective findings.

       a. There is an erythema with fluctuation in the perianal area. Fluctuance may be a late finding.

       b. If the aforementioned is not present, do an anoscopy to visualize an infected anal crypt, which will be oozing from the involved area.

       c. If the aforementioned are not found, have the patient take sitz baths every 4 hours, and re-examine him frequently.

   3. Treatment.

       a. Inject 1% lidocaine with epinephrine intradermally over the abscess.

       b. Allow 5 minutes for the anesthesia to take effect, and supplement if necessary.

       c. Incise the abscess widely.

       d. Use hemostats to open undermined tracts.

       e. Have the patient put ice packs over the incision for 24 hours.

       f. Apply constant, warm, wet compresses during the day after the first 24 hours.

       g. Warn the patient that this may develop into a fistula in ano and require further surgery.

C. Acute fissure in ano.

   1. History and symptoms.

       a. Acute rectal pain during and following defecation may last several minutes to many hours.

       b. Traces of blood may be found on toilet tissue.

   2. Objective findings.

       a. Rectal spasm that increases when the buttocks are separated.

       b. An inverted V-shaped tag with a fiery raw base. Bleeding is not noted on this examination.

       c. Anoscopic examination causes extreme pain and allows the visualization of small hypertrophic anal papillae, in the raw area posteriorly.

    3. Treatment.

        a. Cauterization of anal fissure with 10% silver nitrate on applicator.

        b. Use of Tucks pads for cleansing following defecation and at bedtime.

        c. Dilation of the rectum with a finger cot followed by pramoxine or hydrocortisone suppositories.

        d. Sitz baths for 20 minutes every 4 hours, if possible, in comfortably warm, not hot, water.

        e. Bulk laxative.

D. Acute thrombosed hemorrhoids.

    1. History and symptoms.

        a. Sudden onset of pain followed by a palpable rectal mass.

        b. Not related to the patient's activity but frequently occurs during defecation.

    2. Objective findings.

        a. Purple mass at mucocutaneous line of rectum.

        b. Painful to touch and nonreducible.

    3. Treatment.

        a. Infiltration of hemorrhoid and sphincter with 1% lidocaine or 0.5% bupivacaine.

        b. Elliptical excision of overlying skin and evacuation of clot.

        c. Aftercare.

            (1) Ice bag for 24 hours.

            (2) Sitz bath four times daily for 20 minutes each time.

            (3) Weekly follow-up postoperatively.

        d. It is important not to confuse a thrombosed external hemorrhoid with a prolapsed internal hemorrhoid, because an incision in the latter may result in profuse bleeding.

E. Rectal prolapse.

    1. History, symptoms, and findings.

        a. Generally found in elderly but has also been seen in younger patients.

        b. Large painful mass felt by the patient as a rule

after straining at defecation or severe coughing.

    c. Large purplish circumferential mass protruding 2 to 12 cm from the anus with extreme rectal spasm and pain.

2. Treatment.

    a. Early cases.—With the patient in the knee-chest position, attempt to reduce the edema with gentle digital pressure. If not successful, inject 1% lidocaine into the rectal sphincter, and replace the prolapse manually. Apply a pressure dressing, and then tape the buttocks.

    b. Late cases.—Apply constant, warm, wet compresses. Do not reduce them manually because of the danger of pelvic emboli and sepsis. Allow gangrenous tissue to demarcate with the aid of antibiotics before any surgery is considered.

14

Genitourinary Tract Disorders

The urologic emergencies seen in the emergency department (ED) are trauma (to the kidneys, ureter, bladder, urethra, external genitalia), infections (cystitis, pyelonephritis, urethritis, epididymitis, prostatitis), obstruction (renal colic, acute urinary retention), and external genitalia disorders (testicular torsion, paraphimosis).

I. Genitourinary Tract Injuries

A. Renal injuries.
1. The kidney is injured infrequently due to its mobility, its protection by heavy musculature and the rib cage, and its retroperitoneal position. However, because of its parenchyma's softness and extreme vascularity, it cannot withstand severe blunt or perforating injuries and is liable to be lacerated. Often, the fatty capsule of the kidney acts as a safety valve by limiting the bleeding due to pressure by the confined hematoma.
2. Renal injuries are more common in young persons. The types of renal injuries are simple contusion, minor laceration without urinary extravasation, major lacerations(s) or fracture, and pedicle injuries (Fig 14–1).

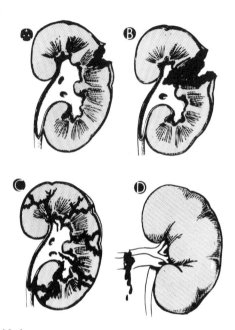

FIG 14–1.
Renal injuries. A, laceration. B, major laceration with rupture
into pelvis. C, "fracture" of parenchyma. D, tear of pedicle.

3. Blunt trauma to the abdomen produces renal injury by transmitting the impact in all directions,
as in a fluid-filled bag, or by impinging the kidney
against a solid structure such as the vertebral col-
umn.
4. Penetrating injuries are often associated with
other visceral injuries.
5. The symptoms of renal trauma may include flank

pain, hematuria, shock, a flank mass that may be expanding, and abdominal guarding or rigidity.

6. Shock should be treated immediately since it is potentially lethal. Early treatment is also important because a patient in shock may not excrete contrast medium, and the resulting nonvisualization of the kidney may be mistaken for a seriously damaged kidney.

7. Diagnosis.

   a. *Urinalysis typically reveals hematuria.* While microscopic hematuria (<100 WBCs/HPF) can be treated by observation and repeat urinalysis, gross (or persistent microscopic) hematuria warrants further evaluation by computed tomography (CT) or intravenous pyelography (IVP).

   b. *CT (with IV contrast material) is the preferred modality* for evaluating the genitourinary (GU) system in any multiple-trauma victim. CT is also indicated if the results of an initial screening IVP are abnormal in patients with isolated flank trauma.

   c. *IVP has a limited role in trauma.* IVP may be used as a screening procedure for isolated flank trauma. However, if such patients are strongly suspected to have sustained renal injury, initial CT scanning may be advisable.

      (1) A negative IVP finding rules out significant renal damage.

      (2) An abnormal IVP result should be followed by a CT, which gives much more information regarding localization and extent of injury.

      (3) A "one-shot" IVP just prior to laparotomy may be useful in patients too unstable to await CT scanning or IVP. Contrast material is injected in the ED or OR, and a single x-ray can then determine the existence

of two functioning kidneys or the presence of gross renal trauma.

8. Treatment.
   a. In less serious injuries, conservative measures are recommended.
      (1) Carefully monitor vital organs, and observe the size of the flank mass.
      (2) Record urinary output and the amount of hematuria.
      (3) Stabilize the blood pressure and pulse with IV fluids and blood.
      (4) Repeat CT or IVP if necessary.
   b. Surgery is indicated when the vital signs cannot be maintained with adequate fluid and blood replacement or when there is an expanding flank mass, falling central venous pressure (CVP), continued inadequate urine output, or continued gross hematuria.

B. Ureteral injuries.
   1. Because of its well-protected position and its mobility, the ureter is rarely injured by external trauma. The most common cause of injury is iatrogenic due to instrumentation.
   2. Symptoms and signs may reflect an increasing mass in the flank or free urine within the peritoneal cavity. CT or IV urography may reveal the site of the rupture or extravasation and may show the dilation of the collecting system above.

C. Bladder injuries.
   1. Rarely does the bladder rupture spontaneously. The most common bladder injuries are due to either direct trauma or associated pelvic fractures. A distended bladder may suffer extensive injury from minimal trauma, whereas an empty, collapsed bladder may escape injury.
   2. Rupture of the bladder may be intraperitoneal but is most often extraperitoneal, depending on the section of bladder wall damaged.
   3. The patient has a history of trauma, tenderness in

the suprapubic region, and often hematuria or the inability to urinate.

4. An IVP or CT usually reveals extravasated dye; however, false-negative IVP results do occur even with large tears. If there is still a strong clinical suspicion, a stress cystogram should be obtained.

5. Large intraperitoneal ruptures often require surgery. Extraperitoneal ruptures can frequently be managed conservatively with an indwelling catheter and anticholinergic medication.

D. Urethral injuries.

1. Posterior urethral injuries (membranous and prostatic urethra) are classic accompaniments of pelvic fractures. Anterior urethral injuries follow direct trauma such as straddle injuries. Iatrogenic damage due to instrumentation is frequent.

2. Depending on the site of the injury, urethral damage may allow urinary extravasation superior to the urogenital diaphragm into the pelvis or below the urogenital diaphragm into the superficial perineal space, scrotum, and lower anterior abdominal wall.

3. Rectal examination may reveal a boggy fullness with loss of the normal landmarks such as the prostatic outline.

4. Blood at the meatus or obvious penile or vulval trauma suggest urethral damage. A retrograde urethrogram should be performed prior to urethral catheterization to avoid further injury.

5. A suprapubic bladder catheter can be inserted in the ED and urologic consultation obtained.

E. Penile trauma.

1. Contusions of the penis are characterized by edema or, in more serious injuries, by ecchymosis that spreads to the scrotum and even to the anterior abdominal wall. The treatment is rest, pressure dressings, ice packs, and an indwelling urethral catheter if there is interference with urination.

2. Fracture of the penis results from severe trauma to the erect organ with resulting rupture of the corpora cavernosa. Bleeding into the subcutaneous tissues is extensive, with severe swelling and pain along the penile shaft.

3. Wounds of the penis are rare, usually due to a gunshot, bite, or stabbing. Occasionally, avulsion occurs when clothing is caught in machinery.

4. Although simple lacerations may be sutured in the ED any significant injury requires accurate surgical repair, usually in the OR.

F. Injury to the scrotum and its contents.

1. The scrotum is commonly damaged by kicks, blows, straddle injuries, gunshot wounds, machinery accidents, and psychiatric patients' self-mutilation. Because of the extreme mobility of scrotal skin over its contents and because of the cremasteric action, the testes are somewhat less liable to trauma. However, when injured, severe testicular swelling due to traumatic orchitis, hydrocele, or more commonly, hematocele may occur. If the testes prolapse through an injury in the scrotal sac, they must be reinserted and the defect repaired.

2. Closed injuries to the scrotum and its contents are generally treated conservatively. Scrotal support is indicated, and ice packs and analgesics are also used. After 48 hours, warm, moist packs may be helpful. Occasionally, evacuation of the hematocele may be necessary.

3. Lacerations of the scrotum are treated by thorough cleansing, debridement, and suturing of the edges, together with adequate drainage if needed. Scrotal skin has a good blood supply and usually heals very well.

4. If a testis has sustained a major injury and physical examination suggests extravasation of testicular tissue into the scrotal sac, immediate operative repair is necessary.

II. Genitourinary Tract Infections

A. Acute cystitis.

1. Cystitis is more common in women. When present in men or if frequent in women, cystitis may reflect an underlying congenital anomaly.

2. Symptoms may include frequency or urgency of urination, dysuria, suprapubic discomfort, backache, or hematuria.

3. Clean-catch, midstream urinalysis will usually reveal WBCs and often red blood cells and bacteria as well.

4. A urine culture and sensitivity determination should be obtained for all men and for all women with frequent or recurrent urinary tract infections (UTIs).

5. Treatment.

a. Recent studies have shown that single-dose therapy for uncomplicated cystitis is effective. Choices include sulfisoxazole (Gantrisin), 2 gm; trimethoprim, 480 mg, and sulfamethoxazole, 2,400 mg (Bactrim DS or Septra DS, 3 tablets); or amoxicillin, 3 gm.

b. Uncomplicated cystitis-type symptoms that do not respond to single-dose therapy may be due to chlamydial urethritis. Treatment for 7 to 10 days is indicated with tetracycline, 500 mg four times a day; doxycycline, 100 mg twice a day; or trimethoprim/sulfamethoxazole (double strength, 160 mg/800 mg) twice a day.

c. Single-dose therapy should not be used for cystitis in males or pregnant women, for UTIs with evidence of renal involvement such as fever or flank tenderness, or if symptoms have been present for more than a few days. A tenday course of antibiotics is then indicated. Sulfa drugs are often used such as sulfisoxazole (Gantrisin), 1 gm four times a day. Alternative agents are nitrofurantoin (Macrodantin),

         50 to 100 mg four times a day; and nalidixic acid (NegGram), 1 gm four times a day.

6. Analgesia may be indicated for significant symptoms. Dysuria can be treated with a local urinary anesthetic such as phenazopyridine (Pyridium), 200 mg three times a day after meals. Anticholinergic agents such as hyoscyamine (Cystospaz), 1 to 2 gm four times a day, can be prescribed for bladder spasm.

B. Acute pyelonephritis.

1. Symptoms are those of cystitis plus flank pain, fever, chills, and often myalgias.

2. Costovertebral angle tenderness is prominent.

3. Outpatient treatment may be sufficient for mild pyelonephritis.

    a. The urine should be cultured.

    b. Oral antibiotics often effective include ampicillin, 500 mg four times a day; cefaclor (Ceclor), 250 mg three times a day; or trimethoprim and sulfamethoxazole, 160 mg/800 mg (Bactrim DS or Septra DS) every 12 hours.

    c. An initial IM dose of an aminoglycoside such as gentamicin, 80 mg, is suggested for frank pyelonephritis prior to discharge from the ED.

4. Admission to the hospital and parenteral antibiotics are indicated for patients with severe vomiting, prostration, high fever, pregnancy, diabetes, or other complicating factors.

5. Perinephric abscess should be considered in any patient with extreme costovertebral angle tenderness, flank muscle rigidity, flank mass, or severe fever, especially if the infection is resistant to antibiotic therapy.

C. Urethritis (See Chapter 15 for a discussion of urethritis in women. This section deals with urethritis in men).

1. Symptoms of urethritis are predominantly dysuria and usually discharge.

2. Bladder infections (UTIs) in men are usually the result of congenital anomalies of the urinary tract. Such men most likely have had several episodes of UTI before puberty. Therefore, any sexually mature man with dysuria, especially with a discharge, who has had no prior history of UTIs, probably has urethritis rather than cystitis.

3. Obtaining a sample of the urethral discharge for Gram stain and culture is preferred. The patient should be asked not to urinate until the discharge specimen has been obtained since urination may wash out any discharge from the urethra. If a discharge is collected, urine studies are unnecessary in the absence of symptoms of epididymitis or prostatitis. (See Item 5.)

4. The prostate should be examined for tenderness or fluctuance and the epididymis evaluated for tenderness (see Sections D and E).

5. If a microscopic examination of the urethral smear from a man shows gram-negative intracellular diplococci, the patient has gonococcal urethritis. If these organisms are not seen, there is strong presumptive evidence for nongonoccocal urethritis (NGU), often chlamydial. The discharge should nevertheless be sent for gonorrheal and chlamydial culture.

6. Gonorrheal and chlamydial infections often co-exist. Because gonorrhea can be identified on Gram stains of urethral exudate but chlamydial infections cannot, it is advisable to treat for both organisms if gonorrhea is found. In the absence of gram-negative intracellular diplococci, treatment for chlamydia alone is probably sufficient. Several treatment protocols have been effective, but they must be revised frequently due to the rapid emergence of resistant strains.

7. Gonococcal urethritis is best treated by the following regimen:

   a. Ceftriaxone, 250 mg IM.

　　 b. Then doxycycline, 100 mg twice daily, or tetracycline, 500 mg four times a day for 7 days, to eradicate chlamydiae.

8. Nongonococcal urethritis (NGU) is usually caused by *Chlamydia trachomitis* or *Ureaplasma urealyticum*. NGU is the most frequent bacterial cause of sexually transmitted diseases in the United States. Uncomplicated urethral NGU in the male can be treated with the following regimen:

　　 a. Doxycycline, 100 mg twice daily, or tetracycline, 500 mg four times a day for 7 days.

　　 b. Or erythromycin, 500 mg four times a day for 7 days.

9. Although any of the aforementioned protocols may eradicate incubating syphilis, it is still advisable to obtain serological tests for syphilis both before treatment and 6 weeks later since patients are often infected with syphilis and gonorrhea simultaneously.

D. Acute epididymitis.

1. Acute epididymitis is most commonly a sexually transmitted disease secondary to urethritis. Older men may acquire epididymitis from a urinary pathogen.

2. The condition is usually unilateral with marked scrotal swelling, pain, heat, tenderness to palpation, and erythema. The testis may be involved and may be enlarged and tender. Epididymitis must be distinguished from torsion, in which the pain often begins more abruptly than with epididymitis (see Section IV, A).

3. If a discharge is present, it should be evaluated as explained before. A urine culture is helpful, especially if no discharge can be obtained.

4. Supportive treatment consists of scrotal support, ice, bed rest, antibiotics, and sometimes anti-inflammatory therapy such as indomethacin, 25 mg three times a day.

5. Antibiotic treatment is similar to that for urethritis, but more prolonged:
   a. Ceftriaxone, 250 mg IM.
   b. Then doxycycline, 100 mg twice daily, or tetracycline, 500 mg four times a day for 10 days.

E. Acute prostatitis.
   1. The prostate may be seeded from a remote source of infection, but more commonly the source is the epididymis and urethra. Prostatitis may be caused by a urinary pathogen in older men but is more often gonococcal or chlamydial in younger men.
   2. Symptoms usually include dysuria, urgency, and frequent urination, often accompanied by a discharge and perineal or suprapubic pain.
   3. Physical examination reveals a tender, boggy prostate.
   4. If a discharge is present, it should be studied as for urethritis. The urine should be cultured.
   5. Treatment consists of tetracycline, 500 mg four times a day; doxycycline, 100 mg twice a day; or trimethoprim and sulfamethoxazole, 160 mg/800 mg (Bactrim DS or Septra DS) twice a day for 10 to 14 days.

III. Urinary Tract Obstruction

A. Renal colic.
   1. Renal or urethral colic is due to the passage of a stone through the ureter with stretching of the urethral smooth muscle and hyperperistalsis proximal to the site of the stone.
   2. The pain is severe, radiates from flank to groin, and is often accompanied by nausea and vomiting.
   3. Abdominal examination is usually unremarkable, but costovertebral angle tenderness is often present.
   4. Urinalysis commonly reveals red blood cells.

However, complete obstruction of a ureter may yield a normal urinalysis.

5. Emergency IVP or ultrasonography are indicated to determine the degree of obstruction and confirm the diagnosis. Recurrent stones may not require repeated diagnostic studies unless the diagnosis is unclear or the stone does not pass within a day or two.

6. Treatment is usually conservative and consists of narcotic analgesics and hydration. Instrumentation and/or lithotripsy (which require general anesthesia) are usually not required for acute renal colic.

7. The urine is strained, and the calculus is chemically analyzed.

8. The patient is admitted to the hospital if continual parenteral analgesics or antiemetics are required.

B. Urinary retention.

1. Acute urinary retention may be caused by benign prostatic hypertrophy, prostatic carcinoma, urethral stricture, acute prostatic infection, vesical or urethral calculus, hemorrhage and clot formation within the bladder, or neurogenic disturbance of bladder function.

2. Immediate relief is achieved by inserting a catheter through the urethra into the bladder.

3. If a catheter cannot be passed via the urethra, a suprapubic cystostomy can be performed with a commercially available suprapubic catheter apparatus.

IV. External Genitalia Disorders

A. Torsion of the spermatic cord.

1. Torsion of the spermatic cord, more frequently called torsion of the testis, is a twisting of the spermatic cord that constricts the blood supply. If untreated, this results in testicular necrosis. It is

more common in children and young adults and in men with undescended testes.

2. The patient experiences the acute onset of pain and scrotal swelling and sometimes nausea, vomiting, and fever. The testis may be palpably rotated as compared with the other one. However, this is not a reliable sign.

3. Differentiating torsion from epididymitis may be quite difficult. Both may be associated with pain, swelling, and fever. Symptoms due to torsion usually begin more abruptly, often during sleep or following exercise. Epididymitis is more likely to cause fever, pyuria, and scrotal erythema. These may be absent, however (refer to Section II, D for a discussion of epididymitis). The differential diagnosis also includes strangulated hernia and testicular tumor.

4. Diagnosis may often (but not always) be achieved with Doppler ultrasonography. Nuclear scanning is not very sensitive and usually requires an excessive amount of time.

5. Treatment consists of prompt surgical intervention when torsion is suspected. The testis is untwisted and anchored to the parietal layers of the scrotum. Because of the risk of torsion on the opposite side, orchiopexy is usually performed on the contralateral side as well.

B. Paraphimosis.

1. Paraphimosis is the result of the retraction of a tight prepucial skin behind the glans penis, which cannot be pulled forward to cover the glans. It frequently results from masturbation. Failure to bring the skin forward immediately results in edema of the glans because of the tight band of constriction formed by the prepuce at the coronal sulcus.

2. The patient has pain, an edematous prepuce and glans, and a tight ring at the corona.

3. The immediate treatment is manual reduction of

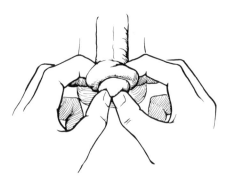

FIG 14–2.
Manual reduction for paraphimosis.

the prepuce (Fig 14–2). The thumbs are placed on the glans, with the index and middle fingers of each hand behind the point of constriction. As the glans is pushed backward, the skin is pulled forward until complete reduction is achieved.

4. If edema is excessive, this type of reduction may be impossible and a dorsal slit may be required. Recurrences are prevented by elective circumcision at a later date.

15

Obstetrics and Gynecology

I. Introduction

A. Gynecologic problems must be differentiated from urinary tract and gastrointestinal (GI) tract disorders, any of which may cause abdominal discomfort. Pelvic and rectal examinations should be performed on all women with lower abdominal pain.

B. Most patients with these disorders experience any or all of the following:
   1. Abdominal pain.
   2. Vaginal bleeding.
   3. Vaginal discharge.

II. Symptoms

The disease entities listed below are only the major causes of the symptoms presented. The list is not necessarily in order of frequency and does not include all the possible disease processes that cause these symptoms.

A. Abdominal pain.
   1. Ectopic pregnancy.
   2. Pelvic inflammatory disease (PID).
   3. Ruptured ovarian cyst.
   4. Urinary tract infection (see Chapter 14).

   5. Appendicitis (see Chapter 13).
   6. Menstrual cramps.
   7. Endometriosis.
   8. Abruptio placenta (in third trimester).
B. Vaginal bleeding.
   1. Not obviously pregnant.
      a. Ectopic pregnancy.
      b. Ruptured ovarian cyst.
      c. PID
      d. Dysfunctional bleeding.
      e. Pregnancy with threatened spontaneous abortion.
   2. Obviously pregnant.
      a. Placenta previa.
      b. Abruptio placenta.
      c. Threatened spontaneous abortion.
      d. Heavy bloody show.
C. Vaginal discharge.
   1. Vaginitis.
      a. Yeast *(Candida albicans,* formerly known as *Monilia albicans).*
      b. Protozoal *(Trichomonas vaginalis).*
      c. Bacterial *(Gardnerella vaginalis,* formerly known as *Corynebacterium vaginale,* or *Hemophilus vaginalis).*
      d. Viral (herpes simplex.)
   2. Salpingitis or cervicitis.
      a. Chlamydiae.
      b. Gonorrhea.
      c. Other bacteria.
      d. Mixed.

III. Specific Diagnostic Entities

A. Ectopic pregnancy.
   1. Symptoms (Any or all of these may be absent).
      a. Menstrual period overdue.
      b. Lower abdominal pain, usually unilateral.
      c. Vaginal bleeding.

        d. Weakness or syncope due to blood loss (often occult intra-abdominal bleeding).

  2. Findings.

        a. Signs of hypotension if significant intra-abdominal or vaginal bleeding has occurred.

        b. Adnexal mass.

        c. Uterus may be slightly enlarged.

        d. Conventional pregnancy tests may be negative in a significant number of ectopic pregnancies.

        e. Newer immunoassay techniques are specific for the β-subunit of human chorionic gonadotropin (β-HCG). Tests that can detect as little as 100 mIU/mL urine or blood and that can be performed within 1 hour are now available. These assays should detect pregnancy by the time of the missed menstrual period and are sufficiently sensitive to be positive at that time in ectopic pregnancy.

        f. If a β-specific HCG pregnancy test is positive—and if the patient is hemodynamically stable—ultrasonography should be performed. Failure to find an intrauterine pregnancy in a patient with a positive pregnancy test result strongly suggests ectopic pregnancy. Detection of an adnexal mass is not necessary for a presumptive diagnosis.

        g. In questionable cases, culdocentesis may be useful by demonstrating nonclotting blood in ruptured ectopic pregnancy.

  3. Treatment.

        a. Replacement of blood loss as needed: intravenous fluids, blood, medical antishock trousers (MAST suit).

        b. Gynecologic consultation and surgery.

B. Spontaneous abortion.

  1. Symptoms.

        a. Any bleeding in early pregnancy must be considered at least a "threatened abortion."

        b. Cramping is often present.

2. Findings.
   a. Blood may be seen at the cervical os.
   b. The os may be partially dilated with tissue extruding ("inevitable abortion").
3. Treatment.
   a. There is no adequate treatment. Bed rest is thought by some to decrease the chance of progression from threatened to inevitable abortion.
   b. If abortion does occur, the process will usually conclude spontaneously with extrusion of all the products of conception.
   c. If bleeding is prolonged or excessive, dilation and evacuation should be considered by the gynecologist.
   d. Blood should be obtained for typing and Rh, and anti-Rh factor antibody given when appropriate.

C. Pelvic inflammatory disease.
   1. *Chlamydia trachomatis* and *Neisseria gonorrhoeae* are the most common causes of PID. However, other pathogens such as GI or genitourinary (GU) flora may also be cultured.
   2. PID may range from infection of only the cervix, through extended involvement of the endometrium, myometrium, salpinges, and peritoneum.
   3. Symptoms.
      a. Symptoms may range from absent to incapacitating, depending upon the acuity and the extent of infection.
      b. Lower abdominal pain is the most common presenting complaint.
      c. Vaginal discharge and sometimes bleeding, along with dysuria and dyspareunia, may also be present.
   4. Findings.
      a. Lower abdominal tenderness is the most common finding on palpation of the abdomen.

b. Cervical motion tenderness is usually present in patients with acute abdominal pain.

c. Adnexal tenderness indicates infection of the salpinges and is usually bilateral.

d. An adnexal mass may suggest a tubo-ovarian abscess.

e. A discharge may be seen extruding from the os in many cases.

f. Fever is usually present but may be intermittent.

g. Leukocytosis is usually present in acute PID and often an elevated sedimentation rate as well.

5. Treatment.

a. Culture of the cervix should be obtained for chlamydial infection and for gonorrhea. Testing of serum for syphilis is generally recommended.

b. If an intrauterine device (IUD) is present, it should be removed. Many authorities recommend 1 to 2 days of antibiotic treatment prior to IUD removal.

c. Mild cases with no significant peritoneal signs may be treated with outpatient therapy so long as there is close follow-up.

   (1) Treatment should include coverage of both chlamydial infection and gonorrhea.

   (2) Ceftriaxone, 250 intramuscularly (IM)—or alternatively a combination of cefoxitin, 2 gm IM, plus probenecid, 1 gm orally, is given in the emergency department (ED).

   (3) The aforementioned parenteral medication is followed by a 10-day course of doxycycline, 100 mg twice daily, or tetracycline, 500 mg four times daily.

d. Patients with significant peritoneal signs or fever should be admitted to the hospital for intravenous antibiotic therapy.

      e. If a tubo-ovarian abscess is suspected, laparoscopy should be considered for further evaluation.

D. Ovarian cyst.

  1. Symptoms.

    a. An intact ovarian cyst may be asymptomatic.

    b. Menstrual cycles may be irregular; vaginal bleeding may range from absent to heavy.

    c. If the cyst ruptures, significant intra-abdominal hemorrhage may occur.

  2. Findings.

    a. Palpation of the abdomen may reveal unilateral tenderness in patients with intact ovarian cysts. The abdomen may be nontender. Rupture of the cyst, however, will lead to significant abdominal tenderness, often diffuse and accompanied by peritoneal signs.

    b. Vaginal bleeding may be present or absent, with either an intact or a ruptured ovarian cyst.

    c. An adnexal mass can usually be palpated with either an intact or a ruptured cyst.

    d. If the cyst has ruptured, there may be signs of significant hypovolemia.

  3. Treatment.

    a. If there is no acute bleeding, gynecologic consultation should be obtained to consider hormonal manipulation.

    b. If there is significant acute bleeding (vaginal or intra-abdominal), immediate evaluation for possible surgery is indicated. Fluid resuscitation should be given as required.

E. Vaginitis (Gonococcal and herpetic infections are discussed elsewhere in this chapter).

  1. Symptoms.—Vaginal discharge, burning, itching, and sometimes dysuria.

  2. Findings.

    a. A vaginal discharge is usually discovered on examination.

    b. Specimens should be obtained for micro-scopic evaluation. Saline and KOH prepara-tions will usually reveal the specific pathogen.

3. Treatment.

    a. Yeast *(C.* or *M. albicans).*

        (1) Miconazole (Monistat) and clotrimazole (Gyne-Lotrimin) vaginal tablets or cream are both effective and are available in dif-ferent concentrations for bedtime use in 1-, 3-, and 7-day regimens. Nystatin (My-costatin) vaginal tablets and cream are less effective and must be used twice a day for 14 days.

        (2) If there is skin involvement, clotrimazole or miconazole cream should also be used twice a day. Nystatin–steroid cream (My-colog), three times a day, is less satisfac-tory.

    b. *Trichomonas*

        (1) Metronidazole (Flagyl), 2 gm in a single dose.

        (2) Teragenicity has not been found in animal studies, but the manufacturer recom-mends withholding metronidazole therapy during the first trimester of pregnancy. Many gynecologists withhold it during the second and third trimesters as well. An al-ternative, though less effective regimen is clotrimazole, 100 mg intravaginally at bed-time for 7 days.

        (3) The sexual partner should be treated also to prevent reinfection of the woman, which may occur even if the man is asymptomatic.

    C. Bacterial vaginosis.

        (1) This disorder is caused by the pleo-morphic rod known as *G. vaginalis,* for-merly *C. vaginale* or *H. vaginalis.*

      (2) The most effective treatment is metronidazole (Flagyl), 500 mg twice a day for 7 days.

      (3) A less effective alternative is ampicillin, 500 mg four times a day for 7 days.

F. Herpes genitalis.

  1. Symptoms.

    a. Local pain and often dysuria and discharge.

    b. Fever, malaise, and even urinary retention may be present.

  2. Findings.

    a. Exquisitely tender vesicles and/or ulcers are found on the external genitalia. Pain may preclude pelvic examination.

    b. Inguinal adenapathy, fever, and bacterial superinfection of viral lesions may be present.

    c. The acute infection will spontaneously resolve usually within 1 to 2 weeks, although recurrence is common.

  3. Treatment.

    a. Oral acyclovir (Zovirax), 200 mg five times a day for 10 days. This drug is moderately effective in shortening the course of initial episodes and may be somewhat helpful for severe recurrent episodes. A topical ointment preparation is less effective. Intravenous acylovir may be required for extremely severe cases.

    b. Local agents such as Burow's solution (Domeboro), may be soothing.

    c. If the viral lesions become superinfected with bacteria, local and sometimes systemic antibiotic therapy will be required.

    d. Urinary tract retention may result from extreme dysuria or periurethral edema. Such patients will require the insertion of an indwelling bladder catheter. Urethral catheterization with a Foley catheter may be adequate, but suprapubic catheterization is often more comfortable.

    e. There is some evidence for an increased incidence of cervical carcinoma in women who have a history of herpes genitalis infections. Therefore, patients should be encouraged to have periodic pelvic examinations and Papanicolaou smears.

    f. Active genital herpes at the time of vaginal delivery can be catastrophic for the neonate. Patients with a history of genital herpes should be instructed to inform their obstetrician so that serial examination and possibly herpes cultures can be considered during the weeks prior to delivery. Active infection would indicate cesarean section.

G. Bartholinian abscess.

  1. Symptoms.—Pain in the vulvar region.

  2. Findings.—Tender, fluctuant mass at the introitus.

  3. Treatment.

    a. Incision and drainage through the mucosal surface of the labia minora.

    b. Irrigation and drain insertion.

    c. Antibiotics if there is fever, adenopathy, or signs of PID.

      (1) Doxycycline, 100 mg twice a day, or tetracycline, 500 mg 4 times a day for 10 days.

      (2) Culture for gonococcal, chlamydial and gram-negative organisms.

H. Third-trimester bleeding. *Caution:* Pelvic and rectal examinations are absolutely contraindicated in the ED. They should be performed only by an obstetrician in a delivery room prepared for immediate cesarean section. Accidental dislodging of a placenta previa by the examiner's finger or by a speculum may lead to a fatal hemorrhage.

  1. Placenta previa.

    The placenta is implanted at or near the cervical os.

    a. Symptoms.

      (1) Vaginal bleeding.

(2) No significant abdominal pain.
    b. Findings.
        (1) Bleeding from the vagina.
        (2) No significant tenderness on palpation of the abdomen.
        (3) Ultrasonography demonstrating a low-lying placenta (to be performed only in stable patients).
    c. Treatment.
        (1) Fatal hemorrhage can result. Intravenous lines should be established, coagulation studies ordered, the blood typed and crossmatched, and fluid resuscitation given as needed.
        (2) Emergency cesarean section may be indicated if bleeding is significant.
2. Abruptio placenta.—Premature separation of normally located placenta.
    a. Symptoms.
        (1) Severe abdominal pain.
        (2) Vaginal bleeding may or may not be present.
    b. Findings.
        (1) Uterine rigidity and tenderness on palpation.
        (2) Blood may or may not be present at the introitus.
    c. Treatment.
        (1) As with placenta previa, the patient should be transferred to the delivery or operating room where the obstetrician will determine the diagnosis and the need for immediate vaginal delivery vs. cesarean section.
        (2) Disseminated intravascular coagulation and amniotic fluid embolism can occur following abruptio placenta. Initial coagulation studies should be drawn.

      (3) Since abruptio placenta and placenta previa cannot always be distinguished, precautions should be taken, including preparation for massive fluid resuscitation if needed.

I. Eclampsia.

  1. Pre-eclampsia refers to the symptom complex during pregnancy that includes edema, proteinuria, and hypertension (>140/>90 or a rise of 30 mm Hg systolic or 15 diastolic over baseline values). The presence of any of these should be called to the attention of the obstetrician and may indicate hospitalization if the blood pressure is significantly elevated.

  2. Eclampsia refers to the aforementioned pattern with the addition of seizures.

  3. The acute seizure may be treated with diazepam (Valium), 10 to 20 mg given intravenously.

  4. Magnesium sulfate is quite effective for the treatment of acute seizures and hypertension as well as for prophylaxis after seizures.

    a. A common regimen is 4 gm intravenously over a period of 4 minutes, followed by 1 to 3 gm/hr by intravenous infusion.

    b. If respiratory suppression or cardiac dysrhythmias occur as a result of excessive magnesium administration, these can often be reversed with intravenous calcium: a 10% solution of calcium chloride (up to 10 cc) or a 10% solution of calcium gluconate (up to 20 cc). These volumes provide equivalent amounts of calcium ion.

  5. Acute hypertension (diastolic pressure above 110 mm Hg) should be treated with intravenous hydralazine, 5 to 20 mg.

J. True vs. false labor.

  1. Abdominal cramping in the third trimester may be due to true labor or may reflect the more spo-

radic symptoms of false labor. Abruptio placenta must also be considered, as discussed earlier.

2. Table 15–1 compares true vs. false labor.

K. Suspected rape.

1. Be sympathetic as well as objective. The physician should offer no opinion as to whether the patient was raped. Legal aspects must always be considered. If the hospital, local government, or police force has a standard protocol for the workup of a suspected rape victim, this should be scrupulously followed.

TABLE 15–1.
True Versus False Labor

Symptom	True Labor	False Labor
Pain	Chiefly in back	Chiefly in abdomen
	Walking intensifies	Walking relieves
	Regular	Irregular
	Strength of contractions increases	Strength of contractions remains constant
	Frequency increases	Frequency remains constant
Bloody show	Often present	Seldom present
Membranes	Often ruptured*	Seldom ruptured
Cervix	Effaced	Often thick
	Dilating, 3+ cm	Closed, not dilating

*If the membranes have ruptured, the patient should be admitted to the hospital, even if contractions have not yet begun.

2. Obtain a good history. Write down what the patient said in her (or his) own words.
   a. Are there other injuries?
   b. Was there actual vaginal or rectal penetration?
   c. Did fellatio or cunnilingus occur?
3. Examine the entire patient for evidence of trauma, especially on the wrists, lower abdomen, buttocks, external genitalia, and rectum.
   a. Inspect the introitus, including the hymen.
   b. Perform a speculum examination.
   c. Obtain secretions from the vaginal vault by aspiration for the following:
      (1) Immediate wet-mount examination for motile and nonmotile sperm.
      (2) Dried smears for similar evaluation by the laboratory.
      (3) Various tests the laboratory may perform such as acid phosphatase and immunologic tests.
   d. Culture for chlamydia organisms and gonorrhea.
   e. Obtain various other specimens such as pubic hair by both clipping and combing.
   f. Send clearly labeled specimens to the laboratory.
   g. Give no opinion.
   h. Never say or write in the chart whether or not the patient was raped.
   i. You may give information to the police with the patient's permission.
4. Consider antibiotic prophylaxis for gonorrhea, chlamydial infection, and syphilis.
   a. The regimens described in Section III,C may be used.
   b. Although incubating syphilis may be eradicated with the aforementioned treatment, serum test for syphilis 6 weeks later is advisable.
5. Consider prophylaxis for pregnancy.

    a. A pregnancy test should be performed if there is any possibility that the patient may already be pregnant.

    b. If there is a significant chance of conception resulting from the alleged rape, hormonal therapy may be given to try to prevent successful implantation. Accepted regimens include:

        (1) Oral norgestrel and ethinyl estradiol (Ovral), 2 tablets initially, repeated 12 hours later.

        (2) Conjugated estrogen (Premarin), 100 mg IM.

        (3) Medroxyprogesterone (Depo-Provera), 100 mg IM.

    c. These agents may be associated with teratogenic risk to the fetus.

        (1) They should be given only if the patient is not already pregnant as determined by a pregnancy test.

        (2) If pregnancy should occur despite hormonal therapy, a therapeutic abortion should be strongly considered.

        (3) The patient must be fully informed of these considerations prior to hormonal therapy.

        (4) She should also be warned not to have unprotected intercourse until after her next menstrual period.

    d. The patient should be advised about the availability of therapeutic abortion whether hormonal therapy is given or withheld.

6. Emotional support is essential.

    a. Rape is a traumatic experience psychologically as well as physically. The physician should be supportive and take time to reassure the patient.

    b. Special social support services are often available to victims of sexual assault, and the patient should be made aware of those in her geographic area.

16
Soft-Tissue Infections

I. General Considerations

A. Types of infections.
1. Cellulitis is the acute inflammation of infected tissue and is characterized by erythema, warmth, swelling, and tenderness. As with any infection, fever may be present.
2. An abscess is a cavity containing pus. Fluctuance is the hallmark of an abscess, although it is not always detectable. Localized warmth, swelling, and tenderness directly over the abscess cavity are also typical.
3. Lymphadenopathy is the tender swelling of regional lymph nodes.
4. Lymphangitis is recognized by red streaks overlying the inflamed lymphatic vessels and extending proximally from the infected area.

B. Principles of treatment.
1. Antibiotics are indicated in soft-tissue infections accompanied by cellulitis, acute lymphadenopathy, lymphangitis, or fever.
2. Incision and drainage (I&D) is the proper treatment for abscesses. Antibiotics are added if there are signs of spreading infection such as cellulitis, acute lymphadenopathy, lymphangitis, or fever. In

the absence of systemic infection, localized abscesses adequately drained may not require antibiotics because the drugs generally do not penetrate into abscess cavities.

3. Elevation and application of heat are suggested for any soft-tissue infection.

II. Traumatic Wounds

A. Prevention of tetanus.
   1. General considerations.
      a. Tetanus organisms cause serious illness by toxin production even when confined to a circumscribed area of tissue damage.
      b. Tetanus prevention is dependent on the following:
         a. Primary prophylactic immunization.
         b. Meticulous surgical care of wounds.
         c. The proper use of *human* tetanus antitoxin and tetanus toxoid.
      c. The identification by smear and culture of this anaerobic, gram-positive, spore-forming bacillus is *not* essential for the use of prophylactic measures or for the diagnosis and management of clinical tetanus.
   2. Immunization.—In patients who have a history of adequate primary immunization, there is no need for routine booster injections more often than every 10 years.
   3. Treatment of patients with no good evidence of complete toxoid immunization.
      a. Patients who have not had the basic series should receive immunization with diphtheria-tetanus toxoid at the time of injury and subsequent injections at 6 and 24 weeks.
      b. For moderately severe wounds, 250 units of tetanus immune globulin (humans) should also be given. Injuries that are grossly con-

taminated, major burns, and major open fractures fall into this category.

c. It is important to remember that tetanus can arise from *minor* injuries that do not receive good local care in persons who have been inadequately immunized.

4. Injured patients with complete tetanus toxoid immunization.

a. These patients should receive toxoid boosters or human antitoxin if they have not had a toxoid booster within the past 5 years.

b. For a severely contaminated wound, especially if neglected for 24 hours, *both* toxoid and human antitoxin should be given.

c. Small penetrating wounds are tetanus prone.

d. Meticulous care of the wound including vigorous irrigation and generous debridement is important to prevent not only tetanus but also other infections.

B. Wound infection.

1. Prevention of wound infection.

a. Cleansing and debridement are the most important means of preventing wound infection. Removal of foreign bodies may require irrigation as well, particularly for deep wounds. Care should be taken not to force irrigating fluid into deep tissue planes.

b. Loose closure of significantly contaminated wounds is suggested in order to allow adequate drainage.

c. Prophylactic antibiotics may be useful for contaminated wounds, especially of the hand, and for bite wounds, particularly human and cat (see Section C). In general, however, prophylactic antibiotics have been demonstrated to be far less important than are adequate cleansing and debridement.

(1) If used, the prophylactic antibiotic should generally be a β-lactamase–resistant agent

effective against coagulase-positive *Staphylococcus aureus*. A typical regimen is a 5-day course of a cephalosporin such as cephalexin, 250 to 500 mg four times daily, or dicloxacillin, 250 to 500 mg four times daily. Erythromycin, 250 to 500 mg four times daily, may be used in penicillin-allergic patients.

(2) Compromised hosts such as diabetics are particularly prone to infection, and prophylactic antibiotics are used more readily in this population.

(3) Infective endocarditis may be caused by the entrance of bacteria through skin breaks, even in the absence of wound infection. People with prosthetic values (mechanical or porcine) or valves previously damaged by rheumatic fever are particularly prone to infective endocarditis.

a Antibiotic prophylaxis in such patients would seem prudent if they sustain significant soft-tissue injuries.

b Regimens might include intramuscular (IM) cephalosporin at the time of suturing (cefazolin, 1 gm IM) plus a 5-day course of cephalexin or dicloxacillin, 250 to 500 mg four times daily.

2. Treatment of wound infections.

a. Antibiotic therapy for actual infection should generally involve a 10-day course of dicloxacillin or cephalexin, 250 to 500 mg four times daily.

b. Opening of the sutured wound by removing some or all of the sutures may be required if there is pus, evidence of abscess cavity formation, or failure to respond to antibiotics.

c. A retained foreign body may cause wound infection. Radiological examination or repeat exploration may be indicated if this possibility exists.

  d. Severe wound infections, particularly those of the hand, may require hospital admission for intravenous (IV) antibiotic therapy.

C. Bite wounds.

 1. Because of their high incidence of infection, bite wounds deserve special mention.

 2. Human bites are most dangerous because they often involve the hand (fist-to-mouth) and because the human mouth is particularly well endowed with bacterial flora.

 3. Cat bites present a high risk of infection because the wounds are typically deep punctures that allow little opportunity for adequate irrigation or drainage.

 4. Cat scratches are also prone to infection because of the feline predilection for licking paws, thereby contaminating them with oral flora.

 5. Dog bites are much less prone to infection. The wounds are usually open tears that can be thoroughly debrided and irrigated.

 6. Debridement and irrigation are crucial. Prophylactic antibiotics will not prevent infection if the wound is left contaminated.

 7. While very minor wounds may be left open, any significant bite laceration should be sutured.

  a. Primary closure is indicated for most animal bite wounds.

  b. Delayed primary closure after 2 to 3 days is the treatment of choice for all human and other primate bite wounds as well as for particularly contaminated bite wounds from any animal. The traditional practice of allowing human bite wounds to heal by secondary intent often results in severe scarring and affords no greater protection from infection than thorough debridement, irrigation, and delayed primary closure.

8. Antibiotic prophylaxis is indicated for human and cat bites. Cephalexin or dicloxacillin, 250 to 500 mg four times daily for 5 days is often used. The combination preparation of amoxicillin and clavulanic acid (Augmentin) may be most effective for cat and dog bites. (See Section C, 11.) Dog bite wounds that are sufficiently open to allow adequate cleansing, do not require prophylaxis.

9. Prophylaxis and treatment of human bite wound infections has traditionally employed penicillin (or clindamycin in penicillin-allergic patients) because human mouth aerobes and anaerobes are most sensitive to these agents. There has been a trend recently, however, to use cephalexin or dicloxacillin to provide staphylococcal coverage.

10. Human bite wound infections, especially of the hand, should generally be treated in the hospital with IV antibiotics.

11. Cat and, to some extent, dog bite infections may involve two separate spectra of organisms, which tend to be differentiated by the time of onset of infection.

    a. Infections arising within 24 hours of the bite are usually caused by *Pasteurella multocida,* a small aerobic gram-negative rod. This organism is most sensitive to penicillin, 500 mg four times daily, and to tetracycline. Several weeks of therapy may be necessary. Surprisingly *Pasteurella* is often resistant to erythromycin and sometimes not very susceptible to cephalosporins or even dicloxacillin.

    b. Infections arising after 24 hours are probably caused by *S. aureus, Streptococcus,* or both. A penicillinase-resistant antibiotic should be used such as dicloxacillin or cephalexin. In penicillin-allergic patients, erythromycin is sometimes effective.

    c. No single antibiotic has been strongly effective against both *Pasteurella* and *Staphylococcus*. However both organisms are susceptible to the recently introduced combination preparations which include a penicillin such as amoxicillin and clavulanic acid (Augmentin).

D. Rabies.

    1. General considerations.

        a. Rabies, caused by an RNA virus, is essentially a uniformly fatal illness in humans.

        b. The prevention of rabies is different from the prophylactic regimens for any other infection in that active immunization usually is given *after* infection has been introduced into the patient.

        c. Wild carnivorous animals, especially skunks, foxes, raccoons, coyotes, bobcats, and bats, are the most important source of rabies infection in the United States.

        d. The presence of rabies in domestic dogs and cats varies from region to region.

        e. Rodents (squirrels, hamsters, guinea pigs, gerbils, chipmunks, rats, and mice) and lagomorphs (rabbits and hares) are rarely infected with rabies and have not caused rabies in the United States.

    2. Evaluation.

        a. Every case must be evaluated individually. Special attention must be paid to the circumstances of the individual exposure, geographic location, species of the animal involved, and prevalence of rabies in that species in the area. Contact state or local health officials.

        b. An unprovoked attack is more likely than a provoked attack to indicate that the animal is rabid. Bites inflicted when feeding or handling an apparently healthy animal should be regarded as provoked.

    c. Any penetration of skin by teeth is a bite exposure, but nonbite exposure occurs in abrasions, open wounds, or contamination of mucous membranes by saliva or other potentially infectious material.

    d. The emergency service record should show the following:

      (1) Whether the animal is known or stray and whether it was caught.

      (2) Where it resides.

      (3) That the local authorities have been notified.

      (4) That tetanus toxoid has been given, unless the patient has received a booster within the last 5 years.

      (5) That an immunization plan, if necessary, has been arranged for the patient.

3. Local treatment of wounds.

    a. Immediate and thorough washing of all bite wounds and scratches may be the most important measure for preventing rabies.

    b. Tetanus prophylaxis and measures to control bacterial infection should be given as indicated.

4. Immunization.

    a. When rabies is suspected, give human rabies immune globulin (HRIG) and vaccine (human diploid cell vaccine [HDCV]) for bite and nonbite exposures, but give vaccine only if prior rabies vaccination and adequate rabies antibody titer are documented.

    b. Always immunize irrespective of the time since exposure.

    c. The recommendations in Tables 16–1 and 16–2 are only a guide. In applying them, take into account the animal species involved, the circumstances of the bite or other exposure, the vaccination status of the animal, and the presence of rabies in the region. *Local and* state public health officials should be consulted if questions arise about the need for rabies prophylaxis.

d. Adverse reactions.
   (1) Local or mild systemic reactions should not interrupt immunization. Use anti-inflammatory and antipyretic agents. Use antihistamines and epinephrine for hypersensitivity and anaphylactic reactions.
   (2) For severe reactions, contact the Center for Disease Control or state or local officials for advice on the interruption of immunization.

III. Abscess

A. Principles of treatment.
   1. I&D is required. Antibiotics are added if signs of spread are present (see Section I,B,2).
   2. A parenteral (needle) drug abuse–related abscess requires admission to the hospital for IV antibiotics if there is any sign of systemic infection such as fever. This is to prevent the development of endocarditis or staphylococcal pneumonia, for which parenteral drug abusers are particularly at risk.
   3. Rheumatic or prosthetic valve patients should be given antibiotics prior to I&D in accordance with the regimen described in Section 11,B,1,c,(3).
   4. Anesthesia is difficult to achieve.
      a. Xylocaine should be injected into the skin above the abscess cavity, but injection into the cavity itself is usually ineffective and unnecessarily painful.
      b. Systemic agents may be helpful such as inhaled nitrous oxide, parenteral narcotics (morphine, 5 to 10 mg, or meperidine, 75 mg IM), or benzodiazepines (diazepam, 5 to 10 mg, or midazolam, 2 to 5 mg IV).

TABLE 16–1.
Indications for Post Exposure Rabies Prophylaxis

Animal Species	Condition of Animal at Time of Attack	Treatment of Exposed Person*
Domestic		
Dog and cat	Healthy and available for 10 days of observation	None, unless animal develops rabies,† then HRIG,‡ and HDCV§
	Rabid or suspected rabid Unknown (escaped)	Consult public health officials. If treatment is indicated, give HRIG‡ and HDCV§
Wild		
Skunk, bat, fox, coyote, raccoon, bobcat, and other carnivores	Regard as rabid unless proved normal by laboratory tests¶	HRIG‡ and HDCV§

Other	
Livestock, rodents, and lagomorphs (rabbits and hares)	Consider individually. Local and state public health officials should be consulted about the need for rabies prophylaxis. Bites of squirrels, hamsters, guinea pigs, gerbils, chipmunks, rats, mice, other rodents, rabbits, and hares almost never call for antirabies prophylaxis

*All bites and wounds should immediately be thoroughly cleaned with soap and water. If antirabies treatment is indicated, both Human Rabies Immune Globulin (HRIG) and Human Diploid Cell Rabies Vaccine (HDCV) should be given as soon as possible, *regardless* of the interval from exposure.

†During the usual holding period of 10 days, begin treatment with HRIG and HDCV at first sign of rabies in a dog or cat that has bitten someone. The symptomatic animal should be killed immediately and tested.

‡If HRIG is not available, use Equine Antirabies Serum (ARS). Do not use more than the recommended dose.

§If HDCV is not available, use Duck Embryo Vaccine (DEV). Local reactions to vaccines are common and do not contraindicate continuing treatment. Discontinue treatment with the vaccine if fluorescent antibody (FA) tests of the animal are negative.

¶The animal should be killed and tested as soon as possible. Holding for observation is not recommended.

TABLE 16–2.
Dosages for Postexposure Rabies Prophylaxis*

Prophylaxis	Comments	Dosage	Route	Frequency
HRIG†	Always give, unless prior adequate HDCV course. Then give only 2 doses HDCV on days 1 and 4	20 IU/kg	Preferably 50% around wound, remainder deep IM injection in buttock or thigh	Once. Give even if delay of weeks between exposure and prophylaxis
ARS†	Used only if HRIG unavailable	40 IU/kg	IM	Once
HDCV†	Dosage similar for children and adults. Only test for antibody response in immunosuppressed patients	5 1-mL doses	IM, not in same site as for HRIG	Repeated on days 3, 7, 14, 28
DEV†	Used if HDCV unavailable. No longer licensed for use in United States	23 1-mL doses	SC	21 daily doses, then on days 31 and 41

*Thorough cleansing to the depth of the wound with a 20% soap solution significantly (up to 90%) reduces rabies risk, especially if the wound is superficial.
†See Table 16–1.

c. Cooling sprays are used by some physicians but generally do not provide sufficient local anesthesia for skin incision.

5. Loculations, if present, should be disrupted by blunt dissection with a hemostat.

6. Irrigation should be continued until all pus is drained. Saline, hydrogen peroxide, or povidone-iodine may be used.

7. Drain insertion (with iodinated gauze) will prevent premature closure while the abscess is still draining. Deep cavities may be packed with the same material.

8. Irrigation and drain replacement should be carried out at 1- to 2-day intervals until there is no more pus formation. If the wound has been packed, progressively less packing should be replaced at each visit to allow closure from the inside out.

9. Diabetes may present initially as a nontraumatic infection such as an abscess. Analyzing urine for glucose may be advisable, especially for a recurrent or refractory abscess.

B. Specific abscesses.

1. Felon.

a. This is an infection of the pulp of the volar pad overlying the distal phalanx.

b. Because the infection often leads to the accumulation of pressure and ischemic necrosis, early drainage is indicated.

c. Under digital-block anesthesia, a central longitudinal incision is made in the finger pulp where the abscess is pointing (Fig 16–1).

d. The digital septa should *not* be disrupted. This does represent a change from the traditional practice, which has often lead to instability of the fingertip.

e. The wound is irrigated with saline and a small drain inserted.

f. The drain can be removed in 1 to 2 days, the

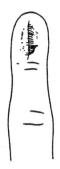

FIG 16–1.
Incision of a felon (distal fat pad infection). (From Way LW (ed): *Current Surgical Diagnosis and Treatment,* ed 7, Los Altos, Calif, Lange Medical Publishers, 1985. Used with permission.)

  tract irrigated, and the wound allowed to close by granulation.

 g. Antistaphylococcal antibiotic coverage is advisable.

2. Paronychium.

 a. This is an abscess of the skin around the base of the nail. It can extend under the nail plate as well.

 b. A longitudinal incision is made over the fluctuant area (Fig 16–2).

 c. The cavity is irrigated and a small drain inserted.

 d. The drain is removed after 1 day and the finger soaked periodically in warm water.

 e. If infection extends under the nail, the lateral third of the nail plate on the side of the paronychium should be removed.

 f. Following surgical drainage, antibiotics are not

indicated unless there are signs of cellulitis, lymphangitis, or felon. However, small paronychia without fluctuance may be treated nonsurgically with warm soaks and an antistaphylococcal antibiotic.

3. Deep infections of the hand.
   a. Infection of the deep palmar space is a major threat to the hand. Hospital admission and surgical drainage are necessary.
   b. Tenosynovitis causes fusiform swelling of the finger and severe pain on passive motion. Surgical drainage is mandatory.
   c. Both types of infection require operative intervention by a hand surgeon and should not be treated in the emergency department.
4. Olecranon bursitis.
   a. Often nontraumatic, this disorder is characterized by painful swelling, fluctuance, and erythema of the extensor surface of the elbow overlying the olecranon prominence.

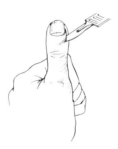

FIG 16–2.

Incision and drainage of a paronychium. (From Rosen P, Sternbach G: *Atlas of Emergency Medicine.* Baltimore, Williams & Wilkins Co, 1979. Used with permission.)

b. The bursitis may be due to a purely inflammatory process or to a bacterial infection.

c. Needle aspiration is indicated. Gram staining and culture of the aspirate should reveal the causative bacteria if infection is present.

d. Nonsteroidal anti-inflammatory agents are used such as indomethacin, 25 to 50 mg three times daily.

e. Antibiotics are added if infection is suggested by fever, elevated serum leukocyte count, or Gram staining of the aspirate. A cephalosporin or dicloxacillin are appropriate, 250 to 500 mg four times daily.

d. I&D is *not* always appropriate, especially if the bursitis is purely inflammatory. Unlike most abscesses, olecranon bursitis is often slow to heal following I&D, whereas a trial of anti-inflammatory and/or antibiotic medication is often successful.

5. Perirectal abscess and pilonidal cysts.

a. A rectal examination should be performed to rule out communication of the abscess with the rectal cavity. If communication is present, surgical consultation is indicated.

b. I&D of the isolated abscess is required. Because this may be quite painful, large abscesses should be drained under general anesthesia.

6. Axillary abscess (hidradenitis).

a. I&D is indicated.

b. Recurrence is frequent, and referral to a surgeon for definitive removal of the recurrently infected sweat glands may be required.

17

Peripheral Vascular Emergencies

I. Acute Arterial Ischemia

The following findings may be present individually or as a full constellation in the event of acute arterial occlusion or injury. All should be sought in the physical examination and documented in the medical record.

    A. Early symptoms and signs.
1. Sudden onset of severe pain in an extremity.
2. Paresthesias followed by the gradual loss of sensation.
3. Gradual loss of motor function.
4. Coolness of the skin below the obstruction.
5. Pallor of the extremity with diminished capillary filling of the fingers or toes.
6. Absence of pulses distal to the anatomic block. The Doppler ultrasound stethoscope is extremely useful for auscultating pulses that are not palpable.

    B. Late symptoms and signs.
1. Violaceous hue of skin.
2. Increased size of an extremity with firm consistency of muscle on palpation.
3. Gangrene.
4. Paralysis of the extremity.

5. Absence of pain or sensation in a distal extremity.
6. Systemic bacteremia.

II. Trauma

A. Laceration, perforation, or contusion of the vessel wall may result in the acute cessation of arterial flow.

B. If the artery is completely severed, the vessel retracts into the surrounding tissues. Usually, constriction of the open vessel edges by contraction of the circular coats of muscle in the media prevents extensive blood loss.

C. A partially transected major artery tends to gape widely and may result in severe hemorrhage.

D. Arterial perforations from knives, ice picks, or low-velocity missiles may not be apparent immediately if the surrounding tissues are filled with blood. Distal pulses may be palpable, and the circulation may appear intact on clinical evaluation. However, if these injuries are untreated, arteriovenous fistulas or pulsating hematomas (false aneurysms) may result.

E. Arterial contusions commonly are caused by the following:
1. Crushing blunt trauma.
2. Fractures (Fig 17–1).
3. High-velocity missiles passing in close proximity to the vessel.
   a. There is damage to the vessel wall, with a hematoma developing between the intima and the media.
   b. As the clot enlarges, the lumen of the vessel gradually becomes occluded (Fig 17–2).

F. In rapidly decelerating vehicular accidents, the origin of the left subclavian artery may be subjected to a shearing force. An absent left radial pulse may be the first indication of injury to the descending thoracic aorta.

G. Treatment.
1. The patient should not be anesthetized unless

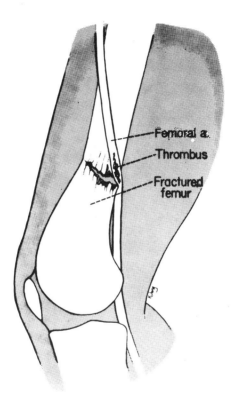

FIG 17–1.
Arterial contusion caused by a fracture.

there is a severe intra-abdominal or intrathoracic hemorrhage.
2. Intravascular volume must be restored and hypoxia and acidosis corrected.
3. Arterial bleeding from a limb wound should be

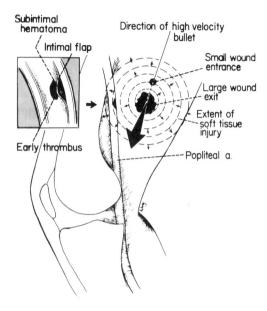

FIG 17–2.
Arterial occlusion produced by high-velocity penetrating injury.

      controlled by bulky compression dressings reinforced with an elastic bandage.

  4. No attempt should be made to control bleeding by blindly clamping in the depths of the wound.

    a. Tourniquets should be used only if absolutely necessary because they occlude collateral circulation and promote distal intravascular thrombosis.

    b. If a tourniquet is the only way to stop the bleeding, it must be loosened every 20 minutes.

5. To avoid additional injury to adjacent vessels, fractures should be stabilized by splinting before the patient is transported.

6. Preliminary arteriography may be helpful to show the extent and exact point of injury.

7. If there is any question of arterial integrity, the patient should undergo surgical exploration. Exploration should also be considered for an injury in which a high-velocity missile penetrates an area adjacent to a major vessel.

8. Arterial repair should be performed in an operating room where adequate anesthesia, light, instruments, and assistance are available.

III. Arterial Embolization

A. Most arterial emboli arise from an intracardiac thrombus. Atrial fibrillation, mitral stenosis, or a recent myocardial infarction is frequently associated with the formation of a cardiac thrombus. Rarely a left atrial myxoma may appear as an acute arterial embolus. Atherosclerotic major vessels and aneurysms are also sites from which particles may embolize.

B. The embolus commonly lodges at major vessel bifurcations. The findings of acute ischemia are present.

C. The pulse above a distal extremity obstruction is usually stronger than a pulse in the normal contralateral limb.

D. Arteriography is useful in anatomic localization. In the elderly, it may reveal associated obstruction secondary to arteriosclerosis obliterans.

E. Treatment is directed toward expeditious extraction of the clot in the operating room. An initial dose of 5,000 units of heparin should be administered intravenously.

IV. Arteriosclerosis Obliterans

A. Occlusion in this arterial disease of aging is a gradual, progressive process. It is usually accompanied by the development of collateral circulation. Occasionally, the narrow-vessel lumen will become thrombotic suddenly or be obstructed by an embolus, thereby causing acute ischemia.

B. The lower extremity is most commonly involved. In addition to the findings characteristic of acute ischemia, the patient often has a history and signs of the following:
   1. Leg claudication.
   2. Trophic skin changes.
   3. Ulceration.
   4. Areas of gangrene.

C. Management.—As soon as the diagnosis of arterial occlusion is made, the patient should be admitted to the hospital. Arrangements should be made for immediate arteriography.

V. Acute Venous Disease

A. Trauma.
   1. Major vein injury is usually associated with arterial trauma. Occasionally, however, a penetrating wound may involve a large vein exclusively.
   2. As in arterial trauma, active bleeding is controlled by compression dressings; blind clamping in the depths of the wound should be avoided.
   3. Since direct repair of injured veins has been introduced, the incidence of post-traumatic extremity edema and phlebitis has markedly decreased.

B. Ruptured varicosities.
   1. Hemorrhage of a thin, dilated superficial vein in patients with varicose veins of a lower extremity may occur spontaneously or following injury.
   2. The area where the greater saphenous vein

crosses the medial malleolus is most commonly involved.

3. Subcutaneous and intradermal rupture of a varix results in an ecchymotic patch or a hematoma that, if untreated, can lead to a stasis ulcer.

4. Blood loss is usually minimal but may be extensive enough to require a transfusion. Bleeding is easily controlled by the application of a compression dressing and an elastic bandage from the toes to the tibial tubercle.

C. Thrombophlebitis.

1. Acute superficial thrombophlebitis.

a. This occurs spontaneously in patients with varicose veins, in women during and following pregnancy, in women taking oral contraceptive agents, in patients following trauma, and in patients with carcinoma or blood dyscrasias.

b. The lesions are painful, erythematous cords that follow the course of superficial veins. The inflammatory reaction usually subsides in 7 to 18 days.

c. If there is proximal progression of skin coolness or evidence of a decrease in motor activity or sensation, immediate surgical intervention is necessary.

d. Treatment includes bed rest with elevation of the extremity and warm, moist packs and analgesics.

2. Deep thrombophlebitis.

a. The urgent nature of this condition stems from the often fatal complication of pulmonary embolism.

b. Thrombophlebitis most commonly involves the deep veins of the calves, the iliofemoral system, the pelvic veins, and the axillary vein.

c. Venous stasis is the underlying cause of deep thrombophlebitis.

d. Signs and symptoms.

(1) There is usually a rapid onset of pain and swelling of the limb.

(2) There is diffuse muscular tenderness on manual compression.

(3) Forcible dorsiflexion of the foot causes pain in the calf. There may be increased resistance to such passive dorsiflexion (Homans' sign).

(4) Calf tenderness on palpation and a firmness of the calf muscles may be the only signs.

(5) Iliofemoral thrombophlebitis causes swelling of the thigh and tenderness along the common femoral vein beneath the inguinal ligament.

(6) The calf and thigh circumferences of the involved extremity may exceed those of a normal contralateral extremity by 2 cm or more.

(7) Clinical diagnosis of deep-vein thrombosis may be extremely difficult.

e. Diagnosis

(1) Venography is the definitive diagnostic procedure, but it is invasive and involves the potential complications of radiographic contrast material.

(2) Radioactive fibrinogen scanning is useful in the diagnosis of *fresh* calf vein thrombosis. It is not useful in the diagnosis of thrombi of the upper part of the thigh or pelvis, which are the most likely to cause embolization to the pulmonary circulation.

(3) Impedance plethysmography is a noninvasive technique for the diagnosis of popliteal, femoral, and iliac vein thrombosis. There is an associated incidence of 1% to 4% false-positive results but a negligible false-negative rate.

    f. Treatment.
      (1) The patient should be admitted to the hospital and restricted to bed rest with the involved extremity elevated.
      (2) A priming dose of 5,000 units of heparin should be administered intravenously. Prior to this, blood should be drawn for a baseline activated partial thromboplastin time.
      (3) Following this, a continuous infusion of heparin via infusion pump should be begun at 1,000 units/hr, with the dose adjusted to maintain the activated partial thromboplastin time at 1.5 to 2.0 times the baseline level.

VI. Aortic Aneurysm

A. Thoracic.
  1. Most thoracic aortic aneurysms are due to atherosclerotic vascular disease and involve the descending aorta. Some are the result of cystic medial necrosis, like Marfan's syndrome, but aneurysm formation due to syphilis is now uncommon.
  2. Dissection of an aneurysm results when blood enters an intimal tear. There is then extravasation into the vascular media and dissection of the hematoma between the layers of the vessel. Dissection may proceed distally and involve the subclavian and even the renal vessels or proceed proximally and cause aortic insufficiency or cardiac tamponade. The aneurysm may rupture into a bronchus and cause hemoptysis, into the gastrointestinal tract and result in hematemesis, or into the left pleural space.
  3. Clinical presentation.—Most patients with aortic dissection experience pain. The pain is usually in

the anterior chest or the epigastrium, is excruciatingly severe, and may radiate to the interscapular area. Occasionally the event is painless; the patient may have syncope or signs of hypovolemic shock. If dissection involves the left subclavian artery, the amplitudes of the pulses in the arms may differ. A murmur of aortic insufficiency or signs of cardiac tamponade may be present. Of patients in whom a rupture has not occurred, most are hypertensive. When hypotension is present, it may be due to hypovolemia or cardiac tamponade.

4. Diagnosis.—The diagnosis is suggested by a widened mediastinal silhouette on the chest x-ray. Definitive diagnosis is by arteriography.

5. Treatment.

   a. If the patient is in hypovolemic shock or cardiac tamponade, he should be treated appropriately (see Chapter 1).

   b. If the patient is hypertensive, the blood pressure should be reduced to a systolic level of 110 to 120 mm Hg. The agent of choice is sodium nitroprusside, 40 mg in 250 mL of 5% dextrose in water. It should be infused via infusion pump, the infusion rate titrated to the effect on the blood pressure.

   c. In addition, propranolol (Inderal) should be administered intramuscularly, 1 mg every 4 to 6 hours to a maximum of 6 mg in the first 12 hours, to reduce the pulsatile nature of aortic flow.

   d. Both cardiology and vascular surgery specialists should be consulted.

B. Abdominal.

1. An abdominal aortic aneurysm is seen predominantly in older men with atherosclerotic vascular disease. Many are initially asymptomatic, with a pulsatile mass found on routine physical examination.

2. Rupture of an aortic aneurysm is generally retro-

peritoneal. This results in the abrupt onset of severe, constant, mid- or lower-abdominal pain, with radiation into the back or groin. A pulsatile abdominal mass may or may not be palpable. Hypotension or shock may be present.

3. The walls of the aneurysm frequently calcify, and the aneurysm may be visible on a lateral x-ray of the abdomen. The presence of an aneurysm can also be determined by computed tomography or abdominal ultrasonography.

4. Treatment.—The patient should be treated for shock (see Chapter 1) and prepared for emergency surgery. A pneumatic military antishock trousers (MAST) suit may be particularly useful in the treatment of a ruptured abdominal aortic aneurysm because it provides for external counterpressure to the abdomen.

18
Bone and Joint Trauma

I. General Considerations

A. Priorities.
1. Priorities for treatment must be established for any patient with multiple injuries. An adequate airway must be established and maintained and gross hemorrhage controlled. Injuries to the chest, abdomen, or great vessels require priority treatment since they may be critical.
2. A check of neurological function as well as the circulation and pulses distal to a fracture is essential, as is complete documentation of such assessment.

B. X-rays.—Adequate roentgenograms of the area of injury are imperative.
1. Standard radiographic (usually posteroanterior, lateral, and oblique) views must be obtained.
2. Additional special views may be needed such as "mortise" or oblique views in ankle injuries.
3. For extremity injuries in children and adolescents, the opposite side is available as a control if there are any questions in interpreting the film.
4. Obtain comparison films, especially for children.
5. Films should include the joints proximal and distal to the area traumatized.

6. Always obtain postreduction x-rays following manipulation.

C. Casts.

1. A well-padded plaster cast is less comfortable and allows more mobilization than a lightly padded cast that is well molded to the contours of the limb.

2. If the cast must later be split and spread, the padding must be divided down to the skin; otherwise, underlying strands of sheet wadding may remain to impair circulation.

3. To prevent "window edema" of the soft tissues through cuts in the cast, fill the gap with fresh sheet wadding held in place loosely with an elastic bandage.

4. If a patient is not hospitalized after the cast is applied, be certain that he returns immediately if the extremity becomes cold or numb or if there is increased pain.

5. Application of a plaster splint to immobilize a fracture until swelling subsides may be indicated in the acute setting.

II. The Upper Extremity

A. Clavicle.—Nonunion of fractures of the clavicle is uncommon. Hospitalization is necessary if there is marked displacement or neurovascular injury. A sling may relieve much of the pain of undisplaced fractures. An active person will be most comfortable in a clavicular figure-eight brace.

B. Scapula.

1. Fractures may be caused by direct trauma or avulsion of muscle origins or insertions.

2. The patient should be examined closely for other associated injuries such as a rib fracture or pneumothorax.

3. For simple fractures and most avulsions, sling and

swath immobilization during the time of acute pain is sufficient.

C. Dislocation of the shoulder.

  1. Dislocation is anterior in 90% of cases and is apparent clinically. The lateral aspect of the shoulder is flat instead of rounded, and a deep sulcus is palpable between the head of the humerus and the acromion laterally.

  2. Examination for associated brachial plexus injury is mandatory. The radial pulse should also be palpated and its presence noted in the record.

    a. Injury to the axillary nerve is common.

    b. It may be impossible to check for motor nerve injury to the deltoid because of pain, but hypoesthesia over the deltoid prominence indicates some compromise of sensory branches.

  3. Have adequate roentgenograms to demonstrate any associated fractures prior to any attempt at reduction.

  4. The dislocation can often be reduced without active manipulation.

    a. The patient is given an appropriate dose of intravenous meperidine, morphine, or diazepam (see Chapter 28).

    b. He then lies face down on the examining table with a shoulder over the edge and the affected extremity dependent.

    c. Ten to 15 lb of weight is tied to the wrist with gauze bandages.

    d. The dislocation may be reduced aftr 10 to 15 minutes of this traction.

  5. Method of Hippocrates.

    a. Exert slow, gentle longitudinal traction on the extremity, with countertraction exerted on the axilla.

    b. Then, slowly and without force, bring the extremity to the midline while maintaining traction.

  6. After the dislocation is reduced, immobilize the

extremity by applying a swath (Velpeau) dressing with the arm on the chest. Prior to application of the dressing, place a gauze pad in the axilla to prevent skin maceration.

    a. A bias-cut stockinette is good for this dressing.

    b. Always obtain postreduction films.

    c. Three weeks of immobilization allows sufficient healing of the soft tissue to lessen the chances of recurrent dislocation later.

D. Acromioclavicular separation.

    1. The patient complains of pain localized just medial to the acromioclavicular joint. The mechanism of injury is a fall on the point of the shoulder.

    2. The injury may involve torn acromioclavicular ligaments only or, in more severe injuries, a tear of the coracoclavicular ligaments also—a complete acromioclavicular separation.

    3. In the second instance, the upwardly displaced distal end of the clavicle is much more prominent.

    4. The only finding on examination may be local tenderness, but roentgenograms of the acromioclavicular joint with the patient holding about 10 lb of weight in his hand should readily demonstrate disruption of the joint.

    5. Either injury may be treated conservatively.

        a. Circumferential strapping extending around the flexed elbow up over the angle of the shoulder and the clavicle may be used to hold the separation reduced. This is difficult to maintain, however. Frequent visits will be necessary to tighten the strapping.

        b. Alternatively, a commercially produced acromioclavicular splint may be applied.

    6. For in complete separation, reduction and internal fixation may be indicated.

E. Humerus.

    1. Fracture of the surgical neck.

    a. Manipulation usually will not appreciably improve the position, especially with marked comminution. The position is often satisfactory, although manipulation or open reduction is sometimes needed.

    b. Function is the most important factor. Start early circumduction motion in a sling collar or cuff.

    c. If the fracture is associated with a brachial plexus injury or dislocation of the head, open reduction and exploration may be indicated.

2. Shaft fractures.

    a. In the elderly, it is often elected to apply a posterior plaster splint and sling and start early circumduction exercises to preserve function.

    b. In young patients, nonunion or malunion is fairly common. A hanging arm cast or sling and swath dressing should be applied.

    c. Radial nerve injury is common; it may appear some hours after the initial injury from motion at the fracture site.

    d. Early exploration usually is not indicated.

3. Supracondylar fracture.

    a. This fracture requires immediate attention.

    b. The possibility of Volkmann's ischemic contracture following these fractures makes them extremely dangerous injuries. Examine the patient for the onset of pain, pallor, no pulse, paresthesias, and paralysis, the classic findings in ischemic injury.

    c. The extension-type fracture is by far the most common.

        (1) The distal fragment of the humerus lies posteriorly.

        (2) Reduction is by longitudinal traction with the elbow in hyperextension.

        (3) The elbow is then flexed to beyond a right angle to maintain the reduction.

        (4) If signs of impending Volkmann's contrac-

ture persist after adequate reduction, reduce the degree of elbow flexion until the
pulse returns.

(5) If there is no improvement, immediate arteriography is indicated.

F. Elbow.

1. Central subluxation of the head of the radius, also
known as "nursemaid's elbow."

a. This is a very common injury, and its history is
important; typically, a sudden longitudinal
traction has been exerted on the upper extremity of a young child, usually under the age
of 3.

b. There is pain when passive flexion or extension of the elbow is attempted.

c. The forearm is held in pronation; attempts at
passive supination aggravate the pain.

d. Obtain x-ray films of the elbow before manipulation.

e. Quick supination of the forearm by using very
little force is all that is needed to thrust the
radial head back through the annular ligament
and relieve the painful disability completely.

f. A sling with a posterior plaster splint may be
applied to hold the forearm in supination after
the reduction. Young children may, however,
not tolerate the application of a splint.

2. Dislocation of the elbow.

a. Always check for associated neurovascular injuries, especially brachial artery and ulnar or
median nerve damage.

b. Reduction is by the application of longitudinal
traction on the forearm with countertraction
on the arm. Reduction may be difficult to
achieve, and general anesthesia may be required.

c. Following reduction, immobilize the arm in a
posterior plaster splint with the elbow flexed

beyond a right angle. Check the distal pulses, and observe the circulation of the hand.
  d. If the elbow is left at a right angle, redislocation is possible.
  e. For stable reductions, mobilization should begin in 3 to 4 days.
3. Radial head fractures.
  a. Most will do well with immobilization in a posterior plaster splint until the acute pain subsides.
  b. Selected cases need surgical treatment.
    (1) Marked angulation that is not corrected by manipulation.
    (2) Cases with marked comminution.
    (3) Displaced medial marginal fractures (where osteoarthritic changes may be anticipated at the proximal radioulnar joint).
4. Olecranon fractures.
  a. If undisplaced, the extremity may be immobilized with the elbow in 90 degrees of flexion.
  b. Even the slightest displacement is unacceptable, and open reduction with internal fixation is indicated.
5. "Tennis" elbow.
  a. The patient often gives a history of repetitive use of the extremity.
  b. He complains of pain localized over and distal to the lateral epicondyle of the humerus near the origin of the extensor muscles.
  c. The pain may radiate down the forearm and is aggravated by pronation of the forearm, flexion of the wrist, and strong grip.
  d. Roentgenogram findings are normal.
  e. Local injection of hydrocortisone and application of a sling for several days usually relieve the pain.
  f. Analgesics should be prescribed for several days, and the extremity should not be used.

g. Pain often returns after subsequent use, and the extremity may require prolonged rest.

G. Forearm: radius-ulna fractures.

1. If pronation and supination are to be preserved in the forearm, close to an anatomic reduction of both fractures is necessary.

2. In children, with their great potential for growth and remodeling, some degree of displacement may be acceptable.

3. In adults, very little short of anatomic reduction can be accepted.

4. Open reduction with internal fixation is indicated if an excellent position obtained by closed reduction cannot be held by plaster.

5. This is so difficult that open reduction is the usual and accepted form of treatment for this fracture.

H. Wrist and hand.

1. Distal radius (Colles' fracture).

a. There may be an associated ulnar styloid fracture.

b. Anesthesia for reduction may be achieved by hematoma block or Bier block.

c. For reduction, apply longitudinal traction with countertraction to the elbow. Increase the deformity by forcible dorsiflexion of the wrist. In this position of hyperextension, the distal fragment can be pushed toward the palm to the proper relationship with the proximal radius. The wrist is then flexed, and the distal radial fragment is molded toward the palm and the ulna to correct angulation and radial displacement.

d. A well-molded short-arm cast or sugar-tong splint is usually adequate to relieve discomfort in an older patient, but a long-arm cast may be desirable for the comminuted fracture. The cast should be split to prevent the development of ischemia due to swelling.

e. It no longer is accepted practice to place the hand in extreme palmar flexion and ulnar deviation; this may help maintain a reduction, but it leaves the wrist stiff, a poor position in the older patient.

2. Navicular fractures.

a. The mechanism of injury is usually a fall onto the outstretched hand. The patient complains of pain in the wrist, especially over the region of the anatomic snuffbox. There is pain on extension and ulnar deviation of the wrist.

b. Initial roentgenograms of the wrist may fail to demonstrate the fracture.

c. In confirmed navicular fractures or those suspected on clinical grounds, apply a short-arm cast incorporating the thumb to the interphalangeal joint in a position of abduction and opposition.

d. If initial films are normal, repeat x-rays out of plaster after 2 weeks. Callus and resorption of bone at the fracture site may then be apparent.

3. Metacarpal fractures (boxer's fracture).

a. Fractures occur at the neck of the second to fifth metacarpals from direct trauma, as in a blow with the fist.

b. The most common fractures are of the fourth and fifth metacarpals. There is palmar angulation of the metacarpal head.

c. Local infiltration of the fracture hematoma with 1% lidocaine usually provides sufficient anesthesia for reduction.

d. Flex the metacarpophalangeal and proximal interphalangeal joints to 90 degrees, and exert strong pressure over the proximal interphalangeal joint dorsally along the axis of the proximal phalanx. This may correct the angulation in a recent injury.

e. Immobilize the hand with the metacarpopha-

langeal and proximal interphalangeal joints of
the injured finger in the functional position in
a short-arm finger cast.

f. A good functional result can be obtained with
less than anatomic reduction. Up to 40 degrees
of volar angulation is acceptable.

III. The Hip

A. Fractures.
1. These may occur with relatively minor trauma in
the elderly.
2. Classically, the shortened lower extremity lies in
external rotation (greater in intertrochanteric than
in neck fractures).
3. Movement at the hip causes groin or knee pain.
4. There is pain on pressure over the greater trochanter.
5. The intertrochanteric type may result in several
units of blood extravasating into the thigh, an increase in the thigh's circumference, and shock.
6. Most neck and intertrochanteric fractures are best
treated by open reduction and internal fixation.

B. Hip dislocation.
1. This injury is the result of severe violence. Automobile accidents are the most common cause. On
physical examination, the hip is flexed and ad-
ducted; the leg is shortened and internally rotated. Sciatic nerve injury is sometimes associated.
2. Early reduction is imperative and lessens such
complications as late aseptic necrosis of the femoral head and pressure injury of the sciatic nerve.
3. Evaluate for associated fractures to the femoral
shaft and pelvis.

C. Trochanteric bursitis.
1. This may be confused with hip joint disease or
with a herniated intervertebral disk.
2. Either the subcutaneous or, more commonly, the

deep trochanteric bursa may be involved. The bursitis is usually aseptic.

3. Direct pressure over the bursa duplicates the pain.

4. If there are no signs of infection, 5 mL of 1% lidocaine with 10 mg of triamcinolone intra-articular suspension can be injected into the bursa. Pain relief is usually immediate and dramatic.

IV. The Lower Extremity

A. Femoral shaft.
1. Diaphyseal fractures.
    a. As in intertrochanteric hip fractures, there may be appreciable blood loss into the thigh. Signs of hemorrhage can be easily missed if the patient is not carefully monitored.
    b. Initial management includes immediate immobilization in a traction splint, evaluation of the extent of volume loss, and administration of intravenous fluids and blood, as indicated.
2. Supracondylar fractures.
    a. Popliteal artery injury may be a complication. A careful evaluation of distal circulation is imperative. Early consultation with a vascular surgeon and arteriography should be obtained in any case in which circulatory impairment is suspected.
    b. The best functional result usually is obtained by meticulous traction with a tibial pin and balanced suspension.
B. The knee.
1. Patellar fractures.
    a. Undisplaced fractures, especially longitudinal ones, may be immobilized with the knee in extension in a cylinder cast or knee immobilizer.
    b. If the fragments are separated as they fre-

quently are in horizontal fractures, surgical reduction is required.

2. Patellar dislocations.

   a. Most frequently, these occur laterally. Adolescent girls and young women are most often affected.

   b. They may be reduced spontaneously and leave only slight swelling and pain on pressure around the medial margin of the patella.

   c. Reduction is achieved by applying medialward pressure over the lateral side of the patella while slowly extending the knee.

3. Nonbony injury.

   a. A common injury is a torn medial meniscus, sometimes associated with anterior cruciate and medial collateral ligament tears. A typical history is the sudden onset of pain following internal rotation of the femur upon the fixed tibia and foot.

   b. If the development of swelling was slow (over a period of hours), a serous effusion is likely; anticipate a cartilage injury only.

   c. If swelling was rapid in onset, anticipate ligament tears or a fracture with a hemarthrosis. However, complete ligament tears may not result in significant effusion.

   d. Arthrocentesis should be performed if a large effusion is present.

      (1) Always aspirate the knee under strict aseptic conditions.

      (2) Note whether the aspirated fluid is serous or bloody.

      (3) Let the tube into which the joint fluid is injected stand. If globules of fat (marrow) rise to the surface, anticipate an osteochondral fracture, which may not be apparent on roentgenograms.

   e. Any acute knee injury may cause sufficient pain to prevent a thorough examination. The patient may require examination under anesthesia or non–weight-bearing conditions.

(1) With the knee flexed at 30 degrees, check for abnormal mobility with medial or lateral pressure applied to the lower part of the leg. If a medial or lateral collateral ligament is torn, excessive motion will be felt, and a fingertip on the joint line will feel the joint rock open on the injured side.

(2) Test for excess anteroposterior motion of the head of the tibia with the knee flexed to 90 degrees. Excessive anterior motion of the tibia is possible with a torn anterior cruciate ligament, and excessive posterior motion is possible with the much less common tear of the posterior cruciate ligament.

f. Many tests demonstrate torn cartilages, but none is exceptionally reliable. The leg may be held in full internal or external rotation with the knee acutely flexed.

(1) A snap or click is sometimes felt or heard as the knee is then brought into full extension while the leg is rotated. There are many variations and eponyms for such tests.

(2) Abnormal laxity, "pops," "clicks," or other findings may be bilateral and unrelated to the injury.

g. Obtain adequate roentgenograms of the knee; these should include "tunnel" or intercondylar notch views and "skyline" or tangential views of the patella if indicated.

h. Early surgical repair is usually advised for torn collateral ligaments or a torn meniscus.

i. If adequate examination is prohibited by excessive pain or swelling, the patient must have follow-up arrangements made for re-examination in several days.

4. Chondromalacia of the patella.
   a. The patient may have a history of recent or old trauma to the patella, but the disease can occur with continued normal use.
   b. The pathological process is a degenerative change of the articular surface of the patella, which is really part of a more generalized change in the entire knee.
   c. The patient complains of pain fairly well localized to the anterior aspect of the knee. The pain is aggravated by climbing and descending the stairs and often does not appear until late in the day.
      (1) With the patient relaxed and supine and the knee extended, crepitus may be felt as the patella is passively glided over the femoral condyles.
      (2) Pain is felt if the patella is pulled distally, pressure is applied in a posterior direction on the patella, and the patient is then asked to contract the quadriceps.

C. Tibial shaft fracture.
   1. Most can be treated satisfactorily by closed reduction. These fractures should be reduced under general anesthesia if the position is not satisfactory. Associated vascular injury probably occurs more often than is suspected clinically.
   2. Proximal shaft fractures are through cancellous bone and usually heal with no difficulty. Fractures through the distal third are in an area of poor blood supply; delayed union is common, and nonunion is by no means rare. Prolonged immobilization may be necessary in this case, sometimes for 6 to 9 months.

D. The ankle.
   1. Sprain.
      a. The anterior talofibular ligament is the most commonly injured, and there is point tenderness anterior to the lateral malleolus.

    b. For the uncomplicated sprain, elastic bandages and taping are used in treatment along with elevation and crutches.

    c. Immediate application of a short-leg walking cast will allow the patient to bear full weight painlessly, with minimal fatigue from the altered gait.

    d. Local heat is never indicated in the acute stage of the injury. It will only increase the swelling.

  2. Fractures.

    a. The history of the injury is very helpful. If the mechanism of injury is reversed, adequate reduction is often obtained even after gross displacement.

    b. Films must include anteroposterior, lateral, and mortise (oblique) views. The "joint line" around the talus should be the same width on both sides and top.

    c. Early reduction before significant swelling occurs is important. Some cases require open reduction.

E. The foot.

  1. Calcaneal fractures.

    a. Check for associated compression fractures of the spine if the mechanism of injury was a fall from a height.

    b. Opinion is divided on whether open or closed reduction is indicated.

    c. The best results seem to follow elevation of the extremity after the application of pressure dressings. Early motion of the foot and ankle *without* bearing weight for 4 to 8 weeks usually gives a good functional result.

  2. Fracture of the base of the fifth metatarsal (ballet fracture).

    a. The peroneus brevis muscle inserts at the base of the fifth metatarsal. The mechanism of injury of the fracture is the avulsion of the base of the metatarsal by a sharp, sudden contraction of the muscle, as sometimes happens during a misstep.

   b. It is a common injury often confused with a sprained ankle. The tenderness and swelling are anterior around the fifth metatarsal base, not around the anterior tip of the lateral malleolus.

   c. These patients are often reasonably comfortable in ordinary shoes. If they experience great pain during walking, they may need a short-leg walking cast.

3. Phalangeal fractures.

   a. Firm, well-fitting shoes relieve much of the pain during walking.

   b. Taping adjacent toes together helps relieve pain but may lead to skin maceration unless there is adequate padding between the toes.

V. The Back

For a discussion of spinal injury, refer to Chapter 12.

VI. Pelvis

A. Pelvic fractures are potentially the most dangerous of bony injuries, being capable of producing exsanguinating hemorrhage.

   1. The source of bleeding is usually the vascular plexus lining the pelvic walls, but there may also be injury to iliac, iliolumbar, or femoral vessels.

   2. When signs of hypovolemic shock are present, early transfusion of blood is mandatory.

   3. Application of the pneumatic antishock garment may be of particular benefit in pelvic fractures.

   4. Reduction of unstable fractures will also diminish bleeding.

B. Fractures with which hemorrhage is most often associated are those of the sacrum or ilium, bilateral pubic rami, separation of the symphysis pubis, and dislocations of the sacroiliac joint.

c. Urinary tract injury accompanies approximately 10% of pelvic fractures.

1. Hematuria is usually present.
2. Urethral injuries in the male usually occur at the level of the prostatic apex.
   a. Gross blood may be seen at the urethral meatus.
   b. Pubic fractures may be palpable at rectal examination, and the prostate may be displaced superiorly and surrounded by a boggy hematoma.
   c. Insertion of a urethral catheter in these patients with meatal bleeding is contraindicated. The diagnosis should be verified by retrograde urethrography and a suprapubic cystostomy catheter inserted if bladder drainage is required.

19
Hand Injuries

Note: See Chapter 18 for a discussion of hand fractures, Chapter 16 for a discussion of antibiotic prophylaxis and treatment of infection, and Chapter 28 for discussion of regional anesthesia.

I. General Principles

A. Evaluation of the patient as a whole must precede diagnosis and treatment of the specific hand injury.
   1. Inquiry must be made as to whether the patient has a chronic systemic disease that may retard wound healing such as diabetes, circulatory insufficiency, or neoplasm.
   2. It should also be learned whether the patient is receiving steroid therapy and what is the status of his tetanus immunization.
   3. Treatment priorities must be established for the patient with multiple injuries. Life-threatening conditions must be dealt with at once.
B. An accurate history of the specific hand injury must be obtained. Important considerations are the time elapsed since injury, how and where the injury was sustained, and the occupation of the patient.
C. Old scars and persistent injuries should be well documented. Sensory, motor, and vascular status must be evaluated. A diagram is useful for describing all lacerations, scars, and deficits.

D. X-rays may be helpful in delineating hand injuries and identifying foreign bodies.

II. Functional Anatomy of the Hand

An accurate diagnosis of injuries and infections requires precise knowledge of the anatomy.

A. Palmar surface of the wrist (Fig 19–1).

1. The palmar surface of the wrist contains three easily palpable tendons: palmaris longus in the middle with flexor carpi radialis and flexor carpi ulnaris to either side. (Palmaris longus is absent unilaterally in approximately 15% of patients and absent bilaterally in 7%.)

2. The median nerve lies just deep to palmaris longus on its radial side. The ulnar nerve and artery lie deep to flexor carpi ulnaris on its radial side. The radial artery lies just radial to flexor carpi radialis.

B. Palm of the hand (Fig 19–2).

1. The transverse carpal ligament forms the roof of the carpal tunnel. This space contains nine tendons and one nerve: the superficialis and profundus tendons to the fingers, the flexor policis longus tendon, and the median nerve.

2. The ulnar artery and nerve occupy a separate compartment formed by the volar carpal ligament.

3. The motor branch of the median nerve leaves the main trunk at the distal edge of the transverse carpal ligament to innervate the thenar muscles and the radial lumbricals.

C. Dorsum of the hand and wrist (Fig 19–3).

1. The extensor tendons of the fingers insert at the base of the middle phalanges.

2. There are two tendons to the index finger and

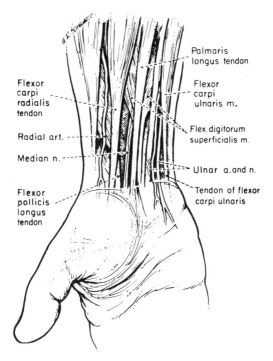

Palmaris
longus tendon

Flexor
carpi
radialis
tendon

Flexor
carpi
ulnaris m.

Flex. digitorum
superficialis m.

Radial art.

Median n.

Ulnar a. and n.

Tendon of flexor
carpi ulnaris

Flexor
pollicis
longus
tendon

FIG 19–1.
Palmar aspect of a wrist.

(with considerable anatomic variation) two tendons to the fifth finger.

D. Radial aspect of the wrist (Fig 19–4).
   1. This region is injured frequently. The long and short extensor tendons and their insertions and

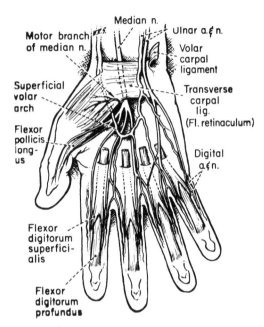

FIG 19–2.
Palm of a hand.

the abductor pollicis longus tendon of the thumb are shown in Figure 19–4.

2. Of greater practical importance is the *sensory* (superficial) branch of the *radial* nerve, which is frequently overlooked in lacerations of this region.

3. If this structure is not repaired, the proximal end can form a neuroma that may become tender and painful.

4. The extensor carpi radialis longus and brevis are

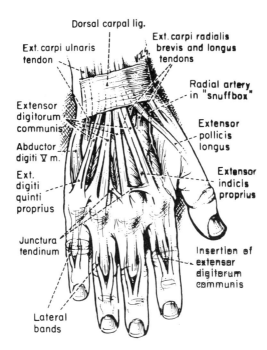

Dorsal carpal lig.

Ext. carpi ulnaris tendon

Ext. carpi radialis brevis and longus tendons

Radial artery in "snuffbox"

Extensor digitorum communis

Abductor digiti V m.

Extensor pollicis longus

Ext. digiti quinti proprius

Extensor indicis proprius

Junctura tendinum

Insertion of extensor digitorum communis

Lateral bands

FIG 19–3.
Dorsum of a hand.

shown in the figure. The brevis is *ulnar* to the longus and is the prime wrist extensor.

III. Diagnosis

Before injection of a local anesthetic, it is crucial to evaluate the vascular status, sensation, and motor function, of the hand.

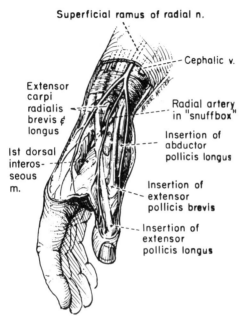

Superficial ramus of radial n.

Cephalic v.

Extensor
carpi
radialis
brevis &
longus

Radial artery
in "snuffbox"

Insertion of
abductor
pollicis longus

1st dorsal
interos-
seous
m.

Insertion of
extensor
pollicis brevis

Insertion of
extensor
pollicis longus

FIG 19–4.
Supeficial ramus of radial nerve.

A. Vascular status.
   1. A cold, pulseless hand indicates severe arterial damage.
   2. Circulation must be restored promptly in the operating room.
   3. Significant bleeding can ordinarily be controlled with a compression bandage.
   4. If bleeding persists, a padded blood pressure

cuff applied to the arm and inflated to above systolic blood pressure will stop the bleeding.

5. The cuff must be deflated every 45 minutes to allow full tissue perfusion.

6. Performance of the Allen test will help delineate vascular status in persons with wrist and forearm injuries.

    a. The hand is elevated, and both the radial and the ulnar arteries are occluded at the wrist by digital pressure.

    b. The patient is asked to open and close the fist repeatedly until venous drainage leaves the hand pale.

    c. Pressure over one artery is then released.

    d. The hand should return to pink within 15 to 30 seconds.

    e. The entire procedure is then repeated as the other artery is tested.

B. Sensation (Fig 19–5).

1. The median nerve carries sensory fibers from the palmar surface of the thumb, index, middle, and radial half of the ring finger, as well as the portion of the palm proximal to these fingers. It also provides sensation to the distal dorsal aspects of these fingers.

2. The radial nerve accounts for sensation over the radial aspect of the same fingers and the dorsal hand proximal to them.

3. The ulnar nerve provides sensation to the ulnar aspect of the ring finger and the entire little finger, as well as to both the palmar and dorsal aspects of the hand proximal to its finger distribution.

4. Anesthesia of the palm or dorsal aspect of the hand is usually accompanied by a loss of sensation to one or more fingers and implies a major nerve injury.

5. Anesthesia of one half of a single finger indicates laceration of a digital sensory nerve.

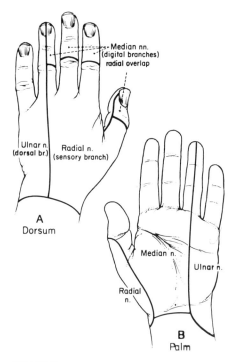

FIG 19–5.
Sensory innervation of a hand.

     6. Hypoesthesia of a given anatomic area is often transient and suggests that the nerve is merely contused rather than transected.

C. Motor function.

     1. Partial tendon transections may leave the patient with sufficient strength to perform a requested

maneuver against gravity. However, if the maneuver is performed against resistance, subtle injuries may be detected.

2. Depending upon the injury, motor function evaluation should include the following:
    a. Flexion of the fingers at the proximal interphalangeal joints (flexor digitorum *superficialis*).
    b. Flexion of the fingers at the distal interphalangeal joints (flexor digitorum *profundus*).
    c. Extension of the fingers.
    d. Opposition of the thumb and little finger.
    e. Abduction of the fingers.
    f. Extension and flexion of the wrist.

3. An inability to flex the distal phalanx with immobilization of the middle phalanx indicates division of the flexor digitorum *profundus* (Fig 19–6).

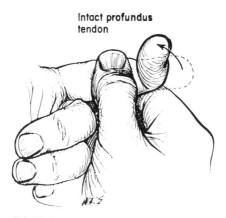

FIG 19–6.
Test for flexor digitorum profundus function.

4. Holding all fingers in extension except the one injured tests the function of the flexor digitorum *superficialis* (Fig 19–7).

5. A laceration over the dorsal surface and the inability to extend the finger fully suggest severance of the following:
   a. The common extensor tendon.
   b. The extensor indicis.
   c. The extensor digiti minimi.

6. Lacerations near the distal interphalangeal joint and droop of the distal phalanx indicate injury of

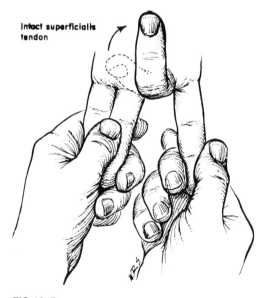

Intact superficialis tendon

FIG 19–7.
Test for flexor digitorum superficialis function.

the extensor complex in this region (mallet-finger deformity).

7. An inability to extend fully the distal phalanx of the thumb suggests division of the extensor pollicis longus tendon.

8. Injuries over the metacarpal of the thumb and the radial aspect of the wrist with the inability to extend and abduct the thumb suggest injuries to the short extensor and long abductor tendons. The long extensor also may be divided.

9. Even small lacerations of the thenar area may divide the motor branch of the median nerve, which innervates the thenar muscles. With such injury, the patient will be unable to oppose the thumb to the base of the fifth finger strongly or to abduct the thumb normally.

10. Damage to the motor branch of the ulnar nerve in the palm will make abduction or adduction of the extended fingers impossible because of the loss of interosseous muscle function.

   a. The best test is to have the patient put his hand palm down on a table and attempt to deviate the index finger radially.

   b. One may observe and palpate the first dorsal interosseous muscle located on the dorsal radial aspect of the second metacarpal bone and assay the extent of movement and muscle tone.

IV. Treatment

See Chapter 28 for a discussion of nerve blocks for hand anesthesia.

A. General principles.

1. Hand lacerations should be sutured within 6 hours of the injury to avoid infection.

2. Single-layer repair is usually sufficient unless a muscle, tendon, or nerve is involved. Multiple-

layer closure on the hand increases the risk of adhesions involving deeper structures.

3. Interrupted stitches should be used. The interrupted vertical mattress technique is often helpful on the dorsum of the hand, an area especially liable to inversion of scar tissue.

4. Inspection of the wound in a bloodless field is important.

   a. A well-padded arm tourniquet can be used. The arm is elevated, and a layer of cast padding is applied. A blood pressure cuff or a commercial pneumatic tourniquet is placed over the padding and inflated to approximately 50 mm higher than systolic pressure. The rubber tubing of the cuff may require clamping to prevent air leakage. The arm will become painful, and the tourniquet should be released as soon as possible, certainly within 45 minutes.

   b. Finger tourniquets can be used. A small rubber catheter or drain or a wide rubber band can be applied to the base of the finger. Since it is theoretically possible for the finger tourniquet to go unnoticed at the end of the repair and be incorporated into the dressing, it is advisable that the tourniquet be secured with a hemostat, which is obviously visible (Fig 19–8). The tourniquet time should be minimized. The laceration can often be repaired after the tourniquet is released so long as adequate inspection was achieved in a bloodless field.

5. Immobilization of the hand is essential to the healing process. If skin overlying joints is involved, those joints should be splinted. In any major hand injury, the entire hand and wrist should be immobilized in a position of function.

6. Elevation of the hand with any significant injury should be encouraged, with a sling used as needed.

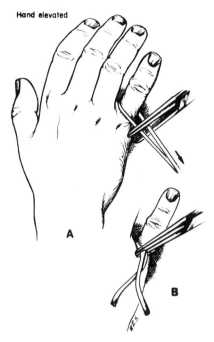

Hand elevated

A

B

FIG 19–8.
Obtaining a bloodless field in a digit.

    7. Hand sutures may generally be removed in 7 to
       10 days.
B. Nerve injuries.
    1. Small areas of numbness over the distal finger
       may be caused by nerve contusion or by the tran-
       section of sensory fibers that are too small to re-
       pair. Many of these deficits resolve spontaneously.

2. Any motor loss or significant sensory loss should be evaluated by a hand surgeon. The skin can be closed primarily and the deficit evaluated in several days if the surgeon is unavailable at the time of the injury.

C. Vascular injuries.
   1. Isolated digital arterial bleeders can usually be controlled with pressure alone. They should not be ligated, if possible, because of their proximity to nerves.
   2. There is usually sufficient collateral circulation so that the loss of a digital artery is of little consequence. However, obvious vascular compromise with decreased capillary perfusion should be evaluated immediately by a hand surgeon.

D. Tendon injuries.
   1. Flexor tendons are generally repaired by a hand surgeon in the operating room. They require extended follow-up and have a high incidence of complications.
   2. Simple extensor tendon transections can be repaired in the emergency department, often by the emergency physician, depending on the practice in the community and the training of the physician. Nonabsorbable suture material should be used and the hand immobilized. The details of tendon repair are beyond the scope of this book.

E. Open fractures.
   1. Meticulous debridement and irrigation will help prevent infection.
   2. Many fractures will heal well with skin closure and immobilization, particularly digital tuft fractures. However, open reduction of fragments, including wiring, will often be necessary.
   3. Prophylactic antibiotics are suggested, such as cephazolin, 0.5 to 1 gm intramuscularly, followed by cephalexin or dicloxacillin, 250 to 500 mg four times daily for 5 days.

F. Avulsions and amputations.
   1. Avulsion of the soft-tissue volar pad over the distal phalanx will usually respond well to split-thickness skin grafting.
   2. Avulsion of the soft tissue over the fingertip often will heal satisfactorily with no repair.
   3. Exposed bone must be covered with soft tissue. A full-thickness skin graft, pedicle flap, or rongeuring of the bone tip with primary skin closure may be necessary.
G. Grease and paint gun injuries.
   1. These may appear to be minimal puncture wounds soon after injury. However, they cause one of the most serious hand injuries. The insoluble organic compound injected into even the fingertip may enter the tendon sheath and be conveyed proximally well into the hand. Delayed inflammatory reaction and swelling are extremely intense, and such injuries often lead to amputation if untreated.
   2. All patients with this type of trauma should be referred immediately to a hand surgeon. Many will require decompression and debridement in the operating room.

20
Facial Injuries

I. Introduction

A. For cases involving multiple-system injury, the entire patient must be evaluated to establish the proper priority of management.

B. Definitive repair of facial wounds can be delayed several hours if necessary. The reduction of facial fractures may even be postponed for several days until soft-tissue swelling has subsided and the patient's general condition permits surgical correction.

C. Adequate anesthesia must always be provided (see Chapter 28). Local infiltration with 1% lidocaine is ideal for closing wounds. Lidocaine with epinephrine, 1:1,000, is appropriate for many facial lacerations.

D. Closing of lacerated wounds.

1. Surgical trauma must be minimized. Plastic surgical instruments should be used and tissue manipulated as atraumatically as possible.

2. Small bleeding points may be controlled by the application of pressure, ligated with fine sutures, or coagulated with electrocautery.

3. Skin edges are approximated with fine interrupted sutures of 5–0 or 6–0 monofilament nylon or polypropylene suture.

4. Interrupted sutures are placed approximately

to 4 mm apart (depending on the thickness of the skin being repaired) for accurate coaptation of the skin edges. Needles must enter and exit perpendicular to the skin.

II. General Wound Care

A. General surgical principles, including the prevention of infection and tetanus prophylaxis, apply to facial injuries as well as to those of other regions. Refer to Chapter 16, which details tetanus prophylaxis.

B. Primary repair of certain facial wounds may be done many hours following initial emergency care.

C. The face must be prepared with an antiseptic solution, and cleansing should include copious lavage of the wound with a sterile saline solution. High-pressure irrigation methods using a syringe or pulsatile hydrostatic nozzles are most effective. The volume of irrigation fluid used should be dictated by the degree of contamination of the wound.

D. Antiseptics that contain alcohol or iodine should not be used for irrigation because they cauterize the healthy wound borders and incite inflammatory reactions in the wound.

E. Facial or scalp hair around the wound may be trimmed closely with a pair of scissors, but the eyebrows should not be shaved since they are valuable landmarks for realignment of tissues and occasionally they will not regrow.

F. Draping with towels helps maintain a clean, unobstructed field (Fig 20–1). The face should be left exposed, as illustrated, in order to reduce patient anxiety, and also to allow the physician to observe the patient's respiratory effort and level of consciousness.

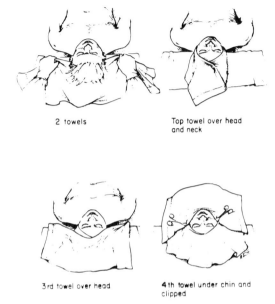

2 towels

Top towel over head
and neck

3rd towel over head

4th towel under chin and
clipped

FIG 20–1.
Draping for facial injuries.

G. Foreign debris and devitalized tissue are removed; however, debridement should be limited
to obviously necrotic tissue, particularly in
wounds near the eyelids and nose.

H. Pressure dressings are generally applied to absorb
wound drainage, control hematomas, and minimize postoperative edema.

III. The Untidy Wound

A. The grossly contused, "untidy," irregular laceration is probably best handled by the following:
   1. Wound excision to obtain precise borders.
   2. Undermining of the wound edges and careful suturing (i.e., with 5–0 or 6–0 nylon sutures) (Fig 20–2).
B. This cannot be done where a feature such as the eyelid is involved; distortion would result.

IV. Suture Technique

A. Suggested suture materials.
   1. Skin.—5–0 or 6–0 nylon or polypropylene.
   2. Subcutaneous sutures and hemostatic ligatures.—4–0 or 5–0 chromic catgut.
   3. Muscle fascia.—3–0 or 4–0 chromic catgut or polyglycolic acid.
   4. Mucosa.—4–0 chromic catgut, silk, or polyglycolic acid.

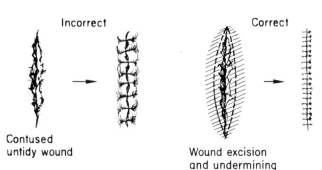

Incorrect

Correct

Contused untidy wound

Wound excision and undermining

FIG 20–2.
Skin laceration.

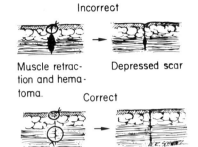

Skin
Fat
Muscle

Incorrect

Muscle retraction and hematoma.

Depressed scar

Correct

FIG 20–3.
Muscle injury.

B. Technical aspects (Fig 20–3).
  1. Fine instruments and meticulous care in handling the tissues are basic requirements.
  2. Sutures must just approximate tissues without constricting (Fig 20–4).
  3. Tight sutures cause tissue necrosis and delay wound healing; they produce "railroad ties" across the scar (Fig 20–5).
  4. Simple sutures that take in sufficient and equal amounts of subcutaneous and dermal tissue usually give good wound approximation. Wound edges should be everted to ensure appropriate healing.
  5. Sutures may be removed from the face in 3 to 5 days. At this time, the wound may be supported with sterile adhesive paper strips.
C. Poor scars result from the following:
  1. Suture material that is too heavy.
  2. Inclusion of too much tissue in the suture.
  3. Sutures that are too tight.
  4. Delayed removal of sutures.

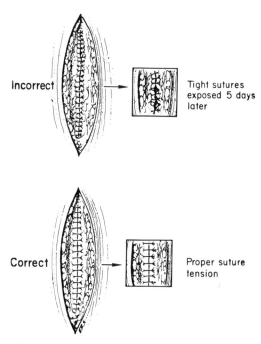

Incorrect

Tight sutures
exposed 5 days
later

Correct

Proper suture
tension

FIG 20–4.
Suture tension in the subcutaneous tissue.

V. Types of Wounds

A. Stellate or V-shaped lacerations may result in an ischemic skin flap if not properly managed.
  1. Care should be taken to avoid strangulation of the tip by sutures.
  2. A "corner suture" through the dermis of the tip may help in alignment (Fig 20–6).
B. Slicing wounds with beveled edges will often heal

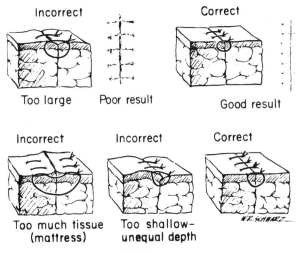

FIG 20–5.
Suture technique.

with contraction along the oblique tract of fibrous tissue and produce a rolled or pouting wound margin (Fig 20–7).

1. This will be even more apparent in the "trap-door" wound where the circular scar also contracts to cause further pouting in the wound margin.
2. Trimming the border to produce vertical edges will result in a better scar (see Fig 20–7).

VI. Tongue and Oral Mucosa

A. Small lacerations of the tongue and lips that are produced by the teeth generally heal satisfactorily without sutures.

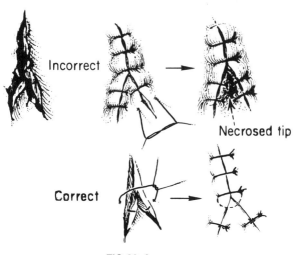

FIG 20–6.
Stellate lacerations.

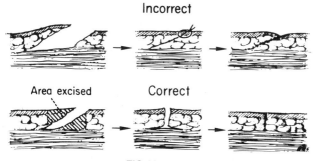

FIG 20–7.
Slicing wound.

B. Through-and-through lacerations of the cheek or lip require the following:
 1. Careful muscle approximation.
 2. Closure of the oral mucosa.
 3. Precise skin approximation.
C. Precise alignment of the vermillion border of the lip is most important (Fig 20–8). This should precede the placement of other skin sutures.
D. Frequent cleansing of the mouth with 3% hydrogen peroxide will prevent crusting and subsequent purulent collections.

VII. Eyelid Lacerations

A. In approximating eyelid lacerations, the most important landmark is the gray line (ciliary margin). This must be approximated as the first step in eye-

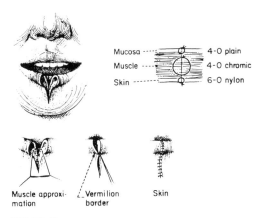

FIG 20–8.
Through-and-through lip laceration.

lid repair. Failure to precisely align the ciliary margin will result in notching of the eyelid. For skin, 6–0 nylon or polypropylene suture should be used, and 6–0 catgut should be used for the mucous membrane.

B. The time of removal of skin sutures will vary with their location and the wound tension.

1. Thin skin such as that of the eyelids heals quickly; hence, sutures can be removed in 2 to 3 days.

2. The somewhat thicker skin of the rest of the face and those areas subject to muscle pull heals more slowly. Sutures should be removed in 4 to 5 days.

3. All sutures must be taken out before any inflammation can develop around them.

4. If sutures are left in place, minor points of inflammation about them invariably lead to local suppuration—the cause of stitch-hold scars.

VIII. Inground Foreign Material

A. After cleansing, the wound is inspected carefully with a magnifying lens or loupe. Close attention is paid to any foreign material.

1. Foreign material must be removed because it becomes fixed rapidly into the tissue edges of lacerations or into abrasions.

2. Failure to remove it will leave permanent pigmentation in the skin, commonly referred to as "accidental tattoo."

B. Foreign material should be removed by irrigation, scrubbing, or surgical debridement. Anesthesia for this procedure may be attained with the topical application of 4% lidocaine. If the material is deep or difficult to dislodge, a motor-driven wire brush may be helpful.

C. When the discoloration is limited to the wound

edges, it may be better to debride these areas with a scalpel.

D. After the abraded wound has been treated, it is dressed by covering it with xeroform and a gauze dressing applied under moderate pressure.

IX. Facial Bone Fractures

A. Clinical diagnosis of facial bone fractures can be made with a high degree of accuracy. Clinical signs of facial bone fracture include point tenderness over the fracture site, bony asymmetry, and mobility of the fractured portion. Malocclusion is one of the most accurate signs of a mandibular or maxillary fracture.

B. Clinical findings should be confirmed with facial radiographs. Lateral and stereo Waters views are the most useful. Other views should be ordered as indicated.

C. An ecchymotic orbit suggests a malar bone fracture (Fig 20–9). Other findings may include the following:

1. Palpable irregularity and depression of the orbital floor.
2. Depression of the level of the globe.
3. Flattening and depression of the malar eminance.
4. Subjective complaints.
   a. Diplopia.
   b. Numbness in the distribution of the infraorbital nerve—the medial portion of the cheek and the upper lip and gums.
5. X-rays may reveal clouding of the maxillary antrum.

D. A blowout fracture of the orbital floor may occur along with other fractures of the malar bone or as a separate entity. It is usually caused by a direct blow to the orbit. This causes an increase in the

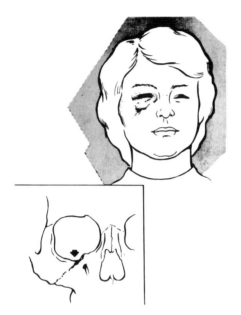

FIG 20–9.
Depressed fracture of the right malar bone.

intraorbital pressure, which in turn causes a fracture of the thin orbital floor.

1. Noting that one eyeball is resting at a lower level facilitates recognition of this fracture. The patient may complain of diplopia, but this may occur in only some directions of gaze, e.g., upward gaze due to entrapment of the inferior rectus muscle.
2. Accurate diagnosis is confirmed by x-ray studies. These may reveal a fracture line, fluid in the maxillary sinus, air in the orbit, or the

herniation of soft tissue into the maxillary sinus.

E. A visible or palpable depression over the zygomatic arch suggests a depressed fracture in this area (Fig 20–10). This fracture is most frequently caused by a direct blow. The diagnosis may be made by palpation of the bony deformity unless there is too much edema. Special underpenetrated views of the zygomatic arches may be obtained to confirm the diagnosis. Other findings include the following:

1. Localized tenderness.

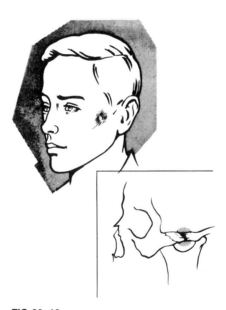

FIG 20–10.
Depressed fracture of the zygomatic arch.

2. Trismus and pain on opening the mouth. These occur when depressed bony fragments impinge upon the underlying mandibular coronoid process and the temporalis muscle.

F. Tenderness along the mandible in one or more areas with irregularity of the lower teeth suggests a mandibular fracture. Other findings include pain on opening and closing of the mouth, malocclusion, mobility of the fractured portion, compounding of the fracture into the oral cavity, and edema or hematoma formation.

1. The condyle is the weakest portion of the mandible (Fig 20–11). Fractures may be associated with bleeding from the external auditory canal if the walls of the canal are disrupted. An open bite suggests the presence of a mandibular dis-

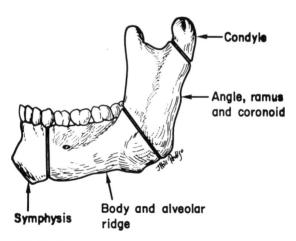

FIG 20–11.
Areas of the mandible.

location or bilateral condylar fractures. Temporomandibular joint views may be required to disclose the abnormality.

2. Fractures of the symphysis are the least common mandibular fractures. If there is injury to or edema around the mental foramen, there will be anesthesia of the chin and lower lip.

G. Fractures of the maxilla fall into several well-defined categories.

1. LeFort I.—This is a transverse fracture across the maxilla (Fig 20–12, A).

2. LeFort II.—This fracture runs through the nasal bones and the frontal maxillary processes (Fig 20–12, B).

3. LeFort III.—In this fracture, the maxilla, nasal bones, and zygoma are separated from their cranial attachments, i.e., there is craniofacial dysjunction (Fig 20–12, C). This type of fracture is usually associated with additional facial fractures.

4. These midface fractures may result in vertical elongation of the midface, malocclusion, and abnormal movement of the maxillary portion of the face. The latter may be demonstrated by grasping the upper teeth and palate and displacing this unit anteriorly.

H. Nasal fractures are usually depressed or laterally displaced. Inspection of the nostrils may reveal a septal cartilage dislocation into either nasal airway.

1. Signs of nasal fracture.
   a. Nasal bleeding.
   b. Deformity.
   c. Septal edema.
   d. Tenderness.

2. X-rays of the nasal bones confirm the diagnosis but are little aid to therapy because nondisplaced nasal fractures without airway obstruction require no treatment.

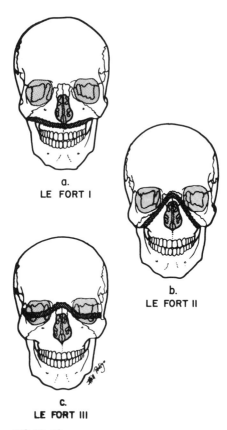

a.
LE FORT I

b.
LE FORT II

c.
LE FORT III

FIG 20–12.
LeFort types of maxillary fracture.

3. The presence of a septal hematoma requires prompt evacuation followed by nasal packing.

I. Tooth avulsion may be managed by reinsertion of the tooth into the socket. The socket should first be irrigated with saline and all clot material removed. An acrylic splint should be placed over the tooth and an adjacent uninjured tooth.

J. Treatment.

1. The reduction and immobilization of facial bone fractures are not necessarily an emergency provided an adequate airway is established.

2. Because extensive soft-tissue swelling usually accompanies facial bone fractures, it may be advantageous to wait 3 to 7 days for this edema to subside. Surgery will be easier, and it will be easier to maintain position.

3. Certain simple mandibular fractures can be treated by interdental wiring or elastic traction.

4. All complicated fractures of the mandible and maxilla require open reduction.

5. Nasal fractures and septal dislocations customarily are treated by closed reduction. It is advisable to manipulate septal cartilage dislocations as early as possible.

   a. A hematoma frequently forms around the cartilage. The hematoma provides an excellent culture medium that in turn leads to a septal abscess.

   b. This is likely to progress to septic chondritis and loss of the septal cartilage and leave the patient with a saddle deformity of the nose.

   c. Therefore, incision and drainage of a septal hematoma are mandatory.

6. Open fractures and fractures extending into the paranasal sinuses will require the administration of antibiotics such as ampicillin, 250 mg four times daily.

7. For all complicated fractures of the mandible,

maxilla, central third of the face, and malar-zygomatic bones, open reduction is indicated.

a. For these cases, it is wise to obtain consultation.

b. Definitive treatment should be delayed several days until facial edema has subsided. Two or 3 weeks' delay is not unusual for severe, extensive injuries.

21

Otolaryngologic Emergencies

I. Acute Airway Obstruction

A. Obstruction due to a foreign body.—If the patient cannot talk, is cyanotic, is in respiratory distress, or is obviously not ventilating, the following measures can be taken:

1. Foreign bodies in the airway can sometimes be dislodged by forceful percussion over the upper part of the back.

2. The Heimlich maneuver may also be successful. The examiner's hands are interlocked and placed over the epigastrium of the supine patient. Forceful pressure is then applied. If the patient is seated or standing, he may be grasped from behind.

3. The patient's pharynx may be swept with the examiner's fingers (with a bite block or an improvised object such as a wallet first placed between the teeth to prevent biting).

4. If the equipment is available, direct laryngoscopy may be used.

5. If the patient cannot be ventilated around the foreign object, intubation should be attempted.

6. If the rapid use of some or all of the aforementioned measures is unsuccessful, an emergency

cricothyrotomy should be performed (see Chapter 5).

B. Obstruction due to laryngospasm.—Laryngospasm may occlude the airway and require cricothyrotomy. If time permits, however, intubation may be possible, with care taken not to traumatize the cords. Sometimes anesthetic spray (Cetacaine) directed at the cords may break the laryngospasm and allow intubation. The best treatment, however, is lidocaine, 75 to 100 mg intravenously (IV).

II. Foreign Body in Air and Food Passages

A. A patent airway must be ensured (see Section I).

B. Etiology.—Certain foreign bodies are common in particular age groups: safety pins, coins, or peanuts in children and dentures, food boli and bones in adults. Fishbones are most often found in the faucial tonsil or at the base of the tongue in the lingual tonsil. Safety pins, coins, and dentures often lodge in the cricopharyngeal area, and smaller objects such as tacks and peanuts are frequently found in the trachea or bronchi. There may be several foreign bodies. Be aware that some previously unrecognized problem such as an esophageal stricture or a psychotic state may exist. Wherever possible, acquire a duplicate of the foreign body or the object from which the foreign body was removed.

C. Symptoms and signs.

1. A foreign body in the airway may cause agitation, pain, stridor, respiratory distress, cough, hoarseness, hematemesis, and possibly cyanosis.

2. A foreign body in the esophagus may cause drooling, localized pain, referred pain (espe-

cially to the jugulosternal notch), odynophagia, and regurgitation.

D. Physical examination.

1. Examine the mouth, pharynx, larynx, neck, and chest. Search for signs of obstruction, hemorrhage, or perforation.

2. Laryngoscopy should be performed as needed. The pharynx is anesthetized with benzocaine spray (Cetacaine) and/or lidocaine gargle (Viscous Xylocaine). Indirect mirror laryngoscopy with the patient in a sitting position may reveal the foreign body. A laryngoscope can be used to perform direct laryngoscopy with the patient supine. Adequate local anesthesia and a gentle touch on the part of the physician are mandatory. If available, fiberoptic laryngoscopy can be extremely useful.

E. X-ray.—Roentgenograms of the neck, chest, and abdomen may reveal a radio-opaque foreign body. Inspiratory and expiratory x-ray films of the chest in frontal and lateral projections are indicated for cases of aspirated nonopaque foreign bodies. Characteristic areas of hyperaeration and/or hypoaeration of the lungs may be demonstrated. Radiographic contrast studies such as barium swallow may be useful, but only after the initial appraisal.

F. Treatment.

1. Visible foreign bodies can sometimes be easily removed.

2. Meat impacted in the esophagus can be softened by drinking small amounts of meat tenderizer (papain) in water.

3. Glucagon (1 cc IV) may relax esophageal smooth muscle and allow passage; often it induces vomiting and regurgitation of the impacted food.

4. There is at least a theoretical risk of esophageal perforation due to papain digestion of isch-

emic esophageal mucosa and to glucagon-induced forceful peristalsis in an obstructed esophagus.

5. Endoscopic removal may be required.

III. Foreign Body in the Nose or Ear Canal

A. Any object small enough to pass into the nostril or external ear openings may be found lodged in these areas. Such objects are frequently wedged in owing to unskilled attempts at removal. The problem in a child may be complicated by his reluctance or inability to cooperate.

B. Signs and symptoms.

1. Nose.—Pain, sneezing, or unilateral nasal obstruction may be present. Later, findings may include bleeding accompanied by fetor and a foul discharge.

2. Ear.—Later signs in the ear may resemble those of external otitis or chronic otitis media.

C. Procedure.—History and examination suggest the diagnosis. Unskilled attempts to remove foreign bodies are to be avoided. Proper illumination of the cavity and suitable instruments are essential for successful removal.

IV. Ingestion of Caustics

See Chapter 29 for a discussion of poisoning. Acids and alkalis used in household cleaning such as lye, ammonia, potassium permanganate, and sulfuric acid are the most common offenders.

A. History.—Ascertain the time of ingestion and the quantity and nature of the material ingested. The reason for ingestion and the past emotional behavior of the patient are important.

B. Physical examination.—Examination of the oral cavity, pharynx, and larynx may reveal marked reddening of the mucosa, denuded areas, or a coagulum of the caustic agent. General status, vital signs, and vital organ functions are to be assessed. Airway evaluation is essential, and tracheotomy eventually may be required.

C. Evaluation.
   1. X-rays of the chest and cervical soft tissues should be obtained in any significant case to help rule out perforation.
   2. Early endoscopy should be performed by an experienced endoscopist.
   3. Contrast studies should be obtained only after endoscopic consultation because contrast material can obscure the findings on endoscopy.

D. Treatment.
   1. Although steroid usage is somewhat controversial, if they are used, they should be given fairly early in the course (e.g., dexamethasone, 20 mg IV every 6 hours).
   2. Antibiotics (penicillin, 1,000,000 units IV every 6 hours) should also be given early to cover the gram-positive oral flora.
   3. Extended in-hospital treatment including surgery is often necessary.
   4. No attempt should be made to induce vomiting because this may re-expose the esophagus to the caustic agent.
   5. Early surgical consultation is mandatory.

V. Trauma

Refer to Chapter 20 for the treatment of lacerations and facial bone trauma.

A. Laryngeal trauma.
   1. Automobile accidents are responsible for most injuries in which the larynx is involved. A large

proportion of these injuries can be prevented by the use of lap and shoulder restraints. The trauma usually occurs to the passenger in the front seat when the extended neck strikes the dashboard.

2. Direct laryngeal trauma may occur after a blow from a baseball bat or golf ball, from a boxing injury, after striking a protruding pipe or tree branch, or from the entanglement of a scarf or necktie in machinery.

3. Symptoms and diagnosis.

   a. Hoarseness, dysphonia, or aphonia following a history of trauma is fairly indicative of nerve or cartilaginous injury involving the larynx.

   b. The airway should be evaluated immediately. Respiratory symptoms range from relatively trivial to progressive stridor, dyspnea, and suprasternal and infrasternal retractions and hemoptysis.

   c. Palpation of the neck in persons with suspected laryngeal trauma may disclose subcutaneous emphysema, pain on palpation, deformity and discoloration or fixation of the thyroid or cricoid cartilages, or fracture of the hyoid bone. Often the thyroid cartilage is flattened, or one ala overlaps the other anteriorly.

   d. Indirect laryngoscopy may reveal hematoma, edema, vocal cord lacerations, deformity of the laryngeal configuration, and impaired mobility of the vocal cords. Lateral and anteroposterior neck x-ray films for soft-tissue detail may reveal air in the soft-tissue spaces or deformity of the structures and should be ordered as soon as possible. Fiber-optic or direct laryngoscopy are indicated for all suspected laryngeal fractures. Early diagnosis and initiation of therapy are crucial.

4. Treatment.
    a. The essence of therapy for laryngeal trauma is the maintenance and preservation of the airway. Cricothyrotomy or tracheostomy may be required. A high index of suspicion and rapid evaluation are important in preventing airway obstruction.
    b. The treatment of minimal soft-tissue injury consists of external hot packs, voice rest, humidification, and surveillance. If the airway is compromised, a low tracheostomy should be performed before it becomes an emergency.
    c. As soon as the patient's general condition permits, fractured cartilages must be reduced, replaced, and maintained in position. This may be done perorally or by open reduction. Failure or inadequate early management results in laryngeal stenosis and the need for a permanent tracheostomy.

B. Nasal trauma.
    1. The history should include, in addition to events relevant to the local nasal injury, an inquiry into lapses of consciousness, history of nasofacial trauma either accidental or surgical, and impairment of sensory and motor function.
    2. The physical findings are pain, swelling, deformity, and impaired function.
    3. There is little medical need for x-rays of isolated, relatively minor nasal trauma. Photographs would actually be of greater value in documenting the degree of deformity. Social and legal requirements, however, may dictate radiographic documentation.
    4. When the swelling is minimal, displaced fractures can be reduced during the first few hours. However, significant swelling can preclude adequate visible evaluation of reduction efforts. In these cases, manipulation should be

deferred for several days to a week until the swelling is reduced.

5. Septal hematoma should always be ruled out by inspection and palpation.
   a. If untreated, infection and necrosis of the septum can develop.
   b. Treatment consists of a local lidocaine (Xylocaine) injection followed by an incision over the inferior portion of the hematoma. A small Penrose drain can then be inserted and the anterior nose packed with petrolatum gauze (see Section VI).

6. Clear drainage from the nose may indicate a leak of the cerebral spinal fluid. (See Chapter 12).

C. Traumatic perforation of the eardrum.
   1. Symptoms.—Frequently there are pain and bleeding from the ear, hearing loss, fullness, and tinnitus. Vertigo, though possible, is not likely. There may be a history of diving, a slap on the ear, head injury, or ear trauma (with a toothpick, needle, cotton swab, or other instrument).
   2. Evaluation.—In a tuning-fork study of an otherwise normally hearing individual, Weber's test will show lateralization to the affected ear; usually the Rinne test will reveal bone conduction dominating air conduction in the affected ear and air conduction exceeding bone conduction in the normal ear. Watch for nystagmus, and check the function of the seventh and other cranial nerves.
   3. Treatment.
      a. Keep instruments and medication out of the ear. Avoid contamination of the ear; secondary infection may cause suppuration. Severe perforations may benefit from immediate otosurgical closure.
      b. The patient should be advised to keep all

extraneous objects from the ear, including fingers, shower water, and over-the-counter medication.

   c. If the perforation is not grossly contaminated, antibiotics are not necessary, but otologic reevaluation should be performed as the wound heals.

VI. Epistaxis

A. Etiology.—Most instances of epistaxis arise from the anterior portion of the nose along the septum. In the young, the cause is usually digital trauma. Epistaxis frequently follows a head cold. The examiner should rule out nasal tumors, trauma, and foreign bodies. Hematologic disturbances should be considered if the skin shows petechiae or ecchymoses. High blood pressure should be ruled out, and if present, controlled. Epistaxis may be a premonitory sign of an impending hypertensive cerebral hemorrhage.

B. Procedure.—Determine the site and cause of the bleeding.

   1. Have a head mirror and adequate light.
   2. Have suction apparatus and nasal aspirating tips.
   3. Position the patient appropriately, seated but slightly reclined.
   4. Protect yourself and the patient with aprons or gowns.
   5. Give the patient a basin into which blood and secretions may be expectorated.
   6. Aspirate all clots and debris from the nose.
   7. Check the pharynx for bleeding posteriorly.
   8. Pack the nose with a large cotton pledget dampened lightly with a suitable topical anesthetic (cocaine, tetracaine [Pontocaine], etc.). These agents also provide vasoconstriction

and may decrease bleeding. Additional topical catecholamines are not usually necessary.

9. If the bleeding has stopped and the site has not been identified, light abrasion of the anterior septum with a cotton applicator may cause renewed bleeding and allow identification of the site.

10. When the bleeding point is identified, chemical cautery may be used with the application of silver nitrate or trichloroacetic acid. This will stop most nosebleeds. Occasionally electrocautery will be required. Injection of the mucosa with lidocaine (Xylocaine) beforehand is advisable.

11. If the bleeding is stopped, emphasize that the patient should not manipulate the nose or engage in exceptional activity for several days. Be sure the general medical condition is satisfactory.

12. Attempt repeatedly, with the nose anesthesized, to locate and cauterize a bleeding point prior to packing lubricated gauze.

13. If the patient is still bleeding after the aforementioned procedure, anterior packing of 1-in. lubricated gauze stripping is layered from the floor to the roof of the nose.

14. If the patient is still bleeding or if the examination demonstrates that the bleeding is posterior in the nose, insert a posterior nasopharyngeal pack and pack anteriorly against it through the nose.

C. Method of inserting a posterior nasal pack.

1. Commercially available epistaxis balloons are excellent. If not available, a 30-cc Foley catheter can be used (nos. 14 to 16 for adults, no. 12 for children).

2. Anesthetize the pharynx and soft palate with anesthetic spray (e.g., Cetacaine). Use a cotton pledget dampened with anesthetic (e.g., cocaine) to anesthetize the nose.

3. Lubricate the catheter with antibiotic ointment and pass it through the anterior nares until it is visible in the oral pharynx.

4. Inject 8 cc of air, and withdraw the catheter until it is engaged in the choanae. Then inflate another 2 to 4 cc of air.

5. While an assistant maintains traction on the catheter, firmly pack petrolatum gauze into the nose anteriorly against the Foley balloon.

6. Protect the nostril and columella with soft gauze or cotton and anchor the catheter.

7. A significant incidence of hypoxia occurs in patients with posterior packs. The patient should be admitted to the hospital, given penicillin, and closely observed.

VII. Infection

A. Throat.
  1. Pharyngitis.
     a. Viral infections account for the majority of sore throats.
     b. Bacterial infections of the pharynx and tonsils can be caused by a number of organisms, but *Gonococcus* and group A β-hemolytic *Streptococcus* are the only types that require antibiotics. Untreated streptococcal infections can be associated with the later development of rheumatic fever or glomerulonephritis.
     c. Diagnosis.
        (1) Both viral and streptococcal infections can cause pharyngeal erythema, mucosal petechiae, tonsillar exudate, and cervical adenopathy. It is generally felt that the greater the number of the aforementioned findings, the greater the possibility of streptococcal infection. It is noteworthy, however, that the

mononucleosis virus is often associated with all these signs in full panoply. An additional finding is a high frequency of posterior cervical adenopathy in mononucleosis.

(2) Definitive diagnosis is made by examining a culture. Full "culture and sensitivity" of the throat is unnecessarily expensive. A culture to rule out *Streptococcus* infection is preferred. If gonorrhea is suspected by history, an anaerobic gonorrhea culture is suggested.

d. Treatment.

(1) Ideally treatment should await culture results. Sociological problems with adequate follow-up of emergency department visits or particularly severe symptoms may favor the initiation of antibiotic treatment, which can then be discontinued if the *Streptococcus* culture is negative.

(2) Rapid latex streptococcal screens are now available in many EDs, and can give fairly accurate results in less than an hour.

(3) For streptococcal pharyngitis, use one of the following regimens:

a Bicillin (procaine plus benzathine), 1.2 million units intramuscularly.

b Penicillin G or VK (phenoxymethyl), 250 mg four times a day for 10 days

c If the patient is allergic to penicillin, administer erythromycin, 250 mg four times a day for 10 days

(4) For gonococcal pharyngitis, use one of the following regimens:

a Ceftriaxone, 250 mg intramuscularly.

b Probenecid, 1 gm given orally, plus

procaine penicillin G, 4.8 million units intramuscularly

B. Peritonsillar abscess.
   1. Symptoms.—Prominent complaints are severe sore throat, worse on one side, with severe pain on swallowing (odynophagia). Weakness, thirst, chills, fever, ear and neck pains referred from the throat, and trismus are common. Trismus may prevent the patient from opening his mouth to allow adequate inspection.
   2. Objective findings.—The patient is toxic and febrile; also noted are thick speech, drooling, trismus, contralateral displacement of the edematous uvula, and a tonsil that is beefy red and advancing to the midline. Respiratory obstruction may, in fact, occur. There is fullness at the juncture of the soft palate and the lateral margin of the palatine tonsil, and asymmetry is usually noticeable. Cervical adenopathy frequently is present.
   3. Treatment: aspiration, incision, and drainage.
      a. Spray the tonsil area lightly with a topical anesthetic (e.g., Cetacaine). Aspiration of the peritonsillar space may relieve some of the trismus, provide suitable bacteriologic material, and aid in excluding the possibility of incising into a great vessel.
      b. Incision and drainage is then usually performed, although there has been a recent trend toward aspiration alone.
      c. Intramuscular penicillin (e.g. procaine penicillin, 1.2 million units) should be given, preferrably prior to the surgical procedure.
      d. Hospital admission should be considered for any significant abscess.
C. Croup and epiglottis.—See Chapter 24.
D. Ear.
   1. Serous otitis media.
      a. Symptoms.—The ears feel "stopped up,"

and there may be a sensation of "fullness." Hearing may be decreased. Otalgia may eventually develop.

b. Physical findings.—The tympanic membrane may at first be retracted, with alteration of the light reflex. As fluid accumulates in the middle ear, the drum becomes dull. Bubbles may occasionally be seen in the fluid behind the drum.

c. Treatment.—The goal is to decrease swelling around the eustachian tube to allow the fluid to drain. Oral and nasal decongestants are used. Since the infection is viral, antibiotics are not indicated.

2. Acute otitis media.

a. Symptoms.

(1) The symptoms of serous otitis are experienced, but otalgia is the prominent complaint. Fever is common.

(2) In young children who cannot verbalize the complaint of ear pain, fever and vomiting may be the only obvious symptoms.

b. Physical findings.

(1) Early in the course, the eardrum may exhibit only dilated vessels.

(2) Eventually the entire drum becomes red with altered landmarks.

(3) The light reflex is lost, and the drum may bulge.

c. Treatment.

(1) The infection is bacterial, and antibiotics are necessary. Decongestants have traditionally been prescribed, but no definitive study has proved them effective.

(2) Adults and children over 6 are often treated with oral penicillin for 10 days.

Erythromycin can be used in patients who are allergic to penicillin.

(3) In areas where *Hemophilus* infection is a frequent cause of otitis, older children and adults may be given ampicillin or amoxicillin.

(4) Because children younger than 6 are often infected with *Hemophilus* organisms, this age group has traditionally been treated with ampicillin or amoxicillin. Erythromycin is an alternative.

(5) If the infection does not respond in several days in a young child, the organism may be ampicillin-resistant *Hemophilus.* Therapy should then be changed to cefaclor or one of several combined preparations: trimethoprim and sulfamethoxazole (Septra or Bactrim), erythromycin and sulfisoxazole (Pediazole), or amoxicillin and clavulanic acid (Augmentin).

(6) In areas where ampicillin-resistant *Hemophilus* is common, one of the aforementioned medications may be used initially.

(7) If the patient is quite ill, if there is severe ear pain, or if the infection is resistant to antibiotic treatment, myringotomy may be necessary.

3. Acute external otitis.
   a. Symptoms.—At first only itching may be present, but eventually pain develops, especially with chewing. A sense of fullness and hearing loss may also occur.
   b. Physical findings.—
      (1) Manipulation of the auricle causes pain.
      (2) The canal may at first be only red. Eventually there is swelling.

      (3) Pus may occlude the canal.

      (4) Otitis media may be present as well.

      (5) Periauricular adenopathy may occur.

  c. Treatment.

      (1) Gently wipe or aspirate the pus, and send it for culture.

      (2) If there is significant swelling or pus, a ¼-in. gauze wick should be gently inserted into the canal.

      (3) Antibiotic drops should be prescribed (e.g., Cortisporin).

      (4) Systemic antibiotics should be used if there is fever, significant periauricular adenopathy, or accompanying otitis media. Decongestants may also be used.

E. Acute sinusitis.

  1. History.—Onset often follows an upper respiratory tract infection, facial trauma, or a tooth extraction.

  2. Symptoms.—Nasal blockage, pain over the involved sinus, fever, chills, malaise, dry throat, and vague orbital discomfort are common; symptoms may be unilateral.

  3. Objective findings.—Tenderness to percussion over the involved sinus is usually present. Swelling, warmth, and erythema may occur as well. The infected sinus may fail to transilluminate. Intranasal examination may reveal injected swollen tubinates and mucous membranes. There is seldom any pus in the very acute stage. The teeth may be sensitive to percussion. Check for a dental focus of infection, especially if toothache is an early symptom.

  4. If the diagnosis is not obvious from physical examination, x-rays can be helpful by revealing clouding of the sinus and thickening of the sinus mucosa.

  5. Treatment.—The principle to be applied is to provide for better nasal and sinus ventilation

and drainage. Culture of the nasal secretions will usually not reveal the correct pathogen. If accurate cultures are required, it is necessary to aspirate the infected sinus. Pneumococci and *Hemophilus influenzae* are the most common organisms. Antibiotic therapy may include ampicillin or amoxicillin, tetracycline, trimethoprim-sulfa, or cefaclor. Also suggested are systemic and local nasal decongestants, high fluid intake, and humidification of the environment. Drainage and irrigation are occasionally required.

VIII. Dental Emergencies

A. Trauma.

  1. Oral soft-tissue trauma.

    a. Lacerations of the tongue, gum, and lips may require suturing. See Chapter 20 for a full discussion. While a multilayer repair may be required for through-and-through wounds, most shallow injuries require only a single-layer repair. Absorbable suture material is used, and a loose closure is performed to allow for drainage. Epinephrine may be added to lidocaine anesthetic to control bleeding if necessary. (The frenulum does not require repair.)

    b. Bleeding inside the mouth can often be controlled with cold water rinsing. The application of ice (a popsicle is ideal) is also useful. A wet tea bag can also control bleeding because tannic acid has some coagulating effect.

    c. Electrical burns of the mouth are usually due to a child's biting on an electrical cord or plug. While such injuries may initially seem trivial, they can quickly lead to massive swelling and even airway compromise. Hospitalization should be strongly considered.

2. Trauma to the teeth.

   a. Avulsion.

      (1) An avulsed deciduous tooth should not be replaced because this may lead to problems with the eventual permanent tooth.

      (2) Avulsed permanent teeth should be replaced as rapidly as possible, preferably within the first 30 minutes.

         a Care should be taken not to disturb the root or any soft tissue still adherent to the tooth. The tooth should not be wiped or rubbed.

         b If necessary any clot material or debris can be gently rinsed away. Normal saline is the best agent, but outside the hospital, milk is a good substitute because it is also isotonic. Tap water is acceptable.

         c Ideally, the tooth should gently be replaced in its socket prior to coming to the hospital.

         d If this cannot be done, an excellent method of transportation is to place the tooth inside the mouth, either under the tongue or in the buccal vestibule. If the injured child is too young for full cooperation, a parent's or older sibling's mouth can be used.

   b. Displacement.—A displaced tooth that is still in the socket and not grossly unstable should not be manipulated in the emergency department because this may lead to disruption of the blood and nerve supply and eventual death of the tooth. Many displaced teeth eventually return to normal alignment due to gradual pressure from the lip and tongue. Obviously, dental consultation is indicated.

 c. Fracture.

  (1) Immediate dental consultation is indicated for a broken tooth if the nerve is exposed, as may be suggested by bleeding from the broken tooth surface or exposure of the pink-colored pulp.

  (2) Temporarily covering the exposed surface with wax or sugarless chewing gum may provide significant analgesic.

  (3) If both a broken tooth and an oral laceration are present, the wound should be thoroughly explored for the missing tooth fragment.

  (4) The alveolar ridge should be examined to rule out a fracture.

B. Infection.

 1. Caries commonly present to the emergency department with toothache. Analgesics may be given and the patient referred to a dentist.

 2. An abscess may be suggested by the presence of fever, swelling, acute submandibular adenopathy, or tenderness to percussion of the tooth (preferably with a metal instrument). Penicillin should be prescribed (250 mg four times a day) and the patient referred to a dentist for drainage. If there is evidence of facial cellulitis, especially if pointing toward the orbit, hospital admission for IV antibiotics is indicated.

 3. Stomatis presents with ulceration of the gums or tongue.

  a. Etiologic agents may include herpes simplex and the coxsackieviruses. The former is generally more localized, the latter more widespread.

  b. No treatment is ideal. Local application or rinsing with Viscous Xylocaine may be helpful. Severe herpes infections may respond somewhat to acyclovir (Zovirax), one pill five times a day.

C. Temporomandibular joint (TMJ) disorders.

1. Inflammation may be chronic or acute and typically causes pain on jaw motion and chewing. Pain may be referred to the ear. While nonsteroidal anti-inflammatory drugs may help temporarily, referral to a dentist is suggested.

2. Dislocation of the TMJ is caused by displacement of the mandible in an anterior direction. The patient is unable to close the mouth. Reduction is achieved by downward and backward traction on the jaw. (The physician's fingers are placed over the patient's lower teeth—after being wrapped with a thick layer of gauze.)

22
Ophthalmologic Emergencies

I. General Considerations

A. In all patients with eye problems except those for whom intervention must be initiated without delay (e.g., caustic burns), visual acuity should be tested prior to diagnostic or therapeutic manipulation. Each eye should be tested separately and the results noted in the medical record. If the patient wears glasses, the acuity may be recorded with the glasses in place and the notation "corrected" made.

B. The standard Snellen eye chart should be used whenever possible, and the smallest line discernible by the patient recorded. A pinhole can be used for patients who did not bring their corrective lenses. If the patient is unable to read even the largest figures on the chart, he should be asked to count the number of fingers the examiner holds in front of him, to detect finger movement, and to perceive light, in that order.

C. Examination of the eye should be complete in each instance. It should include a funduscopic examination and an examination with the slit lamp if one is available. Tonometry should be performed if increased intraocular pressure is suspected. This is easily done with the Schiotz tonometer. Following the instillation of a topical anesthetic in the eye, the tonometer is lowered onto the eye until the footplate rests on the cornea. The reading on the tonometer scale is converted by means of the table that accompanies the tonometer. Normal intraocular pressure is 12 to 20 mm Hg.

D. The use of topical corticosteroid preparations for the emergency patient can be dangerous because of the ophthalmologic complications these drugs may produce. These include the enhanced activity of herpes simplex virus, development of open-angle glaucoma, and fungal superinfection. Topical corticosteroids should, therefore, be used only with specific indications, at the recommendation of an ophthalmologist, and with the assurance of prompt ophthalmologic follow-up.

II. Chemical Burns of the Conjunctiva or Cornea

A. The offending agents are mostly detergents, window cleaning or other cleaning solutions, and strong acids and bases such as battery acid or lye. The most serious injury results from strong alkaline solutions.

B. The severely burned conjunctiva looks white and opaque and breaks down to shreds within a few hours; the cornea turns dull white. The moderately damaged conjunctiva appears edematous and hyperemic.

C. Irrespective of the nature of the offending agent, initial treatment consists of copious irrigation of the conjunctival sac with water in the most readily available form. Tap water at room temperature is an excellent irrigating fluid. Tap water used in a washbowl or sink in which the injured person can immerse the top of his head, including the burned eye, should be recommended over the telephone to any person who reports a chemical injury to the eye. While the eye is under water, the eyelids should be moved vigorously so the water can penetrate into the recesses of the conjunctival sac.

D. In the emergency department, the condition must be recognized promptly and treatment instituted immediately. Sterile saline is preferable to unsterile saline, but tap water is preferable when other fluid is not readily available. Intravenous saline solution may be instilled through intravenous tubing. The following points should be remembered:

1. A few drops of a topical anesthetic (tetracaine, proparacaine, or a similar agent) instilled into the conjunctival sac facilitates the treatment for both patient and physician.

2. The stream of fluid going in should be strong, that is, on the order of several milliliters per second.

3. The spasm of the lid muscles elicited by the burn must be overcome by a gentle pull on the eyelids (if necessary, with lid retractors).

4. The tip of the irrigator should never touch the cornea.

5. The recesses (fornices) of the conjunctival sac, particularly the upper one, should be irrigated thoroughly.

6. The first irrigation should last at least 30 minutes or, when there is particulate foreign matter, until no more particles can be dissolved in the effluent. At least 1 L of solution should be used to irrigate the burned eye.

E. Following irrigation and examination, topical antibiotic preparations should be instilled into the eye every 3 to 4 hours for 1 or 2 days.

III. Large, Sharp Foreign Bodies

Splinters of glass, plastic, or metal 5 to 15 mm long with sharp points or edges can cut into the eye in such a way as to anchor but still move with the movements of the lids. The mere opening of the eye, voluntarily by the patient or manually by the examiner, can add severe trauma by pushing the foreign body deeper into the eye. Topical anesthetic such as 0.5% proparacaine or tetracaine should be instilled into the eye to aid examination. If the object has not penetrated the cornea, it may be removed as described in section IV,B. If there is doubt about penetration, orbital x-rays may identify a foreign body. Penetration should be suspected particularly when a metallic foreign body has been driven at high velocity such as particles propelled by a grinding wheel.

IV. Small Foreign Bodies

A. Because of its position and construction, the human eye easily catches small airborne or mechanically propelled foreign bodies. The large majority, fortunately, do not carry much kinetic energy and are therefore stopped by the surface layer of the cornea or conjunctiva. The movements of the eyeball and eyelids tend to press these foreign bodies slightly into the surface layer and thereby contribute to their "getting stuck." This happens most frequently on the cornea and the upper tarsal conjunctiva. Such foreign bodies can be removed from the latter with cotton-tipped applicators after eversion of the upper lid, which is done most easily when the levator muscle is completely relaxed, as in extreme depression (downward rotation of the eye). One or two drops of topical anesthetic may be instilled to obtain greater patient cooperation.

B. Foreign bodies are removed from the surface of the cornea with spudlike instruments or small hypodermic syringe needles under good topical anesthesia (three to four instillations of an anesthetic such as 0.5% tetracaine or proparacaine). A good headrest and good focal illumination are essential. When a slit lamp is available, it should be used.

C. Removal of a foreign body should be followed by the instillation of a topical broad-spectrum antibiotic, the application of a fairly tight eye dressing, and re-examination of the eye 24 hours later. Application of a topical cycloplegic such as 2% or 5% homatropine drops is indicated if significant damage occurred at the time the foreign body was removed.

V. Occlusion of the Central Retinal Artery

A. The history is a sudden loss of vision in one eye. The objective findings are an absence of the direct reaction of the pupil to light, diffuse gray edema of the retina, and poor filling of the retinal vascular tree (compared with that of the other eye). The prognosis with regard to the return of vision depends on the duration and the degree of retinal anoxia. If the vision is limited to light perception in the temporal field and the duration is longer than 12 to 24 hours, the chances of recovery are minimal. If, on the other hand, the patient is seen within 2 hours of the onset of the condition and can count fingers at 2 or 3 ft, the chances of a return of some vision are reasonably good.

B. Initial treatment consists of measures aimed at vasodilation in the area supplied by the carotid arteries. Having the patient breathe into a paper bag is a widely used form of therapy. Alternatively, a commercially available mixture of 95% oxygen and 5% carbon dioxide may be used for 5 minutes of each hour. Since this may cause systemic vasodilation, the blood pressure should be closely monitored during such treatment. Beneficial effects on the intraocular circulation may be obtained by making the eye hypotonic with acetazolamide (Diamox) in 500-mg intravenous doses. Intermittent manual massage of the globe may dislodge an arterial clot. Other measures such as anterior chamber paracentesis are best left to the ophthalmologist.

VI. Acute Angle-Closure Glaucoma

A. Acute angle-closure glaucoma is an ophthalmologic emergency that must be recognized and treated without delay.

B. The patient complains of severe pain in the eye. This is accompanied by blurred vision, nausea, and vomiting.

C. Physical examination reveals the following:
   1. Conjunctival congestion.
   2. Cloudiness of the cornea.
   3. Shallowness of the anterior chamber.
   4. Midpoint-dilated pupils.
   5. High tactile or tonometric tension.

D. Treatment.—Initial treatment should consist of the application of a topical miotic such as 1% or 2% pilocarpine in drop or ointment form (every 15 minutes in the case of drops and every half-hour in the case of ointment for the first 2 hours) aided by Diamox (500 mg given intravenously) and, if available, an osmotherapeutic agent (such as glycerin by mouth, 150 to 180 mL of a 50% solution flavored with citrus fruit juice, or mannitol in doses of 1.5 to 2.0 gm/kg administered intravenously over a period of 30 to 60 minutes).

Care should be taken in elderly patients because osmotic agents may produce vascular overload. After this treatment is instituted, ophthalmologic consultation should be sought and the patient admitted to the hospital.

VII. Corneal Abrasion

A. Intense ocular discomfort with a history of minor trauma is usually due to a corneal abrasion. The cornea is covered by a squamous stratified epithelium resting on a basement membrane. Objects that brush across the cornea can rub off portions of this epithelium and thereby cause a corneal abrasion. By exposing sensory nerve endings, this elicits photophobia, lacrimation, blepharospasm, and an intense subjective sensation described by patients as a foreign-body sensation or pain.

B. The epithelial defect is often minute and demonstrable only by staining the cornea with fluorescein. This is done by gently touching the conjunctiva of the lower lid with the edge of a moistened fluorescein paper strip and examining the eye with a cobalt blue light. Only the exposed deeper layers of epithelium take the stain and turn green, in sharp contrast to the undamaged and, therefore, unstained surrounding surface layer of epithelium. This staining is best seen in a darkened room under blue light.

C. Except for the rare case in which the epithelial defect becomes a portal of entry for bacterial or viral infections, corneal abrasions heal rapidly. Local anesthetics should not be used topically for relief from the intense discomfort because they may inhibit the regeneration of epithelium and delay healing. Routine treatment aims to immobilize the injured eye with a tightly applied eye dressing and the instillation of broad-spectrum topical antibiotics (bacitracin, neomycin, sulfacetamide) every 4 to 6 hours. Twenty-four hours later, the eye should be re-examined. In most cases, the abrasion heals completely or almost completely within that time.

VIII. Injuries to the Eye

A. The distinction between perforating and nonperforating injuries is of utmost importance. Perforating injuries entail the following dangers:
   1. Intraocular infection.
   2. Retention of a foreign body within the globe.
   3. Damage to the deeper, more delicate structures of the eye.

   The differentiation between perforating and nonperforating injuries is made on the basis of a wound or portal of entry in the former and the signs of sudden stretching of the coats of the eyeball in the latter. The portal of entry can be very large and unequivocal in some cases and almost microscopic in others. A careful analysis of the circumstances under which the accident occurred can yield valuable clues. Orbital plain films may be useful in identifying the presence of metallic foreign bodies. Orbital computed tomography (CT) may also clarify foreign-body location and orbital injury.

B. Initial treatment of perforating injuries consists of prophylactic anti-infective therapy and the prevention of further damage to the globe. It is *not* permissible to wait for definite signs of post-traumatic intraocular infection. Since bacteriologic findings usually are not available when the diagnosis of perforation is first made, the anti-infective treatment should be intravenous penicillin G, 50,000 units/kg/day, or cephalothin, 1 to 2 gm/day in divided doses. A metal shield should be applied to the eye to prevent retraumatization and extrusion of intraocular contents. Extensive ocular examination is not indicated after the diagnosis of perforation is made.

C. Blunt injuries to the eye are inflicted by relatively large, blunt, often round objects. During the impact, the eyeball wall is stretched, and some ocular tissues such as the choroid tolerate this less well than others. In some of these injuries, the mechanical stress is so great that the eyeball wall actually ruptures.

D. In milder cases, the cornea and sclera stretch sufficiently to allow for the deformation caused by the injuring object, and intraocular hemorrhages of varying extent are the principal findings a few hours after injury. Blood in the anterior chamber of the eye—hyphema—is frequently the result. Treatment consists of hospital admission and complete rest for several days to a week since recurrence of the hemorrhage is directly related to physical activity. In addition, the patient may be sedated and should have daily examinations by an ophthalmologist.

IX. Injuries to the Eyelids

A. Lacerations of the eyelids are common. Before these lacerations are repaired, three important points should be remembered:

1. The eye should be carefully examined for signs of injury that may require treatment by an ophthalmologist and that may be more important than the laceration.

2. Lacerations including those of the lid border require more than the usual suturing in one or two layers if permanent notching of the border is to be avoided. (See Chapter 20, "Facial Injuries.")

3. Lacerations including those of the lower lacrimal canaliculus are difficult to repair and should therefore be referred to surgeons with special expertise.

B. The following typical fractures of orbital bones should be suspected if the examination reveals a definite downward displacement of the eye or diplopia in the upper field of gaze:

1. Fracture, dislocation, and/or comminution of the malar bone.

2. The "blowout" fracture of the floor of the orbit.

X. Contagious Diseases

A. Epidemic keratoconjunctivitis.—This is caused by an adenovirus and is highly communicable. The early symptoms may be much more impressive to the patient than to the physician. They are conjunctival and lid edema with mild hyperemia and only scanty discharge. There may be swelling and tenderness of the preauricular lymph nodes. The most important consideration is preventing the spread of the disease by carefully sterilizing ophthalmic instruments and warning the patient of the infectious nature of the process.

B. Other viral conjunctivitis.—This may have accompanying upper respiratory tract infection. The eye is injected and uncomfortable, and there may be some discharge. A Gram stain of this reveals monocytes. Although a topical decongestant such as naphazoline (Vasocon) may be administered, these disorders improve without therapy.

C. Bacterial conjunctivitis.—The patient has a conjunctival injection and copious mucopurulent discharge. He may give a history of the lids sticking together. Staining of the discharge reveals polymorphonuclear leukocytes and bacteria. The discharge should be cultured and broad-spectrum antibiotic drips administered such as bacitracin, neomycin, gentamicin, or sulfacetamide.

D. Herpes simplex keratitis. Patients generally complain of unilateral mild eye irritation, photophobia, and occasionally blurred vision. There may be corneal hypoesthesia. The most characteristic finding is irregular dendritic ulcers on the cornea that take the fluorescein stain. Topical corticosteroid therapy may result in corneal perforation. Ophthalmologic consultation should be sought for the patient with herpetic keratitis.

XI. Other

A. Acute anterior uveitis (iritis, iridocyclitis).—The patient usually experiences pain in the eye, blurred vision, and significant photophobia. The eye is red, with particular dilation of the vessels around the limbus. The pupil is miotic and may be irregular. Slit-lamp examination reveals flare and cells in the anterior chamber as well as cellular deposits on the endothelial surface of the cornea. Treatment consists of pupillary dilation and cycloplegia with 1% atropine drops and referral of the patient to an ophthalmologist for topical corticosteroid therapy.

B. Acute vitreous hemorrhage.—This may be traumatic or induced by systemic illness, especially diabetes and hypertension. The patient complains of visual loss or the presence of multiple "floaters" in the eye. The red reflex of the fundus is diminished, and the fundus is obscured. Treatment is bed rest with the head of the bed elevated 45 to 60 degrees to allow the blood to settle in the bottom of the vitreous.

C. Acute retinal detachment.—The patient complains of persistent flashing lights and a "curtain effect" obscuring a portion of the visual field. The detached portion appears gray with white folds in it, but the detachment may not be visible on direct ophthalmoscopy. A patient with suspect history or physical examination results should have an ophthalmologic consultation.

D. Hordeolum and chalazion.

1. A hordeolum (sty) is a staphylococcal abscess of a meibomian gland of the eyelid. It is a tender, erythematous lesion that may be accompanied by significant lid edema. Treatment is the application of hot compresses and the instillation of topical antibiotics four times daily.

2. A chalazion is a lipogranulomatous reaction in an obstructed meibomian gland. It is a nontender localized swelling of the lid. Treatment is hot compresses and referral for elective surgical excision.

23

Acquired Immunodeficiency Syndrome and Oncological and Hematologic Emergencies

I. Acquired Immunodeficiency Syndrome

A. Risk groups.—Only a small percentage of risk-group patients presenting with complaints felt to be acquired immunodeficiency syndrome (AIDS) related will be found to have AIDS or conditions related to human immunodeficiency virus (HIV) infection. The following groups are at risk of acquiring HIV:
   1. Homosexual/bisexual men.
   2. Intravenous drug users.
   3. Recipients of blood or blood products before 1985.

4. Sexual partners of members of other risk groups.
5. Infants of mothers infected with HIV.

B. Definitions.

1. AIDS.—HIV seropositivity and profound cellular immunodeficiency manifested in one or more of the following diseases:

a. Neoplasms.—Kaposi's sarcoma, brain lymphoma, HIV-positive non-Hodgkin's lymphoma.

b. Opportunistic infections.—*Pneumocystis carinii* pneumonia (PCP), central nervous system (CNS) toxoplasmosis, disseminated or esophageal candidiasis, *Cryptococcus* infection, 1 month of herpes simplex, disseminated cytomegalovirus (CMV), cryptosporidiosis with 1 month of diarrhea, disseminated atypical mycobacterial infection, HIV-positive disseminated tuberculosis or histoplasmosis, or HIV-positive bronchial candidiasis.

2. AIDS-related complex (ARC).—HIV seropositivity and persistent generalized lymphadenopathy in two or more noncontiguous noninguinal node groups for more than 3 months or at least two specific clinical and laboratory findings (see Section C).

C. Primary care problems in AIDS and ARC that require modification of the usual diagnostic approach.

1. Fever.

a. Fever is a common antecedent of AIDS and in the high-risk patient and requires fever of unknown origin workup.

b. The presence of clinical findings suggestive of HIV disease include folliculitis or facial seborrheic dermatitis, oral candidiasis, hairy leukoplakia of the tongue, and generalized lymphadenopathy.

c. Nonspecific laboratory findings are absolute lymphopenia, hyperglobulinemia, and cutaneous anergy.

    d. Persistent fever and sweats without these physical or laboratory findings in high-risk patients is an indication for HIV serology. A negative result makes the diagnosis of HIV infection much less likely.

    e. The presence of these clinical or laboratory findings in positive HIV testing necessitates an aggressive search for AIDS-related disease.

    f. The most common diagnostic presentation of AIDS is *P. carinii* pneumonia, and systemic symptoms usually dominate. Arterial blood gases (ABG), carbon monoxide diffusion, and gallium scanning may be abnormal despite normal chest x-ray findings.

    g. In patients with known AIDS, sustained or spiking fever is common. The workup should be initiated when the fever pattern changes or new systemic or localized symptoms develop (Table 23–1).

2. Diarrhea.—Patients with early HIV infection or AIDS frequently have diarrhea, and the workup includes several stool specimens for ova and parasites and cultures with staining for cryptosporidia. Sigmoidoscopy to inspect the mucosa and to obtain better specimens may be helpful (Table 23–2).

3. Headache.

    a. In high-risk patients presenting with a headache, the workup is routine because CNS disease as a primary presentation of AIDS is uncommon.

    b. In known AIDS patients, a new or increasing headache is a serious problem. A spinal tap, computed tomography (CT), and magnetic resonance imaging (MRI) are important diagnostic tools.

4. Lymphadenopathy.

    a. The most common HIV-related syndrome is generalized lymphadenopathy. It usually pre-

TABLE 23–1.
Fever in Patients With Acquired Immunodeficiency Syndrome*

Abnormality	Cause of Fever
Severe oral candidiasis	*Candida* esophagitis
Neurological deficits	Toxoplasmosis or cryptococcal meningitis
Exanthem	Disseminated herpes; disseminated cryptococcal disease or drug fever (especially trimethoprim-sulfamethoxazole)
Deteriorating visual acuity	Disseminated cytomegalovirus
Progressive anemia with or without liver function abnormalities	*Mycobacterium avium-intracellulare*
Increasing lymphadenopathy	Lymphoma or mycobacterial disease

*From Hollander H: Practical management of common AIDS-related medical problems. *West J Med* 1987; 146:237–240. Used by permission.

TABLE 23–2.
Causes of Diarrhea in Patients at Risk for Acquired Immunodeficiency Syndrome*

Proctitis	Herpes simplex
	Chlamydia
	Neisseria gonorrhoeae
	Nonspecific
Infectious enterocolitis	Bacterial–*Shigella, Salmonella, Campylobacter, Aeromonas*
	Parasitic–*Escherichia histolytica, Giardia lambia, Cryptosporidium, Isospora belli*
	Viral–cytomegalovirus
Inflammatory bowel disease	

*From Hollander H: Practical management of common AIDS-related medical problems. *West J Med* 1987; 146:237–240. Used by permission.

sents with minor symptomatology such as folliculitis, low-grade fever, or local discomfort. Secondary syphilis should be excluded.

b. New or progressive lymphadenopathy in AIDS patients suggests new complications such as an infection or a tumor. The most common are Kaposi's sarcoma, non-Hodgkin's lymphoma, and atypical mycobacterial infections. Fine-needle aspiration is useful; if it is nondiagnostic, an excisional lymph node biopsy may be necessary.

5. Oral lesions and dysphagia.

a. Pain or burning on swallowing may be due to viral or fungal infections in the HIV-positive patient without an AIDS diagnosis. KOH preparations, barium studies, and endoscopy are useful.

b. Kaposi's sarcoma can occur on the hard and soft palate without involvement elsewhere.

6. Cough.

a. This is a very common symptom, often accompanied by shortness of breath, fatigue, fever, and sweats.

b. The most common cause is PCP, followed by bacterial pneumonia.

c. The chest examination may be normal. ABG determinations and a chest x-ray are important for diagnosis. A Gram stain of the sputum is often not helpful, and special stains are needed.

D. Precautions for health workers.—The occupational risk is minimal, and adherence to Center for Disease Control (CDC) guidelines reduces the risk further.

1. Educate personnel to fully understand known facts about transmission. There is no evidence to support the transmission of AIDS by routine, casual contact.

2. Ensure that the personnel are healthy and without skin lesions or weeping dermatitis in the direct patient care setting. The environment snould al-

low workers to function with the least-possible distraction or hurry.

3. Strict needle, fluid, and soiled-object disposal policies must be followed, and only proficient venipuncturists should draw blood from high-risk patients.

4. For virtually all actual patient contact in the emergency department (ED), gloves should be worn and changed between patients. When blood or body fluid contact is anticipated, gowns and even masks and goggles are recommended.

5. Disposable resuscitation equipment should be strategically located throughout the department so that mouth-to-mouth ventilation can be avoided.

6. Reserve respiratory precautions (mask and physical isolation) for patients with known or suspected tuberculosis. The infection control department at each hospital should define its policy on the basis of the local epidemiology.

II. Oncological Emergencies

A. General considerations.

1. Emergencies in cancer patients present to the emergency physician in four major ways:
   a. A patient not known to have cancer presents with a life-threatening emergency.
   b. An emergency arises during the course of a patient's cancer therapy.
   c. An emergency arises in a terminal patient.
   d. The emergency is unrelated to the patient's cancer.

2. The event must be assessed in the context of the patient and the specific disease. The following questions should be answered if possible before initiating therapy:
   a. Is the emergency related to the patient's malignant disease?

b. What is the tumor cell type, stage, and present extent?

c. What surgery, radiation, and/or chemotherapy has the patient already had?

d. Does there remain an effective therapy likely to produce a good remission?

e. What is the realistic probability of cure or long-term control?

B. Neurological emergencies.—Treatment for the following conditions should be instituted within minutes to hours.

1. Cerebral herniation.

   a. Intracranial pressure (ICP).—ICP is a nonlinear function of brain, cerebrospinal fluid (CSF), and cerebral blood volume. A small increase in ICP may produce a sudden major deterioration in clinical condition. Similarly, a small reduction in ICP following therapy may significantly alleviate the patient's condition.

   b. Causes.
      (1) Primary or metastatic tumors.
      (2) Cerebral hemorrhage.
      (3) Subdural hematomas.
      (4) Brain abscess.
      (5) Acute hydrocephalus.
      (6) Radiation-induced brain necrosis.

   c. Presentation.
      (1) Headache (see Chapter 9).
      (2) Herniation syndromes (see Chapter 7).
      (3) Altered mental status (see Chapter 7).
      (4) Seizures, focal or generalized (see Chapter 11).
      (5) Focal neurological signs similar to stroke.

   d. Treatment.
      (1) Institute aggressive airway management. Consider pretreatment with lidocaine, 1 to 2 mg/kg intravenously (IV) if intubation is indicated to protect against a raised ICP.

(2) Initiate hyperventilation to reduce the Pa_{CO_2} to 25 to 30 mm Hg.

(3) Consider giving mannitol, 1 to 2 mg/kg IV.

(4) Consider dexamethasone, 20 to 100 mg IV: its onset of effect is slower than that of intubation or mannitol.

(5) Surgical decompression based on CT scan findings may be needed.

2. Seizures.

a. Causes.

(1) Seizures are common as a presenting symptom of neurological involvement in the cancer patient (20%).

(2) A seizure may be due to a primary tumor or from metastatic, metabolic, infectious, or vascular causes.

b. Treatment (see Chapter 11).

3. Spinal cord compression.—This condition requires prompt diagnosis and initiation of treatment to preserve neurological function, especially ambulation. It may be the presenting symptom of cancer or occur up to 20 years later.

a. Causes.

(1) Breast, lung, and prostate tumors and lymphoma are the most common causes.

b. Presentation.

(1) Local or radicular pain occurs in 90% of epidural metastases and precedes other symptoms by weeks or months.

(2) Mild pain is accentuated by percussion, mechanical or valsalva maneuvers, neck flexion, and straight leg raising.

(3) Weakness (75%).

(4) Sensory loss (50%).

(5) In cervical spine metastases, a classic presentation is unilateral high neck pain aggravated by turning, with radiation to the shoulder or occiput.

c. Diagnosis.

(1) X-rays are essential in any cancer patient

complaining of new, persistent, or worsening back or neck pain.

   (2) CT or MRI.

   (3) Myelography as indicated.

  d. Treatment.

   (1) It is important to obtain early consultation with an oncologist or radiation therapist and a neurosurgeon. Weakness can progress rapidly over hours.

   (2) Radiation is the mainstay of treatment. Early initiation thereof reduces ambulatory disability.

   (3) Surgery may be indicated in special circumstances: for tissue diagnosis, diagnostic confirmation to exclude an abscess, relapse in an area of prior radiation, failed radiation, and further clinical deterioration.

4. CNS infections.

  a. Causes.

   (1) Cancer patients are compromised hosts with impaired immune systems due to one or more of the following:

    a Underlying disease.

    b Steroid therapy.

    c Chemotherapy.

    d Splenectomy.

    e Radiation.

   (2) Most CNS infections occur in leukemia, lymphoma, or head and neck cancer. The latter patients are susceptible as a result of fistulas and invasion which allow organisms access to the CNS.

  b. Major types.

   (1) Meningitis.

    a Presentation.—Headache, fever, and an altered level of consciousness are common. Meningismus is uncommon. A diagnostic delay often occurs due to assigning fever to a systemic source, headache to metastases, and the altered mental status to a metabolic or toxic encephalopathy.

b Diagnosis.

  (i) Lumbar punctures should be done after checking coagulation studies including the platelet count. It may be necessary to replenish the coagulation system with fresh frozen plasma and platelets prior to the procedure as indicated. (See Section II, G, 5.)

  (ii) A CT scan should precede the lumbar puncture if there is any suggestion of a mass lesion.

c Treatment. (See Chapter 7, Section II, H.)

  (i) Combination therapy is preferred until the culture results are available. The choice of antibiotics is based on the underlying disease, the white blood cell (WBC) count, and the results of Gram staining (Table 23–3).

  (ii) Ampicillin, 2 gm IV every 4 hours should be added when *Listeria monocytogenes* is suspected.

  (iii) When gram-negative rods and neutropenia are present, initial therapy should include an aminoglycoside (loading dose, 2 mg/kg) plus a third-generation cephalosporin (cefotaxime, 2 gm IV every 4 hours) or a semisynthetic penicillin (carbenicillin, 400 to 500 mg/kg/day given every 4 hours).

(2) Brain abscess.—These usually present in the ED as a herniation syndrome. (See Chapter 7.)

TABLE 23-3.
Organisms Commonly Causing Meningitis in Different Neoplastic Diseases*

Primary Tumor	Organism	
	WBC >2,700/mm³	WBC <2,700/mm³
Lymphoma	*Listeria monocytogenes* *Diplococcus pneumoniae* *Cryptococcus neoformans*	Gram-negative rods
Leukemia		
Acute	—	Gram-negative rods, especially *Pseudomonas aeruginosa*
Chronic	*Cryptococcus neoformans*	
Head/spine	*Staphylococcus aureus* Gram-negative rods	
Others	*Listeria monocytogenes* *Diplococcus pneumoniae*	Gram-negative rods

*From Yarbo JW, Bornstein RS: *Oncologic Emergencies.* Philadelphia, Grune & Stratton, 1981. Used by permission.

       (3) Encephalitis.—This is very unusual, but difficult to diagnose. The CT scan shows cerebral edema, and the spinal tap shows pleocytosis and an elevated protein concentration without any organisms. Herpes zoster and *Toxoplasma gondii* are the most common causes. Patients should be admitted when the diagnosis cannot be excluded.

C. Vascular disorders.

   1. Causes.—For reasons not well understood, the common conditions of thromboembolic strokes from great-vessel atheroma and hypertensive intracerebral hemorrhage occur less frequently in the cancer population than in the general population. A poorly defined state of "hypercoagulability" in cancer patients produces three conditions of importance:

     a. Disseminated intravascular coagulation (DIC).—Agitation, lethargy, seizures, and stupor are common, as are focal deficits such as focal seizures, hemiparesis, aphasia, and cortical blindness. The neurological effects may be seen before laboratory results are abnormal.

     b. Marantic endocarditis.—Bronchiolar or adenocarcinoma of the lung are the most common primary source, and cerebral infarction is the most common cause of death in these patients. Suspect this diagnosis in patients with multiple strokelike events, other evidence of emboli, and negative blood cultures. Cardiac murmurs do occur in one third, but the echocardiogram rarely is helpful.

     c. Sagittal sinus thrombosis occurs with sinus compression or invasion by leukemic or solid-tumor infiltration of the dura or as a nonmetastatic remote effect of the cancer. It can present with acute neurological effects or a slow progression of obtundation. It is difficult to diagnose and may require high-resolution arteriography with a review of the venous as well as the arterial phases.

D. Toxic and metabolic abnormalities.

1. Causes.—Cancer patients are susceptible because the underlying disease can cause organ failure, electrolyte and nutritional disturbances, and drug reactions. Also, impaired liver function and retarded metabolism cause drug side effects.

2. Presentation.

a. Common presentations include acute or subacute changes in mental status, aberrant behavior, and confusion.

b. Even if fever or a headache is present, it is necessary to exclude a toxic or metabolic cause.

c. Consider hypoglycemia and an unintentional narcotic overdose as causes.

d. It is important to first rule out a mass lesion or infection and to check the levels of electrolytes, blood urea nitrogen (BUN), glucose, calcium, and ABGs and results of liver function tests (LFTs).

3. Treatment.—Administer IV glucose and naloxone both as a diagnostic and therapeutic measure. These patients usually require hospital admission.

4. Specific metabolic states.—Tumors and the treatment thereof are often complicated by metabolic abnormalities. The following are the most common:

a. Hypercalcemia (see Chapter 4).

b. Acute adrenal insufficiency (Addisonian crisis); see Chapter 7.

c. Syndrome of inappropriate synthesis of antidiuretic hormone (SIADH) (vasopressin).—ADH, stored in the posterior pituitary gland, is secreted in response to extracellular fluid (ECF) osmolality changes. Secretion increases as osmolality increases. Renal mechanisms then retain water, and the osmolality decreases. This syndrome (SIADH) results from continued ADH release, which causes continued water retention and dilutional hyponatremia. The usual feedback loop is not functional.

(1) Causes.

   a Ectopic ADH production, most common in oat cell carcinoma, primary and metastatic brain tumors, non–small-cell lung carcinoma, and rarely pancreatic carcinoma.

   b Chemotherapy.—The mechanism is unclear. It occurs with cyclophosphamide, vincristine sulphate, and vinblastine sulphate.

   c Following the administration of narcotics, antidepressants, and phenothiazines, commonly used drugs in cancer patients.

   d Pneumonia and meningitis occasionally manifest SIADH, and these infections are fairly common in cancer patients.

(2) Presentation.—This is primarily dependent on the rate of hyponatremia development. Moderate symptoms occur below 125 mEq/L, and below 115 mEq/L they are severe. Nausea, anorexia, and weakness are common early symptoms. Then confusion follows with vomiting, lethargy, and an altered mental status proceeding to stupor and coma.

(3) Diagnostic criteria.

   a Hyponatremia with no evidence of volume depletion and edema.

   b Normal thyroid, renal, and adrenal function.

   c No diuretic therapy.

   d Inappropriately high urine sodium concentration.

    e Decreased plasma osmolality when the urine sodium concentration is high.

  (4) Treatment.

    a Mild hyponatremia.—Water restriction of 500 to 750 mL/24 hr.

    b Severe hyponatremia, especially with seizures.—Rapid correction of hyponatremia with furosemide, 1 mg/kg IV, and a saline infusion to replace urine losses. Check electrolyte levels frequently, and replace them as needed. If necessary, 3% saline may be used. This often requires central venous monitoring. Correct the serum level to no more than halfway to normal over the first 8 hours.

E. Effects of radiation and chemotherapy.—Because of the increasing use of outpatient treatment for cancer patients, the emergency physician will be seeing more of this group.

  1. Radiation therapy.

    a. Irradiation of the pelvis and abdomen produces mild anorexia, vomiting, cramps, and loose stools. Treat with a low-residue diet. Occasionally these patients require opiate-type drugs to control the diarrhea. Sometimes it is necessary to stop treatment, and severe cases may require hospitalization.

    b. Persistent gastrointestinal (GI) problems suggest severe chronic toxicity, and effects include strictures, fistulas, and even obstruction. Perforation may occur.

    c. Hematuria, if mild, may respond to the removal of stimulants from the diet (tea, coffee, alcohol, and spices). Severe hematuria requires admission for Foley irrigation and cystoscopy.

    d. Acute radiation pneumonitis occurs 2 to 3 months after treatment, with the insidious onset of exertional dyspnea, low-grade fever, nonproductive cough, and progressive lung x-ray interstitial findings confined to lung treatment portals.

e. Restrictive lung disease occurs 9 to 12 months after treatment. It presents with pulmonary fibrosis.

f. A lobular or lobar pattern, a pleural effusion, or mediastinal lymphadenopathy are uncommonly due to radiation, and other causes, usually infectious, should be sought.

2. Chemotherapy.

a. GI toxicity.—This is very common with certain drugs. Treatment with antiemetics may require careful combinations of different drugs, and side effects may occur (Table 23–4).

b. Pulmonary toxicity (Table 23–5).—The difficulty is in differentiating drug toxicity from infection and tumor, and a biopsy may be required to make the diagnosis.

c. Cardiac toxicity.—The most common causes are anthracyclines (doxorubicin and dauno-

TABLE 23–4.
Commonly Used Antiemetic Medications

Phenothiazines
   Prochlorperazine (Compazine)
   Thiethylperazine malate (Torecan)
   Chlorpromazine (Thorazine)
Butyrophenones
   Haloperidol (Haldol)
   Droperidol (Inapsine)
Miscellaneous
   Metoclopramide hydrochloride (Reglan)
   Dexamethasone (Decadron)
   Trimethobenzamide hydrochloride (Tigan)

TABLE 23–5.
Chemotherapeutic Agents Causing Pulmonary Damage

Cytotoxic	Noncytotoxic
Busulfan (Myleran)	Methotrexate
Cyclophosphamide (Cytoxan)	Procarbazine hydrochloride
Bleomycin sulfate	Bleomycin sulfate
Nitrosoureas (carmustine, lomustine, semustine)	Cyclophosphamide
Chlorambucil (Leukeran)	
Mitomycin C	
Hydroxyurea	
Procarbazine hydrochloride	

rubicin) and cyclophosphamide. Anthracyclines produce dysrhythmias, conduction defects, and cardiomyopathy.

d. Neurotoxicity.—Virtually any deficit may occur, as may meningeal irritation after the intrathecal administration of drugs.

e. Allergic reactions.—These range from skin rashes, fevers, and chills to exfoliative dermatitis and frank anaphylaxis. Fevers respond to acetominophen and antihistamines. Anaphylaxis, though rare, may occur after prolonged exposure to certain specific drugs.

F. Cardiopulmonary conditions.

1. Cardiac.

   a. Dysrhythmias and cardiac failure do occur from the effects of antineoplastic drugs (see Section E, 2, c). Pericardial effusion and pulmonary embolism are more frequent, as are electrolyte disturbances.

   b. Superior vena caval obstruction presents with shortness of breath; cyanotic swelling of the face, neck, and shoulders; distended neck veins; cough; and pain. Emergency treatment may require cricothyrotomy. Immediate surgical and radiotherapy consultation are mandatory.

2. Pulmonary.

   a. Chemotherapy effect (see Section E, 2).

   b. Respiratory failure occasionally occurs unexpectedly in cancer patients who have received blood transfusions or undergone surgery.

   c. Life-threatening infections due to immunosuppression from chemotherapy or radiation therapy occur very rapidly.

      (1) Sepsis may present with fever or hypothermia.

      (2) Tachycardia and unexplained hypocapnia without radiological changes may be the first signs of respiratory failure. Early ag-

gressive treatment with antibiotics and intubation as indicated is essential.

(3) It is important to watch for a pneumothorax and bleeding disorders and to consider early biopsy for opportunistic infections.

G. Hematologic emergencies.

1. Erythrocytosis.—This condition is usually secondary, and the most common tumor is a hypernephroma. Hyperviscosity causes dizziness, headaches, angina, and transient ischemic attacks. The signs are retinal vein engorgement and facial redness. If the situation is urgent, phlebotomize 1 unit to reduce the red cell mass.

2. Leukocytosis.—In chronic granulomatous leukemia the count may be 100,000 cells/cm³, which produces leukostasis. This blastic crisis produces thrombosis, vasospasm, and hypoxia. Immediate chemotherapy is indicated.

3. Thrombosis and hemorrhage.—Solid tumors have a significant incidence of these events, up to 10%. Thromboembolic events occur with GI tract adenocarcinomas and tumors of the pancreas, ovary, and breast. Compensated DIC is common in these patients, with increased fibrinogen, fibrin, and platelets. When these levels fall, uncompensated DIC is occurring and requires urgent treatment. An immediate consultation with an oncologist or hematologist is mandatory.

4. Thrombocytosis.—Usually not problematic in cancer patients.

5. Thrombocytopenia.—These patients seldom bleed until the platelet level is below 25,000/cm³. Ruling out splenomegaly during the physical examination is important. If the condition is urgent, consider a platelet transfusion. One unit of random-donor platelets will raise the platelet count by 10,000/cm³. Give 4 to 6 units, and check the count after 1 hour.

H. Infections.
  1. Important predisposing factors.
     a. The malignancy itself and its effects.
     b. Surgery, chemotherapy, and radiation alter the anatomic barriers to infection.
     c. Radiation and chemotherapy alter the immune system and the inflammatory responses.
     d. Neutropenia is a very important single factor.
  2. Evaluation.
     a. Carefully examine the lungs and postauricular, perianal, axillary, and inguinal areas in addition to a complete physical examination.
     b. Prior to initiation of therapy, culture blood, urine, throat, and any area suggestive of infection for aerobic and anaerobic organisms and atypical pathogens. X-ray the chest and possibly the sinuses.
     c. Fever is very important. If present, it mandates a full workup, not nonspecific antipyretic therapy. If the temperature is above 101°F without a history of recent blood product administration, there is an 80% chance of infection if the patient has advanced malignancy and neutropenia.
  3. Treatment.—This may require an oncology and infectious disease consultation promptly, broad-spectrum multiple-agent antibiotics, and very close surveillance in a hospital.

III. Hematologic and Coagulation Emergencies

A. Hematologic emergencies.
  1. Emergent anemia.
     a. Causes.
        (1) Blood loss is the most common cause and presents with early signs of shock. Beware

of subtle signs in infants and the elderly, who may decompensate early.

(2) It is important to check the history for bleeding diathesis, drugs, and underlying diseases.

b. Evaluation.

(1) Examine the patient for bruising and petechiae, and look at the palate and conjunctivae. Perform a stool guaiac test, and check the urine for hematuria. Look for vaginal blood, and do a full pelvic and rectal examination.

(2) Type and crossmatch the blood; check the complete blood count (CBC) and smear, prothrombin time (PT) and partial thromboplastin time (PTT), electrolytes, glucose, creatinine; and save serum for later studies.

c. Treatment (see Chapter 1).

2. Red cell destruction anemias (Table 23–6).

a. Causes.—These occur rarely in emergency medicine but require immediate intervention.

(1) If hemolysis is suspected, immediately order a peripheral blood smear, a corrected reticulocyte count, a haptoglobin level, plasma-free and urine hemoglobin levels, a lactic dehydrogenase (LDH) level, fractionated bilirubin, and direct and indirect Coombs' tests.

(2) For a classification and common drugs causing hemolytic anemia, see Table 23–7.

(3) Sickle cell (SS) disease.—In the United States this is the most common type seen in the ED, although it is dependent on the population served. Sickle C disease and thalassemia also produce sickling.

a In SS trait, only one parent has an abnormal gene, and 50% of the hemoglobin is abnormal.

TABLE 23–6.
Classification of Hemolytic Anemias*

Intrinsic
  Enzyme defects
    Glucose-6-phosphate dehydrogenase deficiency
    Pyruvate kinase
  Membrane abnormality
    Spherocytosis
    Elliptostomatocytosis
    Paroxysmal nocturnal hemoglobinuria
    Spur cell anemia
  Hemoglobin abnormality
    Hemoglobinopathies
    Thalassemias (discussed with microcytic anemias)
    Unstable hemoglobin
    Hemoglobin M
Extrinsic
  Immunologic
    Alloantibodies
    Autoantibodies
  Mechanical
    Microangiopathic hemolytic anemia
    Cardiovascular such as prosthetic heart valve disease
  Environmental
    Drugs
    Toxins
    Infections
    Thermal
  Abnormal sequestrations as in hypersplenism

*From Rosen P, et al: *Emergency Medicine,* ed 2. St Louis, CV Mosby Co, 1988. Used by permission.

    b In SS disease, all the hemoglobin is abnormal because both parents contribute the abnormal gene.
    c The trait occurs in 10% of American blacks. It is rarely symptomatic, although

TABLE 23–7.
Drugs Associated With Hemolysis in G-6-PD Deficiency*

Analgesics and antipyretics: acetanilid, aspirin, phenacetin

Antimalarials: primaquine, quinacrine, quinine

Nitrofurans

Sulfa drugs: sulfamethoxazole, sulfacetamide

Sulfones

Miscellaneous:; napthalene, fava beans, methylene blue, phenhydrazine, nalidixic acid

*From Hamilton GS, in Rosen P, et al: *Emergency Medicine*. St Louis, CV Mosby Co, 1988, p 1635. Used by permission.

it can cause renal-concentrating problems, spontaneous hematuria, and at high altitude, splenic infarction.

d SS disease presents with severe abdominal and chronic bone pain, commonly in the back, ribs and long bones, and often is precipitated by cold, stress, and infection. It mimics embolism, infection, and colic (Table 23–8).

e SS disease patients have an increased susceptibility to infection, especially to *Pneumococcus, Salmonella, Staphylococcus,* and *Hemophilus.*

f If no infection is present, treatment is symptomatic and supportive: IV fluids, oxygen, and pain relief. Recent studies suggest that oral narcotics and fluids are better than parenteral fluids and drugs are because of psychological factors.

g Proper disposition and close supportive follow-up are crucial to the successful management of this disabling disease.

TABLE 23–8.
Organ Damage Seen in Hemoglobin Sickle Cell Disease*

Organ or System	Injury
Skin	Stasis ulcer
Central nervous system	Cerebrovascular accident
Eye	Retinal hemorrhage
Cardiac	Congestive heart failure
Pulmonary	Intrapulmonary shunting, embolism, infarct, infection
Vascular	Occlusive phenomenon at any site
Liver	Hepatic infarct, hepatitis secondary to transfusion
Gallbladder	Increased incidence of gallstones caused by bilirubin
Urinary	Hyposthenuria, hematuria
Genital	Decreased fertility, impotence, priapism
Skeletal	Bone infarcts, osteomyelitis, aseptic necrosis of the hip
Leukocytes	Relative immunodeficiency
Erythrocytes	Chronic hemolysis

*From Rosen P, et al: *Emergency Medicine,* ed 2. St Louis, CV Mosby Co, 1988. Used by permission.

B. Coagulation disorders.—The coagulation cascade is shown in Figure 23–1.
  1. Evaluation.
    a. The evaluation should record the type of bleeding, the site of bleeding, and its pattern. It is important to exclude metabolic diseases, malignancy, and infection. A review of family diseases, and prior transfusions is important.
    b. The useful laboratory tests include the CBC and peripheral smear, PT and PTT, platelet count, and bleeding time. Consider fibrinogen

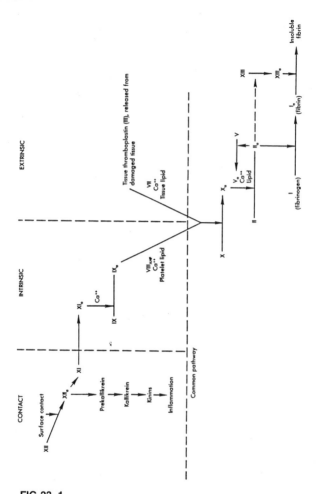

FIG 23–1.
Coagulation pathway. (From Rosen P, et al: *Emergency Medicine*. St Louis, CV Mosby Co, 1988, p 1648. Used by permission.)

levels, thrombin time, clot solubility, and factor levels. Also evaluate the need for selected tests of liver and renal function.

2. Specific disorders.

   a. Vascular disorders.—These are usually acquired (examples are scurvy, meningococcemia), and the effects are due to low platelet levels because of increased consumption or vascular damage.

   b. Platelet disorders.—Usually occurring in women, with mild to moderate bleeding. Epistaxis, menorrhagia, and GI loss are common. The bleeding time is prolonged, and the platelet count can be low, normal, or high.

   c. Thrombocytopenia.—This is usually due to drugs, myelophthisic disease, or alcohol.

   d. Coagulation pathway disorders.—These should be differentiated from platelet disorders by the following:

      (1) Usually they present as soft-tissue or intramuscular bleeds.

      (2) Congenital forms are usually in males.

      (3) Bleeding is usually delayed for 72 hours, although it can follow immediately after trauma or surgery.

      (4) Hematuria and hemarthrosis are more common.

      (5) The bleeding time is normal except in von Willebrand's disease.

      (6) Evaluation.—The PT and PTT are the basic tests for evaluation of these disorders.

         a If the PT is abnormal and the other test results are normal, there is an extrinsic pathway abnormality via factor VII deficiency. The most common causes are liver disease, coumarin use, and vitamin K deficiency.

         b If the PTT is abnormal and the other test results are normal, this represents the major portion of inherited clotting disorders. The factor VIII assay is most important. Two forms of factor VIII deficiency are as follows:

(i) Hemophilia A.—This has a normal factor VIII level but lacks proper clotting function. Most of these cases result from the sex-linked recessive form, while the remainder appear to be spontaneous. Factor VIII activity levels below 1% carry a

TABLE 23–9.
Sample Protocol for Cryoprecipitate Therapy*†

Obtaining cryoprecipitate
    One bag of cryoprecipitate equals 80 units of factor VIII
    Fill out the form as for blood (order in bags), and record the weight of the patient in pounds
    If patient's blood type is known to the blood center, no blood sample is needed. If the blood type is not known, a 10-mL red-topped tube is sent for typing
    If possible, ABO type-specific cryoprecipitate is used. Full crossmatching is not necessary
    After cryoprecipitate has been thawed and pooled, it has an expiration time of 4 hours and must be transfused within this time
Administration of cryoprecipitate
    Cryoprecipitate must be administered through a blood filter. If preferred, a platelet concentration infusion set may be used instead of the regular blood filter. This set allows for administration by an intravenous push
    The details for nursing and physician roles in administration may be detailed in this protocol

*From Rosen P, et al: *Emergency Medicine,* ed 2. St Louis, CV Mosby Co, 1988. Used by permission.
†Similar protocols may be made for the use of fresh frozen plasma or single-donor plasma.

TABLE 23–10.
Dosage of Factor VIII$_{AHF}$*

Bleeding Risk	Desired Factor VIII Level (%)	Initial Dose (units/kg)
Mild	5–10	12.5
Moderate	20–30	25
Severe	50 or greater	50

Standard calculation

1. Patients plasma volume (50 mL/kg × weight in kg) × (Desired level of factor VIII in percent) − (Present level of factor VIII in percent) = Number of units for initial dose
2. In emergency therapy, the present level of factor VIII is assumed to be zero
3. One unit is the activity of the coagulation factor present in 1 mL of normal human male plasma
4. Because the half-life of factor VIII is 8 to 12 hours, the desired level is maintained by giving half the initial dose every 8 to 12 hours
5. Cryoprecipitate is assumed to have 70 to 80 units of factor VIII per bag; factor VIII concentrates list the units per bottle on the label

*From Rosen P, et al: *Emergency Medicine,* ed 2. St Louis, CV Mosby Co, 1988. Used by permission.

high risk of spontaneous bleeding. Between 1% and 5%, the risk persists following trauma or surgery, and between 5% and 10% the spontaneous bleeding risk is small, although in trauma and surgery the risk still persists. The most common bleeding sites are in deep muscle, joints, the urinary tract, and

TABLE 23–11.
Laboratory Diagnosis of Disseminated Intravascular Coagulation*

Test	Finding	Pathophysiology
Peripheral smear	Low platelets, schistocytes, red blood cell fragments	Red blood cell fragmentation on fibrin strands; schistocytes not always seen
Platelet count	Low (usually <100,000/mm^3)	Consumed in clotting; lower numbers are reflected in bleeding time
Prothrombin time	Prolonged	Factors II and IV consumed
Partial thromboplastin time	Prolonged	Factors II, V, and VIII consumed
Thrombin time	Prolonged	Decrease in factor II and fibrin degradation products
Fibrinogen level	Low	Factor II consumed; may be difficult to interpret because this is an acute-phase reactant
Fibrin degradation products	Zero to large	Dependent on the amount of secondary fibrinolysis
Serum creatinine or urinalysis	May be abnormal	Functional assessment of organ most commonly injured by fibrin deposition

*From Rosen P, et al: *Emergency Medicine*, ed 2. St Louis, CV Mosby Co, 1988. Used by permission.

the CNS. For therapy see Tables 23–9 and 23–10. An allergy to cryoprecipitate may require diphenhydramine, 25 to 50 mg IV.

(ii) von Willebrand's disease.—The absence of a specific type of factor VIII activity affects platelet function. It is milder than hemophilia A is and usually presents with mucosal and cutaneous bleeding. Factor VIII (antihemophilic factor [AHF]) levels are in the 60% to 50% range. Treatment is with cryoprecipitate.

(iii) Hemophilia B (Christmas disease).—It is clinically indistinguishable from hemophilia A, but much rarer. It is diagnosed by a factor IX assay and treated with a special plasma prothrombin complex (Proplex) using a similar schedule to that for hemophilia A.

c If the PT and PTT are abnormal, this results from any deficiency of the common coagulation pathway. The most common cause is DIC, diagnosis of which is based on tests shown in Table 23–11. The treatment depends on whether hemorrhage or coagulation dominates the clinical picture.

(i) For hemorrhage, administer platelets, fresh frozen plasma, and blood.

(ii) For coagulation, i.e., fibrin deposition, consider heparin, although its effectiveness varies with the etiology. Prompt hematology consultation is mandatory.

24

Pediatric Emergencies

I. Evaluation of the Febrile Child

Serious illnesses in the child, especially in the young infant, are often characterized by an extremely abrupt onset that may have as the only sign the presence of fever. Important accompanying symptoms may be a refusal to eat, vomiting, unusual fussiness, or lethargy. If physical examination fails to reveal a focus of infection, the following approach is suggested.

   A. Newborn infants.
      1. Sepsis, meningitis, or urinary tract infection should be strongly suspected, and such infants should be admitted to the hospital.
      2. Appropriate diagnostic studies (including lumbar puncture, blood culture, chest x-ray film, urinalysis, and a complete blood cell count [CBC]) should be done and therapy instituted promptly.
      3. Specific clinical signs and symptoms are often absent in the infant under 3 months old.
      4. It is strongly recommended that the infant be admitted to the hospital for observation and/or a repeat spinal tap. Although the white blood cell count and the differential can be misleading in determining whether a fever is of bacterial or viral origin, the CBC may often aid in selecting further diagnostic studies.

B. Older infants and children under the age of 3.
   1. The inability to communicate symptoms, e.g., headache, earache, sore throat, or abdominal pain, is characteristic of children in this age group.
   2. If the physical examination has normal results but it is nevertheless thought that the child is severely ill, investigation should include the following:
      a. Chest x-ray film since auscultatory findings may be nondiagnostic even with bronchopneumonia.
      b. Microscopic examination of a clean voided urine sample.
      c. Microscopic examination, culture, and Gram stain of cerebral spinal fluid.
   3. Tepid water sponging is indicated for a temperature higher than 38.5°C. Acetaminophen (65 mg per year of age) is a useful treatment while the child is being evaluated.
C. Older children.—The older child with fever often is able to relate a specific complaint. While meticulous attention to the details of the history and physical examination is essential, diagnostic laboratory studies are less important in the older child. They should, however, be done as indicated.

II. Management of Specific Symptoms in Children

A. Dehydration.
   1. Dehydration, often with an accompanying electrolyte imbalance, may result from a variety of causes in previously well children, especially decreased fluid intake due to acute illness or gastrointestinal tract loss from vomiting or diarrhea.

2. Dehydration is defined as isotonic (serum sodium concentration, 130 to 150 mEq/L), hypotonic (serum sodium concentration less than 130 mEq/L), or hypertonic (serum sodium content more than 150 mEq/L). The type of dehydration is dependent on the source of the fluid and salt loss as well as the type of fluid used to replace the deficit.

3. Unless there is good evidence of excessive fluid intake or a high solute load that leads one to suspect either hypotonic or hypertonic dehydration, it is reasonable to assume initially that dehydration is isotonic.

4. The amount of fluid deficit in mild dehydration is approximately 30 to 50 mL/kg; for moderate dehydration, 50 to 100 mL/kg; and for severe dehydration, 100 to 150 mL/kg.

5. Start intravenous fluids in the most accessible vein, and obtain a blood sample to measure electrolyte levels and perform the other laboratory tests indicated.

6. Administer normal saline or lactated Ringer's solution, 20 mL/kg rapidly (30 to 60 minutes).

7. Replacement of fluid losses should then be begun, with half the calculated deficit infused in the first 8 hours. One-third or one-quarter normal saline should be used, with 15 to 20 mEq of potassium added to each liter if needed.

8. The sodium deficit in hyponatremic dehydration should be calculated by the following formula:

$$\text{mEq sodium deficit} = (135 \text{ mEq/L} - \text{Measured serum sodium}) \times 0.6 \times \text{kg weight}$$

The number 0.6 is the distribution coefficient for sodium. Normal or two-third–normal saline should be used.

9. In hypernatremic dehydration, the amount of

fluid administered should be calculated to reduce the serum sodium level to 145 mEq/L. The amount of free water necessary to do this may be calculated by the following formula:

Free water = (Measured serum sodium
− 145 mEq/L) × 4 mL × kg weight

The amount of free water necessary to lower the serum sodium concentration by 1 mEq is 4 mL/kg. It is essential that the sodium concentration not be reduced too precipitously because cerebral edema will result. Therefore, quarter-normal saline in 5% dextrose should be infused slowly, with an aim of returning the serum sodium level to 145 mEq/L over a period of approximately 48 hours.

10. Vital signs and urinary output should be monitored to determine the effectiveness of fluid replacement. Periodic serum electrolyte and arterial blood gas determinations should also be obtained.

B. Seizures.

1. Convulsions at the onset or during a febrile illness occur frequently in young (less than 2 or 3 years) children and may or may not indicate a central nervous system infection. If the temperature is higher than 38.5°C, it should lowered by the administration of acetaminophen, 65 mg per year of age every 4 hours, and by tepid water sponging.

2. A convulsion in an afebrile child can be due to a variety of causes, including the following.

   a. Metabolic disorders.
      (1) Electrolyte imbalance.
      (2) Hypoglycemia.
      (3) Hypocalcemia.

   b. Intoxication.
      (1) Lead.
      (2) Phenothiazine.

    c. Intracranial hemorrhage.
      (1) Vascular accidents.
      (2) Coagulation disturbances.
    d. Brain tumor.
    e. Cerebral defects.
    f. Degenerative diseases.
    g. Infection.
    h. Trauma.
    i. Idiopathic epilepsy.

3. Immediate management of the child during the convulsion consists of the following:

    a. Protecting with a mouth gag, suctioning secretions, and padding and restraining when necessary.

    b. Most seizures are brief and self-limiting. If major motor seizure activity persists, treatment with one of the following agents is warranted:

      (1) Diazepam, 0.2 to 0.3 mg/kg intravenously (IV) at a rate of 1 mg/min. The maximum dose for children under 2 is 4 mg; for older children, it is 10 mg.

      (2) Phenobarbital, 5 to 10 mg/kg IV or intramuscularly.

      (3) Paraldehyde, 1 to 1.5 mL per year of age deeply intramuscularly or 0.3 mg/kg via rectal tube to a maximum dose of 7 mL.

4. Further information regarding the control of seizures is given in Chapter 11. Febrile children with a history of febrile convulsions should be examined carefully and a lumbar puncture performed unless the cause of the fever is apparent.

5. As soon as the seizure is controlled or if the child is first seen in a postictal condition, a thorough history and physical examination are performed to determine the cause of the convulsion.

6. In addition to a lumbar puncture, consideration should be given to admitting the child with a

first convulsion to the hospital for diagnostic studies. The clinical appearance of the child, the results of examination and diagnostic tests, and the response to temperature-lowering measures should be used as guides for the necessity for hospitalization.

C. Croup and epiglottitis.

1. Croup in infants and children usually is due to a viral upper respiratory tract infection. Parainfluenza virus is a common cause. Children affected are usually younger than 2 years old. The onset of the disease is gradual, occurring over 1 to 8 days. Symptoms include a barking cough, hoarseness, and difficulty breathing. Children display a varying amount of respiratory distress. Muscular retraction and stridor are frequently present. There is no preferred body position. There is frequently fever but rarely a temperature higher than 39°C.

2. Treatment of croup.

a. Humidity.—Humidification of inspired air by face mask, croup tent, or simply hot water running in a room in which the child is kept is the mainstay of therapy.

b. Racemic epinephrine.—The use of this substance is controversial. Delivered by intermittent positive-pressure breathing or nebulizer, 0.5 mL of 2% racemic epinephrine may be beneficial. The treatment should last 15 minutes and the heart rate, rhythm, and blood pressure monitored during this time.

c. Corticosteroids.—The use of these agents is also controversial, but children who are ill enough to require hospitalization may benefit from their administration. Dexamethasone, 1 mg/kg for the initial dose, is recommended.

d. Croup can usually be managed on an outpatient basis, but children in severe respiratory distress should be admitted to the hospital.

For these severely ill individuals, endotracheal intubation or tracheostomy may be necessary.

3. Epiglottitis is a less common cause of stridor than is croup. The causative organism of this supraglottitic infection is usually *Haemophilus influenzae,* but streptococci or staphylococci may be involved. Children 2 to 6 years old are most commonly affected, but epiglottitis may involve any age group. The onset of illness is rapid, usually progressing over several hours. The child is usually acutely ill, with stridor, severe respiratory distress, high fever, and drooling. The upright position is preferred by the patient. A cough is not usually present. The child may be cyanotic.

4. Diagnosis of epiglottitis.
   a. The diagnosis should be made on the basis of the clinical picture. The oropharynx should not be examined because this may precipitate acute airway obstruction.
   b. A lateral x-ray of the neck may reveal enlargement of the epiglottis or narrowing of the airway. This study should not be done if the diagnosis is obvious on clinical grounds.
   c. Blood cultures are frequently positive for the causative organism.

5. Treatment of epiglottitis.
   a. No effort should be made to place the child supine or otherwise interfere with ventilation.
   b. Humidified oxygen should be applied, if tolerated.
   c. The child should be taken to the operating room where direct laryngoscopy and, if necessary, endotracheal intubation or tracheostomy will be carried out.
   d. Antibiotics may be administered parenterally, but they are not the mainstay of therapy. Am-

picillin, 50 mg/kg in divided doses, is recommended.

D. Asthma (for the treatment of adult asthma, see Chapter 25).—Mild to moderately severe wheezing frequently can be controlled with the following:

1. Aqueous epinephrine (1:1,000), 0.01 mL/kg per dose subcutaneously (maximum single dose not to exceed 0.5 mL). The onset of action is rapid, and the duration of action is approximately 20 minutes. Injection may be repeated every 15 to 20 minutes to a total of three doses. If this fails to terminate the attack, other medications will be necessary.

2. The concomitant administration of oral or IV fluids to liquify mucus is beneficial and is especially important if the child is dehydrated.

3. Isoetharine (Bronkosol) is a selective β_2-stimulator that is administered by inhalation. The dose is 0.5 mL in 1.5 mL of saline administered over 20 minutes. The treatment may be repeated every 2 to 4 hours.

4. If the patient needs further treatment, IV aminophylline should be administered. A loading dose of 5 to 6 mg/kg is given over a period of 15 to 20 minutes; this is followed by a maintenance drip of 1.1 mg/kg/hr. A full loading dose should not be administered to the child taking theophylline preparations. Determination of theophylline levels is useful in monitoring therapy.

5. If the aforementioned measures do not abate the attack, the patient should be admitted to the hospital.

6. If the asthmatic attack responds to treatment, the child may be discharged. Sustained-release epinephrine (Sus-Phrine), 0.005 ml/kg, should be administered subcutaneously.

E. Bronchiolitis.—This frequent manifestation of viral respiratory tract infection in infants under 2 is characterized by the following:

1. The rapid development of dyspnea, respiratory distress, prolongation of expiration with wheezing, and occasionally rales.
2. Small infants can rapidly develop severe respiratory distress with poor ventilatory exchange. Signs of hypoxia may be subtle and nonspecific: restlessness and apprehension.
3. X-rays may reveal hyperinflation.
4. Since differentiation from acute asthma may be difficult, a single dose of 1:1,000 epinephrine, 0.01 mL/kg, may be administered. (Refer to Section II, D,1.)
5. The course of illness is usually benign. Treatment consists of the administration of humidified oxygen and fluids. Specific supportive measures to ensure high humidity and adequate hydration are necessary. Hospitalization is recommended if respiratory distress is severe.
6. Indications for admission to the hospital include dehydration, severe respiratory distress with a respiratory rate faster than 60 per minute, and age under 6 months.

F. Cardiopulmonary arrest (See Chapter 3).
   1. Cardiac arrest in children is often due to disorders that are different from those that commonly cause cardiac arrest in adults. Disorders that cause childhood cardiac arrest are trauma, sudden infant death syndrome, drowning, upper airway obstruction, fluid and electrolyte deficits, congenital heart disease, sepsis, anoxia, and meningoencephalitis.
   2. External cardiac compression.
      a. Infant.—With two to three fingers positioned over the midsternum, compress the sternum ½ to 1 in. 100 times per minute.
      b. Child.—With the heel of one hand, compress the sternum 1 to 1½ in. 80 times per minute.
   3. Ventilation.
      a. Infant.—20 times per minute.
      b. Child.—15 times per minute.

4. Drug dosages.
    a. Sodium bicarbonate.—1 mEq/kg as an initial dose and half this dose every 10 minutes or as dictated by arterial pH.
    b. Epinephrine.—0.01 mL/kg (1:10,000, 1 mg in 10 mL). This may be repeated at 5-minute intervals as indicated.
    c. Atropine.—0.02 mg/kg, repeated as needed to a maximum of 1 mg.
    d. Calcium chloride.—25 mg/kg per dose.
    e. Calcium gluconate.—60 mg/kg per dose.
    f. Lidocaine bolus.—1 mg/kg per dose; maintenance, 30 μg/kg/min.
    g. Dopamine.—1 to 5 μg/kg/min, β-effect; 5 to 12 μg/kg/min, mixed effect; more than 15 μg/kg/min, effect.
    h. Norepinephrine.—Begin α = the infusion at 0.1 μg/kg/min.
    i. Isoproterenol.—Begin at 0.1 μg/kg/min to 1.5 μg/kg/min.

III. Diabetes

A. Hypoglycemic coma.
    1. Hypoglycemia in childhood can be caused by a variety of enzymatic deficiencies, endocrine disorders, and hyperinsulinemic states. In addition, malnutrition, malabsorption, poisoning with ethanol or salicylates, and Reye's syndrome may result in hypoglycemia.
    2. Children may have coma, seizures, apathy, or restlessness.
    3. After a blood sample is drawn to determine the glucose level, IV glucose should be administered. In neonates, 2 mL/kg 25% dextrose should be given, followed by an infusion of 10% dextrose. Older children should be given 50% dextrose, 1 mL/kg. This should also be followed by an IV drip of 10% dextrose.

B. Diabetic ketoacidosis.

1. Ketoacidosis may occur in a known diabetic or be the presenting syndrome in an undiagnosed one. Dehydration, hyperpnea, mental status alteration, vomiting, and abdominal pain are hallmarks. The serum glucose level is elevated, ketones are present in the blood, and both glucose and ketones are found in large concentrations in the urine.

2. Baseline laboratory studies should include urinalysis, and a determination of the levels of serum glucose, ketones, electrolytes, and arterial blood gases.

3. Treatment.

   a. Fluid replacement.—In moderate to severe cases of ketoacidosis, initial fluid replacement should consist of 20 mL/kg lactated Ringer's solution or normal saline for the first hour. This should be followed by the administration of half-normal saline for the next several hours at a rate consistent with the degree of dehydration. The potassium deficit is usually about 6 to 10 mEq/kg. Half of this should be replaced during the first day. No potassium replacement should be instituted until renal function is established.

   b. Insulin.—Regular insulin, 0.1 units/kg, should be given as an IV push, followed by a constant IV infusion of 0.1 units/kg/hr. A solution containing 5% dextrose should be administered when the serum glucose level falls below 300 mg/dL to prevent the development of iatrogenic hypoglycemia.

   c. Sodium bicarbonate.—For persons with profound acidosis (pH 7.1 or less or serum bicarbonate level less than 8), sodium bicarbonate, 2 mEq/kg, should be administered over a period of 1 to 2 hours. No bicarbonate should be given for more moderate acidosis because treatment with fluids and insulin will result in a return to a normal pH.

IV. Infectious Diseases

A. Meningitis.
   1. The classic signs and symptoms of meningitis are fever, headache, nuchal rigidity, Kernig's and Brudzinski's signs, and a bulging fontanelle. Any combination or none of these may be present, especially in the child younger than 6 months in whom lethargy, irritability, and poor feeding may be the only clues to the diagnosis.
   2. Bacteriology.
      a. Gram-negative organisms, especially *Escherichia coli* and streptococci, are the most common cause in the first 2 months of life.
      b. In older children, *Haemophilus influenzae, Meningococcus,* and *Pneumococcus* are the primary causes, with *H. influenzae* less frequently encountered after the age of 6.
   3. Lumbar puncture is the diagnosis procedure of choice and should be performed early in the workup of any patient in whom the diagnosis of meningitis is considered. Fluid should be evaluated for the following:
      a. White blood cell count and differential.
      b. Gram stain and bacterial culture.
      c. Protein.—Normal is 12 to 25 mg/dL.
      d. Glucose.—Normal is two thirds times the simultaneous serum glucose level.
   4. Treatment prior to bacterial identification.
      a. Less than 2 months.—Ampicillin, 200 mg/kg/day IV, and gentamicin, 7.5 mg/kg/day intramuscularly.
      b. Older than 2 months.—Aqueous crystalline penicillin, 300,000 units/kg/day IV and chloramphenicol, 100 mg/kg/day IV.

5. Treatment for specific bacterial pathogens.
   a. *Meningococcus* or *Pneumococcus.*—Aqueous crystalline penicillin, 300,000 units/kg/day IV.
   b. *H. influenzae.*—Ampicillin, 200 mg/kg/day, or chloramphenicol, 100 mg/kg/day, depending on sensitivity.
   c. *Staphylococcus.*—Methicillin, 100 mg/kg/day IV.

B. Pneumonia.
   1. Pneumonia may be particularly difficult to diagnose, especially in an infant in whom fever, respiratory distress, irritability, and poor feeding may be the primary findings.
   2. Subtle physical signs of flaring nasal alae, costal retractions, and tachypnea are often present but may be obscured by crying. Slightly diminished breath sounds may be the only finding.
   3. The older child is more likely to have physical findings of lobar consolidation.
   4. Causative organisms are frequently viruses. Bacterial pneumonias are frequently due to pneumococcus. *H. influenzae* is a common organism in children younger than 6 years old.
   5. Whenever possible, a sputum sample should be obtained for culture and Gram staining. Blood culture often contains bacterial pathogens.
   6. If pneumonia is present, hospitalization is indicated for the following:
      a. Infants less than 1 year of age.
      b. Any infant or child with severe respiratory distress or pleural effusion.
      c. Any child under the age of 3 years with a history of pneumonia.
      d. Any child with a predisposing illness such as sickle cell anemia, fibrocystic disease, diabetes mellitus, or immune system deficiency.
   7. Antibiotic therapy.
      a. Pneumococcus.—Penicillin V, 100 mg/kg/day

in divided doses, or penicillin G, 100,000 units/kg/day.

  b. *H. influenzae.*—Ampicillin, 100 mg/kg/day.

C. Tonsillitis and Pharyngitis.—These are among the most frequently encountered pediatric illnesses. An accurate diagnosis (viral vs. streptococcal) cannot be made on the basis of the clinical impression alone.

  1. Obtain a throat culture.

  2. Treat symptomatically with acetaminophen until the culture results are reported.

  3. If β-hemolytic *Streptococcus* (group A) is found, treat with the following:

    a. Benzathine penicillin, 600,000 units intramuscularly, for children who weigh less than 27 kg, 1,200,000 units for those who weigh more.

    b. Alternatively, phenoxymethyl penicillin (penicillin V) may be given, 50 mg/kg/day in four divided doses.

    c. In patients who are allergic to penicillin, erythromycin, 40 to 50 mg/kg in four divided doses daily for 10 days, is the drug of choice.

D. Otitis media.

  1. Otitis media is a common childhood infection. The distinction between purulent otitis and serous otitis media may be difficult.

  2. On examination, the tympanic membrane may be dull, thickened, or erythematous. The fluid-filled ear will not allow the tympanic membrane to move on pneumatic otoscopy.

  3. The causative organism is usually *Pneumococcus* or *H. influenzae,* the latter being more common in children younger than 6 years.

  4. Treatment should be a 10-day course of ampicillin, 50 mg/kg/day in divided doses. If the patient is allergic to penicillin, give erythromycin, 50 mg/kg/day, and sulfisoxazole, 100 mg/kg/day. In cases of known ampicillin-resistant *Haemophi-*

lus, cefaclor, 20 mg/kg/day in three divided doses, or trimethoprim-sulfamethoxazole, 8 mg/kg trimethoprim and 40 mg/kg sulfamethoxazole daily in two divided doses, should be used.

V. The Battered Child

A. During the past several years, there has been a growing appreciation of the problem of the physically abused child (the so-called battered child). Such children commonly are identified by the finding of multiple bone injuries on x-ray film in the absence of specific bone disease, a history of trauma, or multiple ecchymoses in the absence of a blood dyscrasia. There often is evidence of neglect.

B. The parents of such children have severe emotional problems that require professional help, and the children require protection while the family situation is assessed. The mortality and incidence of permanent physical and mental damage are high in physically abused children.

C. Children who are suspected of being physically abused should be hospitalized immediately and the case referred to the appropriate social service and legal agencies. In many states, such reporting is required by law.

D. When child abuse is suspected, a detailed physical examination should be undertaken to ascertain the presence of additional injury. Skeletal x-rays may reveal skull or long-bone fractures.

VI. The Pediatric Dosage of Drugs

See also section II,F.

A. Aminophylline.
1. Loading dose.—4 to 6 mg/kg IV over a period of 20 minutes.

      2. Maintenance dose.—1.1 mg/kg/hr IV.
B. Bretylium.—5 mg/kg IV up to a maximum of 30 mg/kg.
C. Diazepam.—Seizures, 0.2 mg/kg per dose IV up to a maximum of 10 mg.
D. Diazoxide (Hyperstat).—3 mg/kg.
E. Digoxin.
    1. Digitalization.
      a. Younger than 2 years.—60 µg/kg/day orally, 50 µg/kg/day IV.
      b. Older than 2 years.—40 µg/kg/day orally, 30 µg/kg/day IV.
      c. Administer half the digitalizing dose in the initial dose, and give the remainder in two divided doses.
    2. Maintenance.
      a. Oral: 12 µg/kg/day.
      b. IV.—10 µg/kg/day.
F. Furosemide (Lasix).—1 mg/kg per dose.
G. Glucose, 50%.—1 gm/kg.
H. Hydralazine (Apresoline).
    1. Oral.—0.25 mg/kg every 8 hours.
    2. IV.—0.3 mg/kg every 4 hours.
I. Methyldopa (Aldomet).—10 to 40 mg/kg/day IV in four divided doses.
J. Morphine 0.1 mg/kg/dose.
K. Naloxone (Narcan).—5 µg/kg IV.
L. Sodium nitroprusside.—1 to 8 µg/kg/min IV, titrated to effect.
M. Pancuronium (Pavulon).—0.05 to 0.1 mg/kg IV.
N. Phenobarbital.
    1. Loading dose.—5 to 10 mg/kg IV.
    2. Maintenance dose.—5 to 8 mg/kg/day to maintain a therapeutic level of approximately 20 µg/mL.
O. Phentolamine (Regitine).—0.1 mg/kg IV.
P. Phenylephrine (Neo-Synephrine).
    1. IV.—0.005 to 0.1 mg/kg.
    2. Intramuscular.—0.01 mg/kg.

    Q. Phenytoin (Dilantin).
        1. Loading dose.—10 mg/kg by IV drip.
        2. Maintenance dose.—5 to 8 mg/kg/day to maintain a therapeutic level of 10 to 20 µg/mL.
    R. Procainamide.
        1. Loading dose: 2–6 mg/kg IV.
        2. Maintenance dose: 20–80 mg/kg/min.
    S. Propranolol.—0.01 mg/kg over a period of 10 minutes.
    T. Succinylcholine.—1 mg/kg/IV.
    U. Verapamil 0.1–0.2 mg/dose IV.

VII. Surgical Conditions in Children

    A. Pyloric stenosis.—Characteristically, pyloric stenosis occurs at the age of 2 to 6 weeks in a firstborn male infant, and the vomiting is described as projectile. However, pyloric stenosis can occur in an infant from 1 week to several months of age and may occur in girls as well as boys. The initial vomiting may not be projectile, and the infant who has been weakened with prolonged vomiting and malnutrition may be too weak to vomit forcefully. Palpate the abdomen only when the infant is completely relaxed, preferably immediately after a vomiting episode. The pyloric mass is elusive and may be located anywhere from the midepigastrium to the right upper quadrant under the liver. If an experienced examiner cannot find the mass on repeated examination, x-ray films should be made with attention to the esophagus to detect chalasia or a sliding hiatus hernia, which may simulate pyloric stenosis. When the diagnosis of pyloric stenosis has been made, the stomach is emptied with a size 12 nasogastric tube. The tube is then left on gravity drainage. When the fluid and electrolyte status have been restored toward normal, the child may be examined for surgery.

B. Intussusception.—Intussusception occurs commonly in infants approximately 6 months of age. The mother will note that the child pulls his knees up to his abdomen, cries with pain, and then relaxes. These paroxysms occur 15 to 20 minutes apart, and the child may sleep in the interval. Vomiting is common, and a stool mixed with blood and mucus is often passed during the first 12 hours of illness. If the infant is seen prior to the development of abdominal distension, a sausage-shaped mass may be palpated in the abdomen. If upright films of the abdomen reveal air and fluid levels diagnostic of an intestinal obstruction, attention should be directed to the treatment of shock, replacement of fluids, and an early operation. On the other hand, if the abdomen is not distended or tender and if the child is seen during the first 24 hours, a barium enema should be given to reduce intussusception.

C. Incarcerated hernia.—Hernias are common in children under 1 year of age. They should be repaired when the diagnosis is made, provided the child is in good general condition. When a child is admitted with a swollen, tender scrotum in which the diagnosis could be an incarcerated hernia, sedate him and put him in the Trendelenburg position, but do not push on the scrotal mass. Insert a nasogastric tube and replace fluid and electrolytes if he has vomited. Surgical repair is performed if the hernia does not reduce spontaneously in 1 to 2 hours.

D. Torsion of the Testis.—Torsion of the testis is suspected when an infant cries out suddenly and is found to have a swollen testis. An operation must be performed within 6 hours if the testis is to be salvaged. At the time of the operation, the testis is untwisted and orchiopexy performed. This operation is also frequently necessary on the opposite side.

E. Gastrointestinal tract bleeding.

   1. In the newborn, small amounts of blood may be vomited or passed in the stool secondary to the ingestion of maternal blood or in hypoprothrombinemia. Close observation and gastric lavage are usually all that are indicated. Occasionally, transfusion is necessary. In older infants, anal fissures cause blood streaking in the stool. A history indicates the passage of a hard stool with crying. Place the infant in the prone position and retract the buttocks to see the fissure. Treatment consists of stool softeners, local application of soothing ointments, and reassurance to the parents.

   2. Bleeding from the duodenal ulcer will usually cease spontaneously in older children. However, if the duodenal ulcer accompanies another disease such as burns or central nervous system lesions, the bleeding may be more severe.

   3. A Meckel's diverticulum is suspected when no other source of lower intestinal tract bleeding is identified. Bleeding from a Meckel's diverticulum usually will stop spontaneously, but a transfusion may be needed. Resection on an elective basis may be required.

F. Appendicitis.—Appendicitis should always be considered in the child with abdominal pain. If the pain is at first vague and diffuse and then settles in the right lower quadrant, the diagnosis can almost be made by history alone. Anorexia, nausea, vomiting, and constipation are usually but not always present. If deep pressure in the left lower quadrant elicits right-sided pain and if there is persistent right lower quadrant tenderness, the diagnosis is ensured. A retrocecal appendix may simulate pyelonephritis, and the abdominal findings may be almost normal. Also, if the appendix is deep in the pelvis, the child will have only rectal tenderness. Repeated examination is the best diagnostic measure. Appendicitis in young children is a rapidly progressive disease that can go on to peritonitis and severe toxicity in a few hours. Many diseases cause abdominal pain in children that mimics acute appendicitis. The common offenders are acute pharyngitis with viral enteritis, mesenteric adenitis, and acute pyelonephritis. The diagnostic workup should include a CBC with differential, urinalysis, and x-ray of the abdomen. A rectal examination should always be done. If uncertainty exists, it is better to err on the side of an occasional unnecessary hospital admission than run the risk of missing the diagnosis completely.

G. Foreign bodies in the gastrointestinal tract.

1. Most swallowed objects are small enough to pass through without difficulty, but some stay in the esophagus or the stomach.

2. If a foreign body lodges in the esophagus, the child will hypersalivate and refuse to swallow. Metallic objects are seen on a plain roentgenogram, but others require a radiocontrast procedure to outline them. Esophagoscopic removal is indicated for all foreign objects in the esophagus when the child is afebrile and well hydrated. More than 90% of foreign bodies that reach the stomach go through the remainder of the intestine uneventfully. Children who have ingested such sharp objects as an open safety pin, needles, or a bobby pin need close observation and repeated roentgen examinations. If the object remains in one place for 5 days, particularly in the duodenal curve, suspect a perforation of the bowel wall. An operation to remove the object is then indicated.

25

Allergic Emergencies

I. Bronchial Asthma

A. Bronchial asthma is a disease of the airways that is manifested by diffuse narrowing of the tracheobronchial tree. This results in episodic attacks of dyspnea, cough, and wheezing, with intervening asymptomatic periods.

B. The following stimuli provoke asthmatic attacks:
1. Airborne allergens.
2. Air pollutants.
3. Drugs.—Aspirin and other nonsteroidal anti-inflammatory agents—indomethacin, phenylbutazone—provoke bronchospasm in susceptible individuals. Although these are usually adults with asthma, nasal polyps, and chronic sinusitis, persons without this triad may be likewise affected.
4. Emotional stress.
5. Exercise.
6. Respiratory tract infection, both viral and bacterial.

C. Clinical appearance.
1. The degree of respiratory distress varies.
2. Signs and symptoms are cough, wheezing, dyspnea, tachypnea, expiratory prolongation, thoracic hyperinflation, hyper-resonance, and the use

of accessory muscles of respiration in severe cases. Cyanosis is a very late sign.

3. The aforementioned may not apply to children younger than 2, who show neither the positional preferences nor the anxiety of older children or adults with asthma. The severely asthmatic infant of this age group can lie comfortably flat on his back and, even if cyanotic, will smile pleasantly when his attention is caught by a toy. Tachypnea is extremely pronounced in this age group, and respiratory rates of 60 to 80 per minute are not uncommon. Respiratory movement is entirely abdominal, and the chest, on auscultation, is often surprisingly quiet.

4. Wheezing is caused by turbulent air flow through narrowed airways. Therefore, severe dyspnea and a quiet chest suggest an ominous prognosis. Wheezing depends on the movement of air through a narrowed bronchiole; if ventilation becomes inadequate, wheezing will cease even though the patient's condition is more grave.

5. Following treatment, even when the patient is entirely asymptomatic and the physical examination results are normal, pulmonary function is likely to remain abnormal.

D. Laboratory studies.

1. Arterial blood gases.—These determinations are indicted in patients who are having a clinically severe attack or in those in whom the degree of respiratory distress is uncertain on clinical grounds. Typical blood gas measurements of asthmatics are listed in Table 25–1. Note that even in a mild attack, the P_{CO_2} is low, not normal. Hypocardia and respiratory alkalosis are the rule in mild attacks. A normal P_{CO_2} value in an asthmatic in respiratory distress is indicative of a severe attack and may be a sign that respiratory failure is impending.

2. Total eosinophil count.—In the adequately

TABLE 25–1.
Arterial Blood Gases During Acute Asthmatic Attack

Severity of Attack	pH	Po_2 (mm Hg)	Pco_2 (mm Hg)
Mild	7.45–7.50	75–90	30–35
Moderate	7.45–7.55	60–75	25–30
Severe	7.35–7.45	55–60	35–40
Very severe	<7.35	<55	>40

treated extrinsic asthmatic, the total eosinophil count is less than 50/mm^3. As the disease becomes more active, the total eosinophil count rises, and an elevated count may indicate the necessity for treatment with corticosteroids.

E. Treatment.
1. Oxygen.—Oxygen should be administered by nasal prongs. It should begin at low concentrations (2 L/min) and the flow rate adjusted in light of the arterial blood gas levels.
2. Hydration.—The hydration status of the patient should be assessed. If the patient is not overloaded with fluid, 100 to 250 mL of intravenous fluids should be administered per hour during the acute treatment phase.
3. Epinephrine.—Aqueous epinephrine (1:1,000) may be administered subcutaneously in a dose of 0.01 mg/kg (with a maximum of 0.5 mg) and may be repeated every 20 minutes to a total of three doses. Treatment with the drug should be avoided for patients older than 40 and used with caution in persons with hypertension or severe tachycardia. Alternatively, terbutaline, 0.25 mg, is administered subcutaneously and may be repeated in 30 minutes. When administered subcutaneously, terbutyline produces less tachycardia than does epinephrine.

4. Aminophylline.—For a rapid effect, this drug should be administered intravenously, with a loading dose of 5.6 mg/kg in 100 mL of saline given over a period of 15 to 20 minutes, followed by an intravenous maintenance dosage of 0.5 mg/kg/hr. The dosage should be adjusted as follows: if the patient is older than 50, the maintenance dosage should be reduced to 0.4 mg/kg/hr and to 0.2 mg/kg/hr in persons with liver disease or congestive heart failure. Patients who are smokers may require higher rates of infusion, up to 0.8 mg/kg/hr, because of enhanced metabolism. If the patient has been taking oral theophylline preparations, the loading dose should be reduced by half. If it is believed the patient has been taking full therapeutic doses (see Section I, H,1), the loading dose may be eliminated. Aminophylline may be administered orally or via rectal suppository in a loading dose of 7.5 mg/kg and a maintenance dosage of 7 mg/kg/6 hr. When the serum theophylline level is readily determined, it may be used to guide therapy. Levels of 10 to 20 mg/L are considered therapeutic. Levels less than 10 mg/L are ineffective in providing adequate bronchodilation, while those greater than 20 mg/L are associated with toxic effects.

5. Inhalation therapy.—Bronchodilating medications may be administered via nebulized inhalation or intermittent positive-pressure breathing (IPPB). These include isoetharine (Bronkosol), 0.5 to 1.0 mL in 1 mL of saline, and metaproterenol, 0.3 mL in 2.5 mL of saline. Inhalation treatment may be repeated in 2 hours as needed. Occasionally patients may not be aided by IPPB and may, in fact, be made worse.

6. Corticosteroids.—The effects of these drugs may not be seen for 6 hours after their administration. However, steroids do play a role in the treatment of severe acute asthma. They should be adminis-

tered early in the treatment period and other medications administered prior to the onset of steroid effects. They may be particularly useful in the patient with a severe attack who has previously taken steroids. A dose of 4 mg/kg of hydrocortisone or the equivalent (Table 25–2) should be administered and repeated every 4 hours as needed.

F. Cautions.

1. Sedation is rarely indicated.—Most sedatives tend to depress the respiratory center and are potentially dangerous.

2. Antihistamine drugs are contraindicated in adults with asthma. They are bronchoconstrictors, and some (e.g., diphenhydramine [Benadryl] or promethazine [Phenergan]) have anticholinergic side effects and tend to decrease the flow of bronchial secretion, which is undesirable.

3. Aspirin should not be given to patients with acute asthma until the nature of the asthma is clearly established (see Section I,B,3).

4. If the patient fails to respond to the aforementioned therapeutic measures, hospital admission and inpatient treatment should be considered and prolonged emergency department therapy avoided.

5. Progressive respiratory insufficiency that is unresponsive to medical therapy will require endotracheal intubation and ventilation with a volume-cycled mechanical ventilator. A rising Pco_2, especially in excess of 55 mm Hg, is an indication for such action. Positive end-expiratory pressure should not be used in the asthmatic patient.

G. Respiratory infection.—The asthmatic patient should be examined carefully for evidence of respiratory infection as a cause of the acute episode of bronchospasm. A chest x-ray to determine the presence of pneumonia should be ordered as indicated. The appearance of purulent sputum should call to mind the

TABLE 25–2.
Relative Potencies of Commonly Used Corticosteroids

Generic Name	Trade Name	
	Oral Preparations	Intravenous Preparations
Hydrocortisone	Cortef	Solu-Cortef
Prednisolone	Delta-Cortef	Metacortelone
Prednisone	Deltasone, Prednisone	—
Methylprednisolone	Medrol	Solu-Medrol
Paramethasone	Haldrone	—
Betamethasone	Celestone	Celestone
Dexamethasone	Decadron, Hexadrol	Decadron, Hexadrol
Fludrocortisone	Florinef	—

*Should not be used as a systemic anti-inflammatory agent due to its salt-retaining properties.

possibility of pneumonia or bronchitis. A specimen of sputum should be Gram stained and cultured. If there is no evidence for pneumonia but the patient is producing purulent sputum, he should be given a 7-day course of tetracycline or ampicillin, 250 mg four times a day.

H. Follow-up care.—After the acute episode of bronchospasm has been relieved, there is, unfortunately, a strong tendency for the symptoms to recur within the next 24 to 72 hours. Adequate symptomatic medication during this period will prevent repeat visits to the emergency department. Maintenance therapy should begin at the time of discharge from the emergency department. A follow-up visit with a physician should be arranged within the next few days. The following medications are useful:

1. Aminophylline orally, 200 to 400 mg every 6 hours or as indicated by serum levels.

2. Terbutaline orally, 5 mg three times a day.

Relative Anti-inflammatory Potency (Glucocorticoid Effect)	Relative Sodium-Retaining Potency (Mineralocorticoid Effect)	Equivalent Dose for Anti-inflammatory Effect (mg)
1	1	80
4	0.8	20–25
4	0.8	20–25
5	0.5	16–20
10	0	8–10
25	0	2–3
25	0	2–4
10	125	*

3. Isoetharine by inhalation, two puffs every 4 to 6 hours.

4. Metaproterenol by inhalation, two puffs every 4 to 6 hours, or orally, 20 mg four times a day.

5. Cromolyn by inhalation, 20-mg capsule four times a day. Cromolyn is a mast cell inhibitor that blocks the release of chemical mediators from mast cells. It is not a bronchodilator and is of no use in treating an asthmatic attack once it is in progress.

6. Steroids.—For the severe case or for the previously steroid-dependent patient, a 7- to 10-day tapering course of prednisone, 30 to 60 mg daily or the equivalent (see Table 25–2), may be indicated. The total eosinophil count may be used to guide therapy (see section I,D,2).

7. Beclomethasone by inhalation, two puffs four times daily. Beclomethasone is an inhalant steroid that has no significant systemic absorption.

II. Anaphylactic Shock

A. Anaphylactic (allergic) shock develops within minutes of the exposure of a susceptible individual to an antigen that is inhaled or injected parenterally. It may occur after a more prolonged period following the oral ingestion of medication or food allergens. Insect stings by the Hymenoptera are a common cause of anaphylaxis.

B. Signs and symptoms.—The symptoms and signs occur in various combinations involving mainly four systems:

1. Cardiovascular flushing and/or pallor; tachycardia; palpitations, hypotension, or complete circulatory collapse.

2. Respiratory dyspnea, with or without wheezing; cyanosis; cough; blood-tinged sputum.

3. Cutaneous urticaria and/or angioedema, itching, erythema.

4. Gastrointestinal abdominal cramps; nausea, vomiting, and diarrhea in various combinations. Symptoms might occur in rapid succession, and death is imminent unless immediate measures are taken.

C. Treatment.

1. Ensure an adequate airway and give artificial respiration until oxygen can be administered under positive pressure by face mask or endotracheal tube. If this is impossible due to laryngeal edema, consider an immediate cricothyrotomy.

2. Epinephrine.—This drug is the mainstay of anaphylaxis therapy, and 0.1 to 0.5 mL of a 1:1,000 solution should be injected subcutaneously, with the lower value used in young children. If the person is in shock, 1 to 5 mL of a 1:10,000 solution should be injected slowly intravenously or sublingually. The dose may be repeated in 30 minutes if necessary.

3. Apply a venous tourniquet proximal to the site of

the sting or injection. Leave it in place until the patient's condition is stabilized.

4. Find an adequate vein, and place as large an indwelling venous cannula as possible; if a vein cannot be found, perform central venipuncture by the subclavian or internal jugular routes, or cut down on a vein. Start an infusion of lactated Ringer's solution or normal saline.

5. Intravenous fluids.—Normal saline or lactated Ringer's solution should be administered for hypotension. Severe hypotension calls for the rapid infusion of fluid or the application of a military antishock trousers (MAST) suit. Therapy may be guided by a return toward normal blood pressure or a rise in the central venous pressure.

6. Aminophylline.—If bronchospasm is prominent, 5.6 mg/kg aminophylline should be administered intravenously over a period of 20 minutes and followed with a maintenance drip of 0.9 mg/kg/hr of aminophylline intravenously.

7. Vasopressors.—If shock cannot be overcome by the administration of fluids and epinephrine, vasopressors may be necessary. Levarterenol, 4 to 8 mg, or dopamine, 400 mg in 500 mL of 5% dextrose in water, is the drug of choice. The administration rate should be titrated against the blood pressure. Dopamine administration should be begun at a rate of 5 to 15 μg/kg/min and adjusted as necessary.

8. Antihistamines.—After an adequate response to the aforementioned measures, oral or parenteral antihistamines may be administered to relieve symptoms and prevent relapse. Anithistamines are *not* the medications of first choice. Diphenhydramine (Benadryl), 25 to 50 mg, or hydroxyzine (Atarax, Vistaril), 50 to 100 mg, should be given orally or intramuscularly.

9. Corticosteroids.—Hydrocortisone succinate (Solu-Cortef), 200 mg, should be administered intrave-

nously or the equivalent (see Table 25–2) administered to the patient who has a persistent bronchospasm or hypotension and repeated every 4 hours as long as it remains.

D. Follow-up care.

1. Patients with severe anaphylactic episodes should be admitted to the hospital, and those with milder forms should be observed for several hours prior to discharge.

2. Several days' course of antihistamines (diphenhydramine, 25 to 50 mg every 6 hours) or corticosteroids (prednisone, 30 to 60 mg daily) should be administered to prevent a relapse.

E. Radiographic contrast reactions.

1. Radiographic contrast material is used in arteriography, intravenous pyelography, computerized tomography, and other procedures.

2. There are three types of adverse reactions.

a. The vasomotor reaction is probably caused by the hypertonicity of the contrast material. It is not life-threatening and does not require treatment. Symptoms are flushing, warmth, paresthesia, nausea, and a metallic taste in the mouth.

b. The generalized or anaphylactoid reaction, although not a true immunologically mediated reaction, has similar findings, and the treatment is the same as for anaphylaxis (see Section II,C). The patient may display urticaria, wheezing, airway occlusion, vasodilation, hypotension, and tachycardia. The presence of tachycardia differentiates the anaphylactoid from the vagal reaction.

c. The vagal reaction is the result of profound discharge of the vagus nerve. The result is vasodilation, hypotension, and *bradycardia*. Treatment is the administration of intravenous fluids and atropine. Atropine should be given in initial doses of 0.6 to 0.8 mg intravenously to a maximum total of 3 mg. The pulse rate should be monitored to determine the response; it should be maintained above 60 beats per minute.

III. Urticaria and Angioedema

A. These conditions are not acute medical emergencies unless they accompany anaphylaxis or unless the edema involves the larynx where sudden obstruction to the airway can be fatal.
B. Treatment.
   1. Patients with impending airway obstruction should have an endotracheal tube inserted without delay.
   2. Antihistamines.—These medications should be administered to relieve symptoms and arrest the further development of lesions. Diphenhydramine (Benadryl), 25 to 50 mg, or hydroxyzine (Atarax, Vistaril), 50 to 100 mg, given intramuscularly will serve this end. These medications should be continued for 3 to 4 days to prevent a recurrence.
   3. Epinephrine.—In severe cases, 0.1 to 0.5 mg of a 1:1,000 solution of aqueous epinephrine may be administered subcutaneously, especially when laryngeal edema is suspected.

IV. Serum Sickness

A. This is a systemic allergic reaction consisting of an urticarial, petechial, or maculopapular rash accompanied by fever, myalgias, arthritis, edema, or peripheral neuropathy. Drugs are the most common allergens. A period of 5 to 14 days usually elapses between the administration of the drug and the onset of symptoms.

B. Treatment.—Since the condition usually develops slowly and is usually self-limited and rarely life-threatening, withdrawal of the inciting drug is usually adequate therapy. If symptoms are severe, a course of antihistamines or corticosteroids (see Section II,D,2) is in order.

26

Dermatologic Disorders

I. Atopic Dermatitis

A. Atopic dermatitis is a recurrent condition frequently associated with allergic diseases such as asthma and allergic rhinitis.

B. The skin is dry and lesions scaly, with itching and excoriations prominent.

C. Lichenification (hyperpigmentation, skin thickening, and accentuation of skin furrows) is typical of chronic involvement.

D. The course of the disorder typically involves remissions and exacerbations.

E. Treatment.—Dryness treated by the application of lubricating ointments such as Vaseline or 10% urea in Eucerin, antihistamines, and similar agents for reducing pruritis. Topical corticosteroids (Table 26–1) are the cornerstone of therapy, the ointment form being preferred. Use a fluorinated preparation when involvement is severe (but avoid the use of these on the face).

TABLE 26–1.
Medications Commonly Used in Treating Dermatologic Problems

Agent	Adult Dose	Pediatric Dose (mg/hg/day)
Antibiotics		
Dicloxacillin	125–250 mg q6h	12.5–25
Erythromycin estolate	250 mg q6h	30–50
Erythromycin ethylsuccinate	400 mg q6h or 800 mg q12h	30–50
Penicillin V	125–250 q6h	15–50
Tetracycline*	250–500 q6h	25–50†

Agent	Concentration	Applications/Day
Topical antifungal agents		
Clotrimazole (Lotrimin)	1%	2

Econazole (Spectazole)	1%	2
Nystatin (Mycostatin)	100,000 units/gm	2
Topical corticosteroids		
Betamethasone valerate (Valisone)	0.1%	1–3
Desonide (Tridesilon)	0.05%	2–4
Desoximetasone (Topicort)	0.25%	3–4
Fluocinolone acetonide‡ (Fluonid, Synalar)	0.025% & 0.1%	2–4
Fluocinonide‡ (Lidex)	0.05%	2–4
Triamcinolone acetonide (Aristocort, Kenalog)	0.025% & 0.1%	3–4

*Do not use in pregnant women.
†To be used in children over the age of 8 only.
‡Fluorinated agents.

II. Contact Dermatitis

A. Contact dermatitis is an inflammatory reaction of the skin to physical, chemical, or biologic agents, either irritant or allergic.

B. Treatment.
   1. Mild dermatitis.—Topical application of antipruritic lotions or cool compresses of Burow's solution.
   2. Moderate to severe dermatitis.—Administration of systemic corticosteroids. Oral prednisone, 60 mg/day for severe cases and 40 to 60 mg/day for moderately severe cases, should be administered, with tapering begun after 3 to 5 days. Therapy should be continued for 2 to 3 weeks.

III. Stasis Dermatitis

A. Stasis dermatitis is a dermatitis caused by a disturbance of normal venous blood flow. Changes may consist of inflammation, edema, pigmentation, and ulceration. Most commonly found on the skin of the lower part of the leg, usually just proximal to the medial malleolus, eruptions may be erythematous and oozing, chronic involvement resulting in scaling, discoloration, lichenification, and edema. Pigmentation is almost invariably present.

B. Treatment for acute inflammation.—The application of normal saline or Burow's solution compresses for 20 minutes every 3 to 4 hours is indicated. Corticosteroid creams may be alternated with wet dressings once the acute inflammatory stage subsides. Reduction of edema is important (diuretics, bed rest, and elevation of the extremity should be used).

IV. Drug Eruption

A. Drugs may cause virtually any type of dermatitis. Skin lesions may even appear after treatment with a drug has been discontinued if it or its metabolites persist in the system.

B. Treatment begins with discontinuation of therapy with the inciting agent. Itching can be controlled by the application of a drying antipruritic lotion such as calamine or the administration of antihistamines. If the condition is severe, systemic corticosteroid therapy should be instituted such as 40 to 60 mg of prednisone daily until improvement is noted, followed by tapering of the dose. This is most likely to be necessary for severe erythema multiforma, drug-induced toxic epidermal necrolysis, or vasculitis.

V. Erythema Multiforme

A. Definition.—An acute, usually self-limiting eruption precipitated by a variety of factors (most common factors are drug exposure and herpes simplex infection) and characterized by the sudden appearance of erythematous macules, papules, vesicles, or bullae.

B. Appearance.—The distribution is symmetrical most commonly on the palms, soles, backs of the hands or feet, and extensor surfaces of the extremities. The hallmark is the target lesion (a papule or vesicle that is surrounded by a zone of normal skin and then by a halo of erythema), commonly seen on the hand or wrist.

C. Stevens-Johnson syndrome.—A severe form is occasionally fatal and characterized by bullae, mucous membrane lesions, and multisystem involvement.

D. Management.—Search for an underlying cause.

Mild forms resolve spontaneously. Severe cases, including Stevens-Johnson syndrome, require hospital admission for intravenous hydration and systemic corticosteroid therapy (equivalent of 80 to 120 mg of prednisone daily).

VI. Febrile Illness With Rash

See Table 26–2.
- A. Gonococcal dermatitis.
    1. Appearance.—Lesions, often multiple with a predilection for periarticular regions of the distal extremities, begin as erythematous or hemorrhagic papules that evolve into pustules and vesicles with an erythematous halo and may have a gray or hemorrhagic center.
    2. Management.—Hospitalization is usually recommended.
    3. Treatment regimens.
        a. Aqueous crystalline penicillin G, 10,000,000 units intravenously per day for at least 3 days, followed by ampicillin, 500 mg four times daily, to complete at least 7 days of antibiotic treatment.
        b. Amoxicillin, 3.0 gm or ampicillin, 3.5 gm, each with 1 gm of probenecid, followed by 500 mg of ampicillin or amoxicillin four times daily for at least 7 days.
        c. Cefoxitin, 1.0 gm, or cefotaxime, 500 mg intravenously four times daily for 7 days, or ceftriaxone, 1 gm intravenously once a day for 7 days.
        d. Patients allergic to penicillin or cephalosporins.—Tetracycline, 500 mg four times daily, or doxycycline, 100 mg twice daily for 7 days. Tetracycline should not be administered to pregnant women.
- B. Hand-foot-and-mouth disease.—Coxsackievirus infection that produces a distinctive syndrome of

TABLE 26–2.
Features of Various Eruptions of Febrile Illness

Eruption	Area of Initial Involvement	Direction of Spread	Other Features
Hand-foot-and-mouth disease	Face or trunk	Extremities	Oral lesions
Measles	Forehead or neck	Trunk, extremities	Koplik's spots
Roseola	Trunk	Neck and extremities	High fever
Rubella	Face	Neck, trunk, and extremities	Lymphadenopathy
Scarlet fever	Chest	Head and extremities	Desquamation

stomatitis and exanthem involving the hands and feet. The rash is maculopapular, begins on the face or trunk, and spreads to the extremities. Oral lesions are bullae that evolve into erosions. All lesions are painful. Treatment is symptomatic.

C. Measles.—Measles (variola) has an onset with fever and malaise. Cough, coryza, and conjunctivitis begin within 24 hours. Koplik's spots (irregular small red spots with bluish white centers appearing on the buccal mucosa) are pathognomonic of the disease. Maculopapular erythematous lesions involve the forehead and upper part of the neck and spread to the trunk, arms, legs, and feet. Koplik's spots begin to disappear coincidentally with the appearance of the rash. Treatment of measles is symptomatic only.

D. Meningococcemia.

1. The severity varies from a mild illness to an acute, fulminant, sometimes fatal infection. Its onset is usually sudden, with fever, chills, myalgias, and arthralgias. A rash develops in three fourths of cases and initially consists of macular nonpruritic erythematous lesions that appear on the trunk or extremities, are 2 to 15 mm in diameter, and blanch on pressure. Petechiae may be present and may coalesce into large intracutaneous hemorrhages.

2. Early treatment is imperative. Penicillin G is the drug of choice. Adults should receive 24,000,000 units daily in divided intravenous doses and children, 250,000 units/kg/day. Chloramphenicol should be administered to patients with penicillin allergy.

3. Household contacts and medical personnel who have had close contact with the patient's secretions should receive treatment with rifampin, 300 mg twice daily for 4 days.

E. Roseola infantum.—A benign illness with a high fever, skin eruption, and a paucity of other physical findings, usually in children 6 months to 3 years of age. The fever typically has an abrupt onset and rises rapidly to 39 to 41°C. Lesions are pink macules or maculopapules 2 to 3 mm in diameter and blanch on pressure. The infant may not appear particularly ill despite the high fever. The cause of the illness is unknown, and the prognosis is excellent, although febrile convulsions may occur.

F. Rubella.—Rubella (German measles) is characterized by fever, skin eruption, and generalized lymphadenopathy. A day prodrome of headache, malaise, sore throat, coryza, and a low-grade fever antedates the rash, which appears on the face and spreads rapidly to the neck, trunk, and extremities. The appearance is pink to red maculopapules that disappear in 3 days. The most severe complication is fetal damage when the illness occurs during pregnancy.

G. Scarlet fever.

1. Caused by a group A β-hemolytic streptococcal infection, the illness has an abrupt onset with fever, chills, malaise, sore throat, and rash. This consists of a generalized papular eruption overlying a hyperemic base that may spare the perioral area. The skin has a rough "sandpaper" texture. There may be erythematous lesions or petechiae on the palate. Desquamation of the involved areas follows resolution. Late complications include rheumatic fever and acute glomerulonephritis.

2. Penicillin is the drug of choice. For children younger than 10 years old, use 600,000 units of benzathine penicillin and 600,000 units of aqueous procaine penicillin intramuscularly. For older children and adults, the dosage of benzathine penicillin is 900,000 units. Patients allergic to penicillin should receive erythromycin, 250 mg four times daily for 10 days. Aspirin should be avoided in these patients.

H. Varicella.—Varicella (chickenpox) begins with a low-grade fever, headache, and malaise. Skin lesions rapidly progress from macules to papules to vesicles to crusting. Vesicles are 2 to 3 mm in diameter and surrounded by an erythematous border. The hallmark of varicella is the appearance of lesions in all stages of development in one region of the body. The illness is self-limited, and treatment is symptomatic only. The disease is contagious until all vesicles are crusted and dried.

VII. Fungal Infection

The dermatophytoses ("ringworm") are fungal infections limited to the skin and are characterized by scaling and pruritis. They may involve the scalp, arms, legs, or trunk and classically produce a sharply marginated annular lesion with raised or vesicular margins and central clearing. Lesions should be scraped and examined under the microscope in a potassium hydroxide preparation. A number of effective topical antifungal preparations are available (including clotrimazole, haloprogin, miconazole, and tolnaftate), and these should be applied 2 to 3 times daily.

VIII. Herpes Virus Infection

A. Herpes Simplex.
1. There are two serotypes of herpes simplex virus (HSV) that cause cutaneous infection. HSV-1 affects predominantly nongenital sites (classically the mouth or lips). HSV-2 lesions appear mainly in the genital area. The hallmark is grouped vesicles on an erythematous base. Tender regional lymphadenopathy may be present. Children are more frequently affected with HSV-1 infection than are adults.
2. Genital lesions in the male usually appear on the penile shaft or glans or in the perianal re-

gion. In primary cases fever, malaise, and headache are common. Tender inguinal lymphadenopathy occurs in about half of the patients. During recurrences, constitutional symptoms are minimal or absent.

3. The infection is much more severe in the female and may involve the introitus, cervix, or vagina and produce severe pelvic pain, dysuria, vaginal discharge, or urinary retention. Hospitalization may be necessary.

4. Treatment of an initial episode of genital herpes is with acyclovir (Zovirax), 200 mg five times per day for 10 days. Such treatment does not prevent the development of recurrent lesions.

B. Herpes Zoster.

1. Herpes zoster (shingles) occurs exclusively in individuals who have previously had chickenpox and is caused by a reactivation of latent varicella-zoster virus present since the initial infection. Pain in a dermatomal distribution may precede the eruption by 1 to 10 days. The rash consists of grouped vesicles on an erythematous base that involves one or several thoracic, abdominal, or facial dermatomes. Although an association with Hodgkin's lymphoma and other malignancies is well known, the majority of cases occur in healthy individuals.

2. Treatment is largely symptomatic, including the administration of codeine-containing analgesics. The administration of acyclovir (see Section VIII, A) is favored by some. Pain that persists after the lesions have healed occurs more commonly in elderly and immunosuppressed patients, may last a number of months, and is often resistant to treatment with analgesic medications. Corticosteroids to treat this postherpetic neuralgia are controversial. Prednisone,

40 mg daily for 10 days with tapering, may be administered.

IX. Impetigo

A. A pustular eruption most commonly caused by group A streptococci, it begins as 1- to 2-mm vesicles with erythematous margins. When these break, they leave erosions covered with a golden-yellow crust. Postpyodermal glomerulonephritis is a recognized complication.

B. Bullous impetigo (a less common form) is caused by phage group 2 staphylococci. The initial skin lesions are thin-walled bullae 1 to 2 cm in size. When these rupture, they leave a thin serous crust.

C. Treatment of impetigo caused by streptococci should be with intramuscular benzathine penicillin (40,000 units/kg for children under 6 years of age and 1,200,000 units for older children and adults) or oral penicillin V (25 mg/kg/day for 10 days). Penicillin-allergic patients may be treated with erythromycin. Bullous impetigo should be treated with a penicillinase-resistant antibiotic such as dicloxacillin. Topical therapy should consist of soaking in warm water 3 to 4 times daily to remove the crusts, followed by the application of povidone-iodine (Betadine) or a topical antibiotic ointment.

X. Infestations

A. Pediculosis.—The diagnosis is made by the identification of louse eggs in the pubic hair. These attach to the bases of the hair shafts and appear as white dots. The patient usually presents with severe itching. Treatment should be with gamma benzene hexachloride (Kwell) shampoo.

B. Scabies.
   1. Scabies is characterized by severe itching that is usually worse at night. The areas of the body most commonly involved are the interdigital web spaces, wrists, axillae, buttocks, lower back, penis, scrotum, and breasts. Typical lesions are reddish papules or vesicles surrounded by an erythematous border. Secondary infection is common. Close personal contact is involved in transmission.
   2. Treatment forms are gamma benzene hexachloride (Kwell) and crotamiton (Eurax) lotion, cream, or shampoo. Clothing and bedding should be treated with boiling or hot water washing.

XI. Pemphigus Vulgaris

A. An uncommon but potentially fatal disorder of unknown cause, it is a bullous disease most common in men 40 to 60 years old. The typical skin lesions are small flaccid bullae that break easily and form superficial erosions. Any area of the body may be involved. Blisters may characteristically be extended or new bullae formed by applying firm tangential pressure to the intact epidermis.

B. Oral mucous membrane lesions typically antedate cutaneous lesions by several months.

C. Patients with suspected pemphigus should be hospitalized. Treatment with oral corticosteroids in doses of 100 to 300 mg of prednisone or the equivalent should be initiated.

XI. Syphilis

A. The chancre is the manifestation of primary syphilis. Chancres usually appear as single lesions, but they may be multiple. They usually appear on the genital mucous membranes. The chancre is characteristically a painless ulcer about 1 cm in diameter with a clean base and raised borders.

B. There are various cutaneous manifestations of secondary syphilis. Lesions may be erythematous or pink macules or papules, usually with a symmetrical, generalized distribution. Pigmented macules and papules classically appear on the palms and soles. Generalized lymphadenopathy accompanies the lesions.

C. The diagnosis of primary syphilis is made by the identification of spirochetes with darkfield microscopy. Serological tests for syphilis are invariably positive in secondary syphilis but may be negative in the primary stage.

D. Primary and secondary syphilis should be treated with benzathine penicillin, 2.4 million units by intramuscular injection. Patients with penicillin allergy should be treated with tetracycline, 500 mg four times daily for 15 days.

XII. Toxic Epidermal Necrolysis

A. There are two forms of toxic epidermal necrolysis (TEN). Both are characterized by the acute loosening of large sheets of epidermis from underlying dermis.

1. One is associated with *Staphylococcus aureus* infections (staphylococcal scalded skin syndrome [SSSS]) and is generally seen in children under 6 years old and has an excellent prognosis.

2. The other is related to the use of medications, infection, or medical illness or is idiopathic. It is associated with a substantial mortality.

3. The two conditions are distinguishable by skin biopsy.

B. Treatment of SSSS is with penicillinase-resistant

penicillins. Intravenous therapy is with nafcillin, 50 mg/kg daily. If the patient can take oral medications, cloxacillin, 50 mg/kg daily, may be administered.
C. Treatment of nonstaphylococcal TEN includes fluid replacement and the administration of systemic corticosteroids (prednisone in a dosage of 100 to 300 mg daily or its equivalent).

XIII. Urticaria

A. Urticaria appears as circumscribed raised wheals ("hives") that may be slightly erythematous or display central clearing.
B. Substances that can cause urticaria by contact with the skin include textiles, animal dander and saliva, plants, topical medications, chemicals, and cosmetics. Almost any drug may produce urticaria, with penicillin and aspirin being the most common. A variety of food allergies may also produce urticaria.
C. The treatment of urticaria involves removal of the inciting factor (when applicable) and the administration of antihistamines or other antipruritics. Hydroxyzine (Atarax, Vistaril) in a dose of 25 to 50 mg is recommended.

27

Environmental Trauma

I. Thermal Burns

A. General principles.
   1. Burn injuries range from relatively trivial to exceedingly complex.
   2. It is important to decide which patient requires hospitalization, what therapy can safely be instituted in the emergency department, and which patient requires initial procedures before being admitted to the inpatient service or transferred to a burn center.
   3. Rigid asepsis (cap, mask, gown, instruments, gloves, etc.) must be the rule in examining and treating the patient with a major thermal injury. Until some type of therapy is instituted, the wounds are open and subject to contamination.
   4. The history should include all details of the accident.
      a. Exact time and duration of contact.
      b. Exact place—closed or open space (greater chance of pulmonary injury in a closed space).
      c. Exact heat source—flame (often deep burn), hot water (less often full thickness), etc.
      d. Presence of noxious substances—gases, plastics, etc.

e. Possibility of associated injuries—explosion with shrapnel or glass, motor vehicle accident, etc.
5. The history should also include nonassociated but potentially crucial factors such as pre-existing diseases or medications.
6. A complete and thorough physical examination is mandatory. Special emphasis should be given to ruling out other injuries.
7. Tetanus prophylaxis should be given if indicated (Chapter 16).
B. Extent of injury.
1. A rough estimation of the extent and depth of the burn is helpful to determine whether the patient requires hospitalization and intravenous (IV) fluid therapy. Table 27–1 represents a standard technique for estimating the extent of the burn.

TABLE 27–1.
How to Estimate the Percentage of Burn

Area	Infant	Child	Adult
Head and neck	20	15	9
Arms			
Right	10	10	9
Left	10	10	9
Legs			
Right	10	15	18
Left	10	15	18
Trunk			
Front	20	20	18
Back	20	20	18
Perineum	—	—	1
Total	100	105	100

(Percentage spans Infant, Child, Adult columns)

2. The depth of the burn is often difficult to determine. Subsequent infection can convert a partial thickness wound to a full-thickness one.
3. Superficial burns usually heal with little if any permanent scarring.
   a. First-degree burns involve only the epidermis and are characterized by erythema.
   b. Second-degree burns involve the epidermis and some of the dermis. Blistering and superficial denudation are prominent.
4. Deep burns heal with permanent scarring.
   a. Deep second-degree burns involve most of the dermis. The burned skin may be inelastic and red.
   b. Third-degree burns are full thickness. All layers of skin are destroyed, and scarring is significant. The burned skin is tough, inelastic, and discolored (white or charred). It does not blanch and is anesthetic because blood vessels and nerves are destroyed.

C. Criteria for admission.
   1. If there is any doubt, admit the patient to the hospital. Critical cases should be transferred to a burn center, but only after several IV lines have been established and adequate fluid resuscitation begun.
   2. Outpatient care is appropriate for superficial burns that involve less than 15% of the body surface area in adults and 10% in children.
   3. Outpatient care of full-thickness burns less than 2% is reasonable. Patients with deep burns greater than 10% are usually admitted.
   4. Other factors that favor admission are extremes of age or involvement of the hands, feet, face, or perineum.
   5. Inhalation injuries and electric burns need careful evaluation for admission.

D. Minor Burns.
   1. Early immersion of the burned area in cool water

or the application of cold packs will relieve pain and decrease swelling. Ice should not be applied directly to the skin.

2. The burn should be gently cleaned and debrided of nonviable tissue such as the nonadherent epidermis of already ruptured blisters.

3. Intact blisters generally should not be debrided. Because they are likely to rupture, large tense bullae over joints may be considered for sterile aspiration.

4. First-degree burns can be treated with antibiotic cream. Bandaging is unnecessary.

5. Second-degree burns should be treated with an antibiotic cream and a closed dressing. One common regimen employs silver sulfadiazine cream applied to the burn, with antibiotic-impregnated gauze (Xeroform) over this. The wound should be inspected and the dressings completely changed at 1- to 2-day intervals. Ideally, the patient might apply the antibiotic cream several times a day, but this is often impractical in outpatient therapy.

E. Severe burns.

1. Airway maintenance is vital. Significant burns of the upper airway may require immediate intubation and perhaps eventual tracheostomy to prevent upper airway obstruction from secondary edema.

2. "Pulmonary burns" are thought to be due to chemical injury caused by the inhalation of toxic chemicals. Water vapor in the upper and lower airways usually cools the inhaled gases so that actual thermal injury to the lower airway (lungs) probably does not occur. (A possible exception is steam inhalation, which can cause thermal injury to at least the larger airways of the lung.) Inhalation injury is suggested by singed nasal hair, soot in the nose or mouth, perinasal and perioral burns, or rhonchi heard on auscultation of the

chest. Inhalation injury may lead to thermal injury to the upper airway or chemical injury to the lower airway, which may eventually cause adult respiratory distress syndrome (ARDS).

3. Escharotomy of the chest may be necessary if a dense third-degree eschar restricts ventilation (Fig 27–1).

4. Escharotomy of the extremities may occasionally be required to restore impeded arterial circulation.

5. The fluid requirements in a significantly burned patient are enormous. IV lines should be inserted

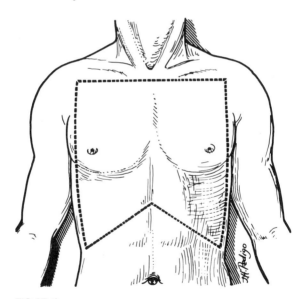

FIG 27–1.

Chest escharotomy.

early and resuscitation begun in the emergency department.

6. Formulas may be used to estimate fluid replacement. It must be emphasized that these are only rough guidelines and care must be individualized.

7. Recent evidence has demonstrated significant capillary permeability to colloid during the first 24 hours. Newer formulas therefore delay colloid replacement. The *Parkland (Baxter) formula* is recommended:

    a. First 24 hours—Crystalloid (lactated Ringer's solution) 4 cc/kg/percent burn. (Burns greater than 50% are considered 50%.)

    (1) Half the volume over the first 8 hours.

    (2) Half over the next 16 hours.

    b. Second 24 hours.

    (1) Five percent dextrose in water in quantities sufficient to maintain the urine output at greater than 30 cc/hr.

    (2) Colloid (plasma) as needed. This can be given in several ways:

    a 0.5 cc/kg/percent burn over the first 8 hours, or

    b 500-cc aliquots as needed to maintain urine.

8. Inpatient wound care involves topical antibiotics and periodic debridement.

9. If the patient must be transferred to a burn center, adequate IV fluid resuscitation should be initiated prior to transfer.

II. Electric Shock

A. Injury can result from several mechanisms:

1. Passage of electric current.

2. Electrothermal heat conduction.

3. Massive tetany of the musculature that leads to bone fractures.

4. Myonecrosis and myoglobinuria from the afore-mentioned mechanisms.

5. Ventricular fibrillation or asystole from current passing through the heart.

6. Asystole secondary to apnea (due to suppression of the cerebral respiratory center from a current traversing the brain).

B. The skin burn can appear deceptively minor, with massive necrosis of deeper structures initially not apparent. Therefore, burn patients with all but the most minor electric burns should be admitted to the hospital.

C. The skin burn is treated like any thermal burn.

D. Underlying injuries must be discovered and treated.

E. If myonecrosis is suspected, the urine should be alkalinized and its volume maintained to reduce the chance of myoglobinuric renal failure. Osmotic diuretics may be helpful.

F. Lightning causes an electric burn that may produce massive injury or surprisingly little damage.

1. Because the duration of lightning current is exceedingly brief, lightning often "flashes over" the victim and causes extensive skin damage but relatively little internal injury. Common internal targets, however, are tympanic membranes, eyes, heart, and brain.

2. Lightning causes death by halting cardiac and brain activity, which leads to cardiac and respiratory arrest. Surprisingly, only one in four patients struck by lightning is killed.

3. Skin burns from lightning are treated like other electric or thermal burns.

4. Underlying injuries should be ruled out.

III. Hyperthermic States

A. Hyperthermic disease entities fall into three categories: heat cramps, heat exhaustion, and heat stroke.

B. Heat cramps are spasm of the voluntary musculature due to the depletion of electrolytes.
   1. Both salt and water are lost in sweat. The patient with heat cramps has usually replaced the water loss by drinking but has not replaced the salt loss.
   2. Treatment.
      a. Place the patient in a cool place.
      b. Replace NaCl orally with high–salt content drinks or IV with normal saline.
C. Heat exhaustion is a loss of both salt and water; either loss may predominate.
   1. Symptoms include headache, nausea, dizziness, and visual disturbance.
   2. The patient may be febrile to 102°F but does exhibit sweating.
   3. Use laboratory values to guide the replacement of salt with isotonic fluids, or water with hypotonic fluids.
   4. Cool the patient as needed by exposure, fanning, and other methods.
D. Heat stroke is severe hyperthermia (above 41°C or 106°F) with a loss of heat regulation.
   1. Symptoms include confusion, coma, and seizures.
   2. Fatigue of hypothalamic and/or sweat gland regulation leads to loss of heat dissipation because *the person does not sweat*. Thus, the skin is warm and dry.
   3. Fluid and salt loss is not usually severe.
   4. Complications may include hyperthermic damage to the brain, liver, kidney, heart, and other tissues.
   5. The treatment is to lower the body temperature rapidly.
      a. Ice packs should be applied to the skin, especially to the axilla, groin, and scalp. Cold water should be splashed on the skin and then evaporated by fanning. A cooling blanket may be helpful.
      b. Cold fluid enemas, gastric lavage, and perito-

neal dialysis, have all been used but are probably of limited effectiveness.

   c. Immersion in a cold water bath is generally impractical and interferes with proper monitoring and care.

   d. Massage may increase vasodilation and heat exchange.

   e. Shivering must be avoided because it will raise the body temperature. Chlorpromazine may also be used to control shivering (50 mg IV) but may cause hypotension.

   f. Complications may follow, including rhabdomyolysis and myoglobinuria or disseminated intravascular coagulation.

   g. Discontinue active cooling measures when the core temperature falls to 101 to 102°F.

IV. Hypothermic States

A. Cold injury may be localized to a peripheral area as in frostbite, or it may be generalized as in hypothermia.

B. Frostbite.

   1. Symptoms include numbness, tingling, pain, and burning, which are particularly apparent with rewarming.

   2. Examination reveals discoloration, with eventual blistering in severe cases.

   3. Treatment consists of rapid rewarming in an agitated water bath at 104 to 108°F (40 to 42°C).

   4. It is absolutely crucial to avoid refreezing. If there is any danger of this, it is better to postpone rewarming until a suitable environment can be reached.

   5. Wounds should be treated open, with initial debridement of only previously ruptured blisters. Frostbitten tissue is quite fragile and must be handled with great care. Massage is contraindicated.

Frostbitten toes and fingers should be gently separated with sterile cotton.

6. Tetanus prophylaxis should be given if indicated (Chapter 16).

7. Unless there is infection, extremities with dry gangrene should be allowed to demarcate and spontaneously autoamputate.

8. In-hospital treatment may include vasodilating medication.

C. Hypothermia.

1. Symptoms include progressive shivering, loss of fine motor control, confusion, and coma.

2. Complications can involve dysrhythmias, electrolyte disturbances, pulmonary edema, and paradoxical vasodilation and shock on rewarming.

3. The electrocardiogram (ECG) may show J or Osborne waves, a notching at the end of the QRS segment that is pathognomic of hypothermia (Fig 27–2).

4. Treatment consists of controlled rewarming of the central core.

   a. Active rewarming of the extremities should be avoided to conserve vasoconstriction until the core temperature is raised.

   b. Rapid warming can cause sudden shifts in electrolyte balance and should be avoided (as opposed to frostbite, for which rapid warming is indicated).

   c. In mild cases, warmed or electric blankets, heated inspired O_2, and warmed IV solutions may suffice.

   d. In severe hypothermia, additional modalities may include gastric lavage, enemas with warm fluid, or peritoneal lavage with isotonic peritoneal dialysate (previously heated through a blood-warming coil to 100°F) at a rate of 2 L every 20 to 30 minutes.

   e. A rectal temperature probe is essential for severe cases.

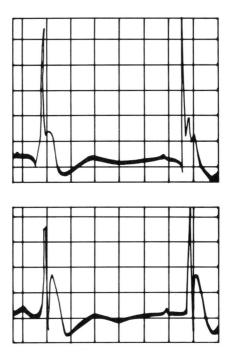

FIG 27–2.
J or Osborne wave in hypothermia.

    f. After the rectal temperature has reached 86°F (30°C), rewarming should be slowed to a rate not exceeding 2°F (1°C) per hour. A warm-water bath or hydraulic water pad can be used.

    g. Dysrhythmias and electrolyte disturbances may occur during rewarming and should be treated as necessary. Ventricular fibrillation or asystole may be refractory to the usual regimens. In such cases, emergency thoracotomy and direct warming of the heart in warm saline may allow successful conversion to a viable rhythm.

h. Severely hypothermic patients may appear dead, with cardiac output and respiration so minimal that blood pressure, pulse, and even heart sounds may not be detected. Because of hypothermic suppression of metabolism, however, many such patients actually recover with little residual deficit. There is wisdon in the old axiom that hypothermic patients should not be considered dead until they are *warm* and dead.

i. The apparently dead hypothermic victim may thus be alive. The cold heart is extremely susceptible to fibrillation due to mechanical irritation. It is therefore often recommended that cardiopulmonary resuscitation (CPR) not be used in such patients unless cardiac monitoring reveals ventriculor fibrillation or true asystole.

V. Decompression Illness (Barotrauma)

A. A rapid decrease in atmospheric or water pressure can lead to inert gases (principally nitrogen) vaporizing out of solution in various parts of the body.

B. Any decrease in ambient pressure can cause decompression illness, including rapid ascent while scuba diving, high-altitude flying with inadequate cabin pressure, or excessively rapid ascent in tunnel workers (caisson disease).

C. Damage may occur in any organ, particularly the lungs, brain, spinal cord, skin, and heart.

1. Nitrogen bubbles may form in the blood and lead to vascular occlusion of any organ.

    2. Nitrogen expanding from the dissolved to the gaseous phase may distend cells sufficiently to cause cellular rupture. Fat cells are particularly liable to such damage, which leads to the release of fat into the blood and a subsequent fat embolus to the pulmonary circulation.

    3. A similar process may disrupt lung cells and lead to pneumothorax or a systemic arterial air embolus.

D. Symptoms and signs will depend on the organ affected and may range from pruritus and joint pain (bends) to paralysis and death.

E. Treatment consists of repressurization in a hyperbaric chamber.

    1. Care should be taken not to decompress the patient even further during transport. If air evacuation is necessary, the flight should involve low altitudes in a pressurized aircraft.

    2. The patient should be kept at total rest and given high-flow oxygen at 100%.

    3. The left lateral decubitus, head-down position will reduce the chance of gas bubbles blocking blood flow through the heart.

    4. Specific measures may be required, for example, treatment of dysrhythmias or pneumothorax.

28
Anesthesia

I. Regional Anesthesia

A. Local infiltration block.
   1. For superficial cuts that need approximation and debridement, this form of anesthesia is the most practical and readily available. The approach is either from within the wound by injecting the local anesthetic centrifugally into the tissues or outside the wound by infiltrating just lateral to the wound edges.
   2. Drug of choice.
      a. A 0.5% or 1% lidocaine (Xylocaine) solution is recommended. Lidocaine diffuses through tissues and tissue planes quickly, and a small amount of epinephrine (1:200,000) might be needed to retain the drug longer in the operative site. Epinephrine should not be used for anesthesia in the area of the end arteries, i.e., fingers, toes, nose, ears, and penis.
      b. Mepivacaine (Carbocaine), 0.5%, does not diffuse as rapidly as lidocaine and may be more useful for longer procedures.
      c. If an operating time of several hours is anticipated, a 0.25% solution of bupivacaine (Marcaine) may be used. The maximum dose is 200 mg.

3. Procedure for infiltrating around a wound.
   a. Raise a small skin wheal by injecting anesthetic into the dermis with a ½-in. or a 25- or 27-gauge needle.
   b. After a short wait, insert the needle through the wheal and inject the anesthetic.
   c. Insert the needle to its full length, and then inject the drug as the needle is withdrawn.
   d. Repeat this step until the entire area has been injected.
   e. Wait until the anesthetic takes effect. This requires 5 to 15 minutes following the injection.
   f. Observe the guidelines for the maximum dose administered. For lidocaine and mepivacaine, the recommended maximum dose is 6 to 10 mg/kg. No more than 500 mg (100 mL of a 0.5% solution or 50 mL of 1.0%) should be administered regardless of the weight of the patient.
4. Sedating the patient may be necessary (see Section III). It may also be helpful to apply a gauze pad soaked in 4% lidocaine (Xylocaine) to the wound prior to local anesthetic infiltration.

B. Regional nerve blocks.
   1. Head and neck.
      a. Trigeminal nerve and its branches.
         (1) For these blocks, 2 to 4 mL of 2% lidocaine or mepivacaine with or without epinephrine is indicated.
         (2) Mandibular nerve.
            a Distribution.—The block provides anesthesia to the anterior two thirds of the tongue, the temporal and mandibular regions of the face, the lower lip, and the lower teeth and gums (Fig 28–1,b).
            b Landmarks.—Intraoral injection of anesthetic is just medial to the mandibular ramus about 1 cm posterior to the third molar. Paresthesias of the tongue or lower jaw are frequent.

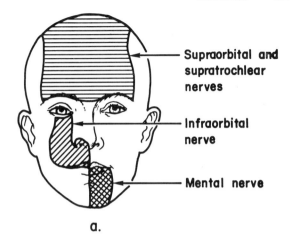

Supraorbital and supratrochlear nerves

Infraorbital nerve

Mental nerve

a.

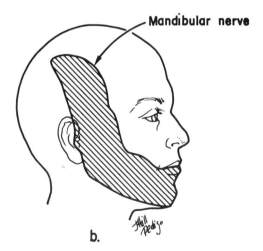

Mandibular nerve

b.

FIG 28–1.
Sensory area distribution of branches of the trigeminal nerve.

(3) Mental nerve.

   a Distribution.—The block provides anesthesia to the chin, lower lip, and gums (Fig 28–1,a).

   b Intraoral landmarks.—Injection is at the junction of the buccal surface of the lower lip and gum at the level of the second bicuspid tooth.

   c Extraoral landmarks.—Injection is percutaneous at the level of the second bicuspid, about 1 cm above the inferior mandibular border and 2.5 cm from the midline.

(4) Infraorbital nerve.

   a Distribution.—The block provides anesthesia to the upper lip, the side of the nose, the medial portion of the cheek, and the lower eyelid (Fig 28–1,a).

   b Intraoral landmarks.—Injection is at the border of the upper gum with the buccal mucosa of the upper lip at the level of the canine tooth. The needle is advanced to about 1 cm inferior to the lower orbital rim.

   c Extraoral landmarks.—Injection is about 1 cm inferior to the infraorbital rim at its midline.

(5) Supraorbital and supratrochlear nerves.

   a Distribution.—The block of the branches of these nerves provides anesthesia to the forehead and the anterior half of the scalp (Fig 28–1,a).

   b Landmarks.—Injection is across the forehead and the bridge of the nose from one lateral eyebrow border to the other.

(6) Superficial cervical plexus.

   a The superficial cervical plexus is accessible at the posterior margin of the sternocleidomastoid muscle midway between the origin and the insertion.

        b Injection of 10 to 15 mL of a 1.0% or 1.5% local anesthetic will provide anesthesia for skin, muscle, and subcutaneous tissues of the front of the neck and the anterior aspect of the chest almost down to the nipple line.

    (7) Great auricular nerve.

        a This nerve supplies sensation to most of the ear.

        b It may be blocked by the infiltration of 1 to 2 mL of local anesthetic at multiple sites over the mastoid process. The initial infiltration should be at the most inferior portion of the mastoid process, just posterior to the inferior portion of the pinna.

2. Upper extremities (see also Chapter 19).

  a. Digital nerve block (Fig 28–2).

    (1) Anesthetic solution containing epinephrine should never be used for a digital block because it can cause severe vasoconstriction and necrosis.

    (2) One of several techniques is presented.

        a A solution of lidocaine (Xylocaine) hydrochloride and a no. 25 hypodermic needle are used.

        b The needle is placed in the web space and advanced toward the palm at a 20-degree angle to the long axis of the finger being anesthetized.

        c The needle is inserted slowly until it encounters the proximal phalanx. It is then withdrawn slightly, and the plunger is pulled back to be sure the needle point is not in a vessel.

        d Two or 3 mL of solution are then injected to produce a ''ballooning'' of the web space. The procedure is repeated through a separate needle puncture on the other side of the digit.

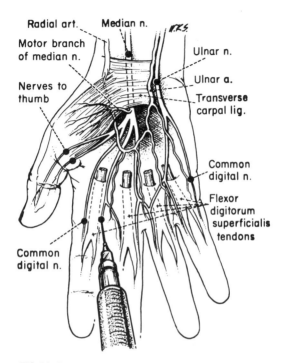

FIG 28–2.
Sites for nerve blocks.

     e Solution is placed in a position corre-
sponding to web space injection for the
radial digital nerve of the index finger
and the ulnar digital nerve of the fifth
finger.

     f The digital nerves of the thumb flank the
flexor pollicis longus tendon. Two to 3

mL of solution is injected on each side of the tendon at the base of the thumb on the palmer surface.

    g If an injury affects the dorsum of the finger, particularly distal to the distal interphalangeal joint, it is advisable to supplement the digital block with a field block on the dorsum. Two milliliters of solution is injected transversely across the dorsum of at the base of the finger.

b. Median nerve block (Fig 28–3).

  (1) If the palmaris longus tendon is present, the needle is inserted radial to the tendon just proximal to the distal flexion crease of the wrist.

  (2) If the palmaris longus tendon is absent, the needle is inserted approximately 1 cm ulnar to the flexor carpi radialis tendon.

  (3) The needle is advanced until resistance by deep fascia is encountered. One milliliter of 2% lidocaine (Xylocaine) is injected.

  (4) The fascia is then penetrated, and an additional 2 mL is injected.

  (5) Paresthesias in the distribution of the median nerve are often elicited as the needle point contacts the nerve. It is preferable to inject the anesthetic *around* the nerve since an intraneural injection may produce painful neuritis.

c. Ulnar nerve block (Fig 28–4).

  (1) At the wrist 2 to 3 mL of 2% lidocaine (Xylocaine) is injected radial to the flexor carpi ulnaris tendon, just proximal to the pisiform bone.

  (2) At the elbow the same amount of anesthetic is injected around the nerve where it is palpable in the olecranon groove along the medial epicondyle of the humerus.

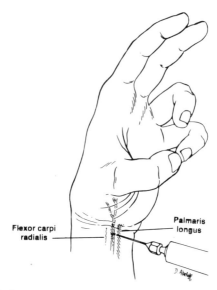

FIG 28–3.
Median nerve block. (From Rosen P, Sternbach G: *Atlas of Emergency Medicine.* Baltimore, Williams & Wilkins Co, 1979. Used with permission.)

    d. Radial nerve block (Fig 28–5).
        (1) The radial nerve at the wrist has already divided into several sensory branches. A modified field block is thus necessary.
        (2) Five milliliters of anesthetic is injected over an area extending from a point just radial to the radial artery, across the radial aspect of the wrist, and onto the extensor surface.

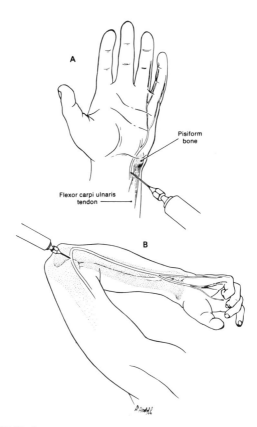

FIG 28–4.
Ulnar nerve block. (From Rosen P, Sternbach G: *Atlas of Emergency Medicine.* Baltimore, Williams & Wilkins Co, 1979. Used with permission.)

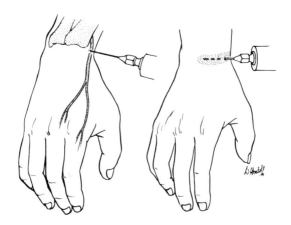

FIG 28–5.
Radial nerve block. (From Rosen P, Sternbach G: *Atlas of Emergency Medicine.* Baltimore, Williams & Wilkins Co, 1979. Used with permission.)

    e. Axillary block.—This may be the ideal anesthetic technique for brief surgical procedures from the midarm down to the fingers.

    (1) The nerves of the brachial plexus within the axillary sheath are superficial and readily accessible at the apex of the axilla immediately under the shelf of the pectoralis major muscle. If the arm is extended at a right angle from the body and supinated and flexed at the elbow, the axillary artery, which is the major guide to the nerves, may be seen to pulsate at the above site. If it is not discernible, its pulse can be felt here.

(2) The artery at this point lies in a hollow formed by the four major nerves of the upper extremity—the median, ulnar, musculocutaneous, and radial. Staying close to the artery with the block needle increases the success of the block tremendously. Care should be taken, however, not to inject local anesthetic intravenously (IV). The other factor that enhances the success of the block is the elicitation of paresthesias to the hand (median and ulnar nerves) and to the wrist and forearm (radial and musculocutaneous).

(3) A ¼-in. rubber tube tourniquet is placed around the upper part of the arm just distal to the pectoralis major muscle shelf and tightened enough to compress the artery slightly. The axillary artery is palpated against the humerus close to the apex of the axilla. A ⅝-in., 25-gauge needle attached to a 10-mL syringe containing 2% lidocaine is inserted through a skin wheal between a gap formed by the finger palpating the artery. Paresthesias are elicited by advancing the needle, and 3 to 5 mL of solution is injected every time a paresthesia is provoked. The needle should always be perpendicular to the humerus, but probing should be done close to, above, below, and behind the artery for the radial nerve. This is always the hardest paresthesia to elicit. Failure to include the radial nerve in the block can be frustrating since the hand and the arm may be paralyzed but some sensation remains around the wrist, the anatomic snuffbox, and the dorsum of the hand, thumb, and index, middle, and ring fingers.

(4) Two to 3 mg/kg of anesthetic should be injected. The total dose should not exceed 500 mg (25 mL of a 2% solution). The tourniquet is left on for 5 to 10 minutes after injection to direct the drug cephalad toward the brachial plexus.

3. IV regional anesthesia with lidocaine (Bier block).—This is one of the simplest and most effective anesthetic procedures for the forearm and hand.

   a. A 20- or 18-gauge plastic IV catheter is inserted into a dorsal hand vein and taped to the skin. The IV line should be attached to a 250-mL bottle of saline or 5% dextrose in water. The injection site on the IV tubing closest to the needle is used to introduce the local anesthetic.

   b. The IV drip is turned off, and an Esmarch bandage is applied to the hand and forearm, used to milk the venous blood proximally, and removed. A padded sphygmomanometer cuff is placed on the upper part of the arm. After the upper extremity has been emptied of blood by the Esmarch bandage, the cuff is inflated to 250 mm Hg pressure. Lidocaine solution, 0.5%, is injected in a dose of 2 to 3 mg/kg. After instillation of the local anesthetic, the IV needle is removed, and bleeding at the site is stopped by local pressure. After anesthesia is achieved (usually after 10 to 15 minutes), the procedure for which the block is being performed may be undertaken.

   c. After 30 minutes, the cuff may be deflated without fear of flooding the systemic circulation with the local anesthetic. At the end of this period most of the local anesthetic has been absorbed into the lipid tissues and will be released slowly to be metabolized by the liver. There is danger of systemic lidocaine toxicity, however, if the cuff is accidentally released before this time.

d. This procedure may also be used on the lower extremity with the double-cuffed tourniquet. Because of the greater bulk of tissue to be compressed, a greater pressure of about 500 mm Hg may be necessary. Cannulation of a vein on the dorsum of the foot would ensure sufficient anesthesia of the foot and toes. The use of the Esmarch bandage to milk the extremity of blood is not obligatory. Holding up the extremity for about 5 minutes may achieve the same objective, though perhaps not so efficiently. Considering the bulk of the lower extremity, a dose of 5 to 8 mg/kg local anesthetic will be needed to achieve the same degree of anesthesia as in the upper extremity.

4. Chest, intercostal nerve block (see Chapter 6, "Thoracic Injuries").

5. Lower extremities.

   a. Sciatic nerve.

   (1) Distribution.—The block provides anesthesia to the back of the thigh, the lateral aspect and the back of the leg, and the foot (Fig 28–6,a).

   (2) Landmarks.—With the patient lying on the contralateral side and the hip flexed about 40 degrees, anesthetic is injected 3 to 5 cm distal to the midpoint of a line from the posterior superior iliac spine to the proximal border of the greater trochanter. A long needle is used. Paresthesias should be elicited and 7 to 10 mL of 1% anesthetic injected.

   b. Femoral nerve.

   (1) Distribution.—The block provides anesthesia to the medial thigh, leg, and foot (Fig 28–6,a).

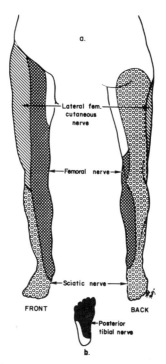

FIG 28–6.
Sensory area distribution of nerves in the lower limbs.

> (2) Landmarks.—Anesthetic is injected at a
> point just lateral to the femoral arterial
> pulse, 2.5 cm distal to the inguinal liga-
> ment. Five to 15 mL of anesthetic should
> be injected in a fanwise manner. Paresthe-
> sias are rarely elicited.

   c. Lateral femoral cutaneous nerve.
      (1) Distribution.—The block provides anesthesia to the lateral portion of the thigh (Fig 28–6, a).
      (2) Landmarks.—Anesthetic is injected 2.5 cm medial and 2.5 cm distal to the anterior superior iliac spine. No paresthesias need to be elicited. The needle should be passed through the fascia lata and 5 to 10 mL of anesthetic injected in a fan pattern.
   d. Posterior tibial nerve.
      (1) Distribution.—The block provides anesthesia to most of the sole of the foot except the most proximal and lateral portion (Fig 28–6, b).
      (2) Landmarks.—Anesthetic is injected posterior to the posterior tibial pulse at the level of the medial malleolus. Paresthesias are occasionally elicited. Five to 10 mL of 1% lidocaine or mepivacaine should be injected.

II. Complications of Regional Anesthesia

A. Except for the intercostal nerve block during which inadvertent entry into the thoracic cavity may produce a pneumothorax, most of the regional procedures described are rarely associated with significant complications. Complications that arise from the procedure itself or from the technique involved are usually minimal.

B. The priorities in the initial treatment of the complications of regional anesthesia are as follows:
   1. Assurance of an adequate airway.
   2. Maintenance of adequate respirations.
   3. Maintenance of adequate circulation. (See Chapter 1 for a more extensive discussion.)

C. Toxic reactions.

1. Systemic reactions may well be the most serious complication of regional anesthetic blocks.

2. They usually are associated with the inadvertent introduction of large amounts of local anesthetic into the systemic circulation.

3. The symptoms are proportional to the amount of local anesthetic introduced.

4. They are usually referable to the following:
   a. Central nervous system (CNS).
   b. Cardiovascular system.
   c. Respiratory system.

5. A mild toxic reaction may be characterized by nothing more than a feeling of warmth, light-headedness, dizziness, and being "high," a form of psychic instability. It is easily managed by the administration of oxygen and reassurance of the patient.

6. More severe toxic reactions cause a more marked stimulation of the CNS that leads to convulsions. These should be managed as outlined in Chapter 11. IV diazepam (Valium) is the drug of choice to control such convulsions.

7. CNS depression (general anesthesia) may occur after an initial CNS stimulation. The barbiturates, diazepam, or narcotics can augment the CNS-depressant action. As depression of the CNS increases, the local anesthetic starts to act as a general anesthetic, and unconsciousness may ensue. Local anesthetics have in fact been used as general anesthetics by IV administration.

8. Respiration may be diminished by action on the respiratory center and possible peripheral curare-like effects of the local anesthetic.

9. The local anesthetic can affect the membrane of the myocardial cell and depress cardiac output.

10. Peripherally, the local anesthetics may depress ganglia and smaller blood vessels and cause dilation and hypotension.

D. Management.
  1. Respiratory failure.
     a. Establish a patent airway by properly positioning the head and mandible, by inserting an oral or nasal airway, or by inserting an endotracheal tube.
     b. Assist ventilations with a bag mask or a mechanical ventilator system.
  2. Cardiovascular problems.
     a. Occasionally bradycardia may be severe, even progressing to cardiac arrest.
     b. Treatment of bradycardia should be with IV atropine, 0.5 mg. This can be repeated every 5 minutes to a maximum of 2.0 mg. If bradycardia persists, a drip of isoproterenol, 2 mg in 500 mL of 5% dextrose in water, should be begun and the infusion rate adjusted to maintain a pulse faster than 60 beats per minute.
     c. Hypotension.—The patient should be placed in the Trendelenburg position, and 200 to 300 mL of normal saline solution is infused IV over a period of 15 to 20 minutes. If the hypotension is refractory to this, dopamine, 400 mg in 500 mL of 5% dextrose in water, should be infused at a dose of 5 to 15 μg/kg/min or levarterenol, 4 to 8 mg in 500 mL of 5% dextrose, with the dose titrated against the blood pressure response.
E. Hypersensitivity.—The response of the patient is very similar to that from a severe systemic reaction (see Chapter 25). The amount of local anesthetic that was administered may be quite small compared with that for a true systemic reaction. The management of this condition is very similar to that of a severe allergic reaction.
F. Reaction to epinephrine.—Epinephrine in small concentrations frequently is used to prolong the duration of a local anesthetic. This is particularly true of lidocaine, which tends to diffuse quickly and be

absorbed rapidly. The addition of epinephrine causes vasoconstriction and slows down the absorption and diffusion of the drug. However, absorption of the epinephrine itself, even in minute amounts, can cause tachycardia, mental excitement, and occasionally piloerection.

G. Fear.—The response of an apprehensive patient may well produce a "reaction" to local anesthetics. No matter how hard one tries to allay the patient's fear and explain the procedure, fear of the needle or the effects of the local anesthetic may provoke severe apprehension. Nausea and vomiting are probably the most common manifestations of this psychogenic reaction. Hypotension, bradycardia, and loss of consciousness may also occur, and these may mimic a severe systemic toxic reaction. These usually respond to elevation of the legs and administration of oxygen. Sedation of the patient may be necessary.

III. Sedation

It is frequently advantageous to administer sedative or analgesic medications to patients prior to repairing a laceration or performing other procedures. This is especially true of children. A number of agents are available.

A. Hydroxyzine (Vistaril).
  1. This antihistamine has CNS-depressant activity, which makes it useful to allay tension and anxiety.
  2. Hydroxyzine has no known adverse respiratory or cardiovascular effects, but it may potentiate the effects of narcotics and barbiturates.
  3. Dose.—1 mg/kg intramuscularly.

B. Narcotic analgesics.
  1. These drugs are frequently necessary when the patient is in severe pain and when a definitive procedure to correct or remedy the source of pain is contemplated. Disadvantages of this group

of drugs are the respiratory center depression and hypotension that may result. However, these and other narcotic analgesic effects can be reversed by narcotic antagonists.

2. Dose and choice of drug.—The commonly used narcotic analgesics are morphine and meperidine (Demerol). For meperidine, the dose is 0.5 to 1.0 mg/kg intramuscularly or IV. The usual adult dose is 50 to 100 mg. This may be accompanied by intramuscular promethazine (Phenergan), 0.25 to 0.5 mg/kg. This drug is useful for its sedative and antiemetic properties. Respiratory depression is dose related with all narcotic analgesics. Morphine is ten times as potent as meperidine, and doses may be computed on the basis of 0.05 to 0.1 mg/kg. IV administration results in transiently high blood levels and excellent analgesia. Small IV doses may be administered and the amount titrated against the degree of pain remaining. Careful monitoring of respirations is necessary.

3. Reversal.—If hypotension or respiratory depression follows the administration of a narcotic, naloxone (Narcan), a narcotic antagonist should be administered IV. The initial dose is 0.4 to 0.8 mg. Additional antagonist may be administered as needed. The duration of action of IV administered naloxone is 1 to 2 hours. Additional treatment for hypotension includes elevation of the legs and infusion of IV fluids.

C. Benzodiazepines.

1. Midazolam (Versed), a short-acting benzodiazepine, is the drug of choice. It has a rapid (2 to 3 minutes) onset of action when administered IV.

2. The dosage is 0.03 mg/kg IV over a period of 30 seconds initially (about 2 to 3 mg in the average adult). Additional medication may be administered as needed and titrated to effect.

3. Respiratory depression and hypotension may be caused. The vital signs should be closely monitored.

IV. Muscular Paralysis

A. Succinylcholine.
1. This is a short-acting muscle relaxant that may be used to facilitate endotracheal intubation.
2. Its onset of action is within 1 minute, and the duration of action is 5 to 15 minutes.
3. When administered in an IV bolus, the usual dose is 40 to 80 mg for an adult and 20 mg for a child. Muscular fasciculations precede relaxation.
4. More prolonged muscle relaxation may be attained by continuous IV infusion. A solution containing 1 to 2 mg of succinylcholine per milliliter of IV solution should be mixed. The administration rate should be monitored by the degree of muscle relaxation present.
B. Tubocurarine.
1. This is a longer-acting agent than succinylcholine. The onset of action when administered IV is within 3 minutes, and the duration is 30 to 40 minutes.
2. The usual dose is 15 to 30 mg for adults and 0.2 mg/kg for children. Reversal may be accomplished by the administration of atropine, 0.2 mg/kg, and neostigmine, 0.08 mg/kg. The usual adult dose is 2.5 mg of neostigmine given IV with 1.0 mg of atropine.
C. Nondepolarizing agents.
1. Pancuronium is a more potent muscle relaxant than tubocurarine is and has a comparable onset of action and duration.
2. The recommended dose is 0.04 to 0.1 mg/kg IV, with repeated injections as needed. The effects

may be reversed with atropine and neostigmine in the doses given in Section IV,B,2.

3. Other nondepolarizing agents include vecuronium and atacurium. Both have rapid onsets of action and have shorter durations of action than pancuronium does. The dose for vecuronium is 0.08 to 0.1 mg/kg; that for atacurium is 0.4 to 0.5 mg/kg.

29

Poisoning, Overdose, and Envenomation Management

I. General Considerations

A. Poisonings and drug abuse constitute a significant portion of the medical emergencies faced by physicians. About 75% of the cases in the United States occur in children under 5, but 95% of the fatalities are in adults. Poisoning is also common in retarded older children. Suicide and homicidal attempts also result in large numbers of poisonings. Occasional accidental ingestions occur in adults.

B. Household products such as bleaches, polishing fluids, and pesiticides are responsible for much of the poisoning in children. The medicine chest and kitchen cabinets are common sources of poison. Studies of poison control centers throughout the United States have shown that more than 1,000 different household products have been responsible.

C. In many cases, the diagnosis of poisoning or overdose is obvious, and a history of ingestion is easily elicited. In other cases, it is difficult to elicit a history of ingestion or pica. In occasional cases, a history of ingestion is never obtained despite clinical and laboratory evidence for poisoning. In puzzling clinical problems in which the cause of the symptoms is not apparent, the possibility of poisoning or overdose should always be considered.

II. Signs, Symptoms, and Physical Findings

A. A large number of symptoms may develop as a result of poisoning. These include vomiting, pallor, convulsions, coma, somnolence, burning in the mouth, fever, collapse, hyperexcitability, and diarrhea.

B. Physical findings suggestive of poisoning include disturbed states of consciousness, constricted pupils, dilated pupils, cyanosis, abnormal odor of tissues, and increased sweating. The urine may be discolored and the skin stained. The specific symptoms and physical findings often suggest the type of poison ingested.

C. Various clinical syndromes may be helpful in identifying the drug or poison involved.

1. Comatose patients with dry skin, dilated pupils, tachycardia and/or dysrhythmias, hyper-reflexia, hypotension, and convulsions suggest anticholinergic drug ingestion. Comatose patients with miotic pupils and cardiopulmonary depression suggest narcotic toxicity. Pulmonary edema, seizures, and miosis suggest propoxyphene toxicity.

2. Patients with cholinergic poisoning show salivation, lacrimation, sweating, pulmonary edema, bronchoconstriction, bradycardia, miosis, muscular weakness, fasciculation, seizures, and coma.

3. Acute cyanosis and hypotension secondary to methemoglobinemia may be due to nitrate, ni-

trite, nitrophenol, nitrobenzine, benzocaine, or phenacetin.

4. A metabolic acidosis with an anion gap may be due to salicylates, methanol, ethanol, ethylene glycol (antifreeze), and isoniazid.

5. Cardiac dysrhythmias may result from tricyclic antidepressants (TCAs) phenothiazines, cocaine, amphetamines, and cardiac drugs.

6. Nystagmus may occur with sedative-hypnotic drugs and phenytoin. Horizontal or vertical nystagmus is characteristic of phencyclidine (PCP) toxicity.

III. Identification

A. Although the general nature of the poison may be indicated by symptoms and physical findings, definite identification of the agent is desirable. Examination of the original container for the product is frequently helpful. As a result of the Federal Hazardous Substances Act, the containers of most dangerous household chemicals are labeled with a list of ingredients.

B. It must be recognized that often the poisoning substance may not be in the original container but in a soda or milk bottle, a fruit jar, or a drinking glass. Examination of the remainder of the tablets or pills from the container will often lead to identification of the poisoning compound.

C. A history of peeling paint or plaster or other environmental hazards in the home, the industrial plant, or a recreation site should be elicited.

D. Toxicology laboratory.

1. Facilities for clinical toxicological examination to provide immediate results for certain substances should be present in every hospital dealing with emergencies.

2. The routine toxic screen is usually of little value

during the initial emergency department (ED) phase of care. It often takes 6 to 8 hours to complete and has poor sensitivity, i.e., a negative result does not rule out intoxication.

3. Recent evidence suggests that determining the acetaminophen level in most possible overdose patients is worthwhile because of the lack of helpful diagnostic symptoms in the early phase and the availability of a potentially lifesaving antidote.

4. Determining the levels for the following drugs and toxins may alter the treatment or disposition:

Acetaminophen
Carbon monoxide (CO)
Digitalis
Ethanol
Ethylene glycol
Iron
Lithium
Methanol
Methemoglobin
Salicylates
Theophylline

5. Always ask laboratories to give units of concentration used, and the usual therapeutic range to avoid incorrect interpretation of reported concentration units.

E. In cases of poisoning, appropriate tests of blood, urine, stomach contents, or vomitus are useful. Direct communication with the toxicology laboratory is helpful with regard to the test required and the urgency of the determination. If a specimen cannot be sent to the laboratory immediately, it should be refrigerated. "Preservatives" should not be added.

F. A flat-plate x-ray of the abdomen may show oblong masses (heroin or cocaine in condoms), pills, concretions, or radio-opaque liquids. The mnemonic useful for this finding is CHIPES. A negative x-ray does not rule out ingestion of these substances.

  C = Chloral hydrate, CCl_4.
  H = Heavy metals.
   I = Iron, iodides.
  P = Psychotropics (phenothiazines, TCAs).
  E = Enteric coated (salicylates, KCl).
  S = Solvents ($CHCl_3$, CCl_4).

G. Nonspecific examinations such as hemoglobin and hematocrit tests for anemia, determinations for methemoglobinemia, and urine for myoglobin and coproporphyrin may be of value in assessing cases of poisoning.

IV. Attempted Suicides

A. Suicide attempts using the ingestion of poisonous substances or excessive doses of medications are common. There is a high frequency of this in adolescent and postadolescent women as well as in older depressed persons. About 50% of adult ingestions are the result of attempts at suicide.

B. In addition to treatment of the poisoning, attention must be given to the psychiatric problems underlying the suicide attempt. Hospitalization is desirable in many such cases. Psychiatric evaluation is essential after the patient has recovered from the immediate effects of the ingestion. If there is suspicion of a homicidal attempt, appropriate legal authorities must be notified. The possibility of child or elder abuse must also be considered.

V. Principles of Management

A. In the management of poisoning, there are three main principles.

 1. The poison should be evacuated and its absorption inhibited if these can be done safely.

 2. Supportive and symptomatic therapy should be instituted promptly, including the administration

of intravenous (IV) fluids and maintenance of an adequate airway. Any patient with an altered state of consciousness thought to be due to poisoning or drug overdose should receive, after blood is drawn for a baseline glucose level, 50 cc of 50% dextrose in water and IV naloxone, 0.8 mg.

3. If there is a specific antidote for the poison ingested, it should be administered. However, for only a small percentage of poisonings are specific antidotes known (Table 29–1). The availability of a specific antidote does not obviate the need for general supportive measures.

B. Early in the evaluation of each case, a decision must be made about the necessity for hospitalization. Not all cases of ingestion require hospitalization. In doubtful cases, however, hospitalization is the safest choice, and it avoids medical-legal problems. Patients with a suicidal risk should be evaluated psychiatrically.

C. For ingestions, a prime consideration is whether evacuation of the stomach is indicated either by the induction of vomiting or by gastric lavage. Evacuation of the stomach is contraindicated in poisonings caused by corrosives such as lye or strong acids. Evacuation is also contraindicated if aspiration of small amounts of the poisonous substance is likely to cause severe aspiration pneumonia. The hydrocarbons are the major groups involved, and recent research has resulted in a more rational approach about when to evacuate the stomach in cases of hydrocarbon ingestion (Tables 29–2 and 29–3).

1. In most cases of poisoning, the induction of vomiting for emptying the stomach is more efficacious and faster than gastric lavage is. For certain drugs (see Section D), it may be useful to give charcoal first and then initiate lavage. Vomiting should not be induced, however, in unconscious, stuporous, or seizing individuals or in patients with deteriorating mental status. Although

vomiting may be induced in a child with a finger or a spoon, the preferred method is ingestion of syrup of ipecac. In fact, a 30-mL bottle of this medication should be in every household that has small children.

2. The initial dose of syrup of ipecac is 30 mL in adults and 15 mL in children, and the medication should be followed by the ingestion of about 200 mL of water or clear fluids. Vomiting usually occurs within 20 minutes. If vomiting does not occur, the dose may be repeated once. A smaller dose of 10 mL should be used in children aged

TABLE 29–1.
Effective Antidotes for Specific Intoxications*†

Specific Agent	Symptoms Requiring Treatment	Antidote
Acetaminophen (Tylenol; Nebs)	Hepatotoxicity (hepatocellular necrosis)	*N*-acetylcysteine
Anticholinergic agents	Central and/or peripheral anticholinergic symptoms and at least one of the following: Hypertension Hallucinations Convulsions Coma Arrhythmias	Physostigmine
Cholinergic agents Physostigmine Neostigmine	Cholinergic crisis Diaphoresis Lacrimation	Atropine sulfate

Continued.

TABLE 29–1 (cont.).

Specific Agent	Symptoms Requiring Treatment	Antidote
Pyridostigmine Pilocarpine Bethanechol Methacholine	Bronchial secretions Excessive urination and defecation Convulsions Fasciculations	
Cyanide (potassium cyanide, hydrocyanic acid, laetrile, nitroprusside sodium)	Cyanosis Cardiopulmonary arrest Convulsions Coma	Sodium nitrite Sodium thiosulfate
Ethylene glycol	Acidosis Oxalate crystals in urine	Ethanol
Haloperidol (Haldol) Loxapine succinate (Loxitane) Molindone (Moban) Phenothiazines Chlorpromazine (Thorazine) Thioridazine (Mellaril) Fluphenazine (Prolixin)	Extrapyramidal symptoms: Dystonia Dyskinesia Oculogyric crisis Parkinsonian symptoms	Diphenhydramine
Iron salts (ferrous sulfate, ferrous gluconate)	Hypotension Shock Coma (free serum iron present)	Deferoxamine

Methanol	Acidosis Methanol blood level exceeding 20 mg/dL	Ethanol
Methemoglobin- producing agents: Nitrates/ nitrites Phenazopyri- dine Phenacetin	Methemoglobin- emia (>30%)	Methylene blue
Narcotic analgesics and related agents (pentazocine [Talwin], propoxyphene [Darvon], diphenoxylate [Lomotil])	Respiratory depression Hypotension Coma	Naloxone
Organophosphate insecticides Malathion Parathion	Cholinergic crisis: Diaphoresis Lacrimation Bronchial secretions Excessive urination and defecation Convulsions Fasciculations Profound weakness Muscular twitching	Atropine sulfate
		Pralidoxime

*From Watanabe A, Rumack B, Peterson R: Enhancement of elimination in poisonings. Aspen Systems Corp 1: 1979. Used with permission.
†See text for dosages.

TABLE 29–2.
Hydrocarbons: General Indications for Emesis*

Agents for Which Emesis Is Generally Recommended	Agents for Which Emesis Is Generally Not Recommended	Agents Generally Considered Nontoxic and Unnecessary to Vomit
The following agents can produce CNS† toxicity or other toxic effects Halogenated aromatic hydrocarbons (trichloroethane, trichlorethylene, carbon tetrachloride, methylene chloride; see also specific managements), aromatic hydrocarbons (toluene, xylene, benzene; see also specific managements), or turpentine if doses of 1 mL/kg or more are ingested Gasoline, kerosene, (e.g., coal oil, deobase), charcoal	There is no evidence that the following are absorbed from the GI† tract, yet they have the highest risk of severe aspiration pneumonitis Mineral seal oil or signal oil (as found in furniture or oil polishes)	The following agents do not generally cause significant CNS or pulmonary problems, although with frank aspiration they may produce low-grade lipoid pneumonia (as opposed to severe, progressive, chemical pneumonitis) Asphalt or tar Lubricants (motor oil, transmission oil,

lighter fluid, petroleum ether
(benzine), petroleum naphtha
(lighter fluid), VM&P naphtha
(paint thinner), mineral spirits
(Stoddard solvent, white spirit,
90% mineral turpentine,
petroleum spirits) if doses of 1
mL/kg or more are ingested
(minimum of 1 oz or 30 mL)
Any hydrocarbon or petroleum
distillate in any amount with
dangerous additives (heavy
metals, insecticides,
nitrobenzene, or aniline)

cutting oil, household
oil, and heavy greases)
Mineral oil or liquid
petrolatum (laxatives,
baby oil, suntan oil,
and white petrolatum)
Fuel oil (gas oil) or
diesel oil

*From Rumack BH: Hydrocarbon management, in Rumack BH (ed): *Poisindex*. Englewood, Colo, Micromedex, Inc, 1975, p 871. Used with permission.
†CNS = central nervous system; GI = gastrointestinal.

TABLE 29–3.
Indications for Emesis*†

Group I.—Emesis indicated for ingestions greater than 1 mL/kg:
   Halogenated hydrocarbons.—Carbon tetrachloride,
      trichloroethane, etc.
   Aromatic hydrocarbons.—Large amounts of benzene, xylene,
      toluene
   Hydrocarbons with benzene fraction greater than 2% to 5%
   All solvents and thinners.—Stoddard solvent, petroleum ether,
      VM&P naphtha, etc.
   Machine oil
   Hydrocarbons containing camphor, insecticides, nitrobenzene,
      or heavy metals
   Moth balls or demothing agents
Group II.—Emesis not indicated for high-viscosity products:
   Grease, petroleum jelly, paraffin wax, lubricating oils
   Fuel oil, diesel oil, mineral or baby oil
   Rubber cement, glues, tar, asphalt
Group III.—Emesis not indicated for low-viscosity products:
   Mineral seal oil or signal oil as found in furniture polish
   Domestically retailed gasoline†
   Charcoal lighter fluid†
   Kerosene†

*From Geehr E: Management of hydrocarbon ingestions. Aspen Systems Corp
1: 1979. Used with permission.
†This reflects the author's opinion. The recommendation of emesis for
   these products remains a controversial subject.

6 months to 1 year. Syrup of ipecac is relatively ineffective after phenothiazine poisonings because of the antiemetic properties of these compounds.

3. Gastric lavage with a large orogastric tube can be used in unconscious or stuporous patients or if induction of vomiting with syrup of ipecac is not successful. Examples include a small volume of vomitus, sustained-release and other pills not coming up the tube, or pills known not to adsorb to charcoal. Lavage may be used in semiconscious patients if the gag reflex is present; the patient should be turned onto his side. In unconscious patients with no gag reflex, tracheal intubation must precede gastric lavage. Gastric lavage is contraindicated after the ingestion of caustics, ammonia, strychnine, and some petroleum products (see Tables 29–2 and 29–3). A lubricated large-bore catheter (large than 28 French) should be used. Oral gastric intubation in the cooperative or unconscious patient is more effective. Physiological saline can be used for lavage, with instillation and subsequent aspiration of 200-mL amounts of the fluid many times until between 2 and 4 L has been used. In the awake uncooperative patient, a nasogastric tube can be passed nasally and ipecac administered. This tube is inadequate for lavage.

D. Activated charcoal.

1. Activated charcoal is useful in many types of poisoning. It adsorbs many poisonous compounds and reduces absorption. Activated charcoal should not be given simultaneously with syrup of ipecac since it adsorbs the latter. However, the charcoal may be given after vomiting has been induced.

2. Substances that are effectively bound by activated charcoal are aspirin, dextroamphetamine, strychnine, chloroquine, phenytoin, phenobarbital,

theophylline, TCAs, and primaquine phosphate. Glutethimide is less effectively bound. There is some evidence that when induction of vomiting has been delayed, the immediate administration of activated charcoal may delay further absorption of these drugs. Activated charcoal is of no value for binding ethyl alcohol, methyl alcohol, caustic alkalis, mineral acids, organic phosphates, iron, or lithium.

3. The dose of activated charcoal is 1 gm/kg body weight initially and given as soon as possible after the ingestion of the poisonous substance. Tap water is added to the activated charcoal to make a slurry. The material may then be administered by a large spoon, glass, or stomach tube. Repeated doses of 20 to 60 gm 2 hours later and then 4 to 6 hours later of certain drugs appear to be useful (Theophylline, and drugs with enterohepatic circulations).

E. Catharsis.—Saline cathartics are preferable—magnesium sulfate, 250 mg/kg orally, repeated every 4 hours until charcoal stools appear. Avoid laxatives except sorbitol: they may adsorb charcoal.

F. Diuresis and dialysis.—Urine output is a good indicator of kidney function, but it may not correlate with the excretion of a drug. In general, drug elimination by renal excretion is independent of urine flow rates. Forced diuresis, often with alteration of urine pH, is useful in certain situations (Tables 29–4 and 29–5). Dialysis effectiveness depends on a number of factors including volume of distribution, protein binding, molecule size, and metabolism. Dialysis is indicated for certain drugs (Table 29–6). The value of charcoal hemoperfusion is now clear in certain situations (Table 29–7).

G. The list of poisonous substances that may be encountered is long. The best sources of information are microfiche texts updated at least every 6 months *(Poisindex)* and regional poison control centers. Lo-

TABLE 29–4.
Forced Diuresis*

Diuresis

Hypertonic or pharmacological diuretics should be given along with adequate fluids. Usual urine flow is 0.5–2 ml/kg/hr and with forced diuresis should be 3–6 ml/kg/hr. Alkaline or acid diuresis should be chosen on the basis of the drug's pKa so that ionized drug is trapped in the tubular lumen and not reabsorbed. Monitoring urine pH is required

Alkaline diuresis

This can usually be accomplished with sodium bicarbonate, 1–2 mEq/kg IV, and observing for potassium depletion. Administration of potassium chloride may also be indicated. Serum electrolytes and pH must be assessed

Acid diuresis

This may be accomplished with ascorbic acid or ammonium chloride, IV or po. Serum and urine pH must be followed. Ascorbic acid may be given in doses of 500 mg to 2 gm IV or po as needed to obtain an acid urine (pH of 5.5). po is less effective than is IV. Ammonium chloride may be used IV or po at a total dose of 2–6 gm/day or 75 mg/kg/day in four divided doses. Caution is advised for patients with renal or liver disease

*From Watanabe A, Rumack B, Peterson R: Enhancement of elimination in poisonings. Aspen Systems Corp 1: 1979. Used with permission.

TABLE 29–5.
Some Drugs Helped by Forced Diuresis*

Toxicant	Type of Diuresis
Alcohol	? Effectiveness
Amphetamines	Acid
Bromides	Saline
Isoniazid	Alkaline
Meprobamate	? Effectiveness
Phencyclidine†	Acid
Phenobarbital	Alkaline
Salicylates	Alkaline
Quinine/quinidine	Acid

*From Watanabe A, Rumack B, Peterson R: Enhancement of elimination in poisonings. Aspen Systems Corp 1: 1979. Used with permission.
†May precipitate or aggravate myoglobinuria

TABLE 29–6.
Dialysis Indications*

Immediate dialysis indicated regardless of condition:
    Ethylene glycol and methanol
        If acidotic, start ethanol, then dialyze
Dialysis indicated on basis of condition:

Alcohols	Chloral hydrate	Quinidine
Amphetamines†	Isoniazid	Quinine
Antibiotics	Meprobamate	Salicylates
Barbiturates	Paraldehyde	Strychnine
(long)‡	Potassium	Theophylline
Bromides		

Dialysis not indicated except for support (therapy is intensive supportive care)

Antidepressants
  (tricyclic and MAO§
  inhibitors also)
Antihistamines
Benzodiazepines
Digitalis and related
  compounds
Diphenoxylate
Ethchlorvynol
Glutethimide

Hallucinogens
Methaqualone
Methyprylon
Narcotics
Propoxyphene
Phenothiazines
Synthetic
  anticholinergics and
  belladonna
  compounds

*Watanabe A, Rumack B, Peterson G: Enhancement of elimination in poisonings. Aspen Systems Corp 1: 1979. Used with permission.

†Amphetamines respond better to acid diuresis, but if not responding, consider dialysis for severe toxicity.

‡While the long-acting (renal cleared) barbiturates are more readily dialyzable than the short (hepatic cleared), dialysis may be helpful if the patient has criteria for supportive dialysis needs (i.e., renal failure, electrolyte imbalance, and hyperthermia).

§MAO = monoamine oxidase.

TABLE 29–7.
Poisonings Reported Treated With Hemoperfusion*

Amanita muscaria
Barbiturates
  Long acting: phenobarbital
  Short acting: secobarbital
Ethchlorvynol
Methsuccimide
Salicylate
Phenytoin
Theophylline
Tricyclic antidepressants

*Modified from Watanabe A, Rumack B, Peterson G: Enhancement of elimination in poisonings. Aspen Systems Corp 1: 1979.

cal zoos, museums, and aquariums are useful in specific situations. Reference books on poisons should be available in each hospital that treats emergencies.

VI. Specific Poisons and Drugs (see Chapter 30, Section VIII)

A. Salicylates.
  1. Salicylate poisoning is common. It occurs in young children as a result of accidental ingestion or from a therapeutic overdose. Salicylates are commonly used in suicide attempts, particularly by adolescents. In young children, a respiratory or other primary illness may be complicated by secondary salicylate poisoning. Salicylates are eliminated primarily by conjugation with glycine to form salicyluric acid. Relative excretion tends to slow as the total amount of salicylates in the body increases. When liver metabolism is saturated, renal excretion becomes the primary route.
  2. Symptoms of salicylate poisoning include tinnitus, anorexia, fever, vomiting, sweating, flushed appearance, hyperventilation, delirium, coma, and convulsions. A history of ingestion usually can be elicited, although chronic overdosage is becoming a more common cause. The Phenistix test of urine is useful (the stick turns brown, and the color is resistant to bleaching by 1 drop of 20N H_2SO_4), as is the ferric chloride test (a purple color after a few drops of 10% $FeCl_3$). The plasma sodium level is usually normal, but the plasma bicarbonate level is usually reduced as a result of hyperventilation. Reducing substances in the urine and ketonuria are common.
  3. Determining the blood salicylate level 6 hours after ingestion and the blood pH is mandatory. Levels above 35 mg/100 mL are considered toxic, al-

though there is no good correlation between salicylate levels and symptoms. The level must be evaluated by considering the time elapsed since the ingestion (Fig 29–1). Toxic doses have much longer half-lives than do therapeutic doses, rising from 4 to 20 hours. Geriatric patients receiving chronic therapy can become poisoned easily when increased doses overload the detoxifying pathways.

4. Treatment.
   a. Vomiting should be induced by syrup of ipecac if ingestion has been relatively recent.

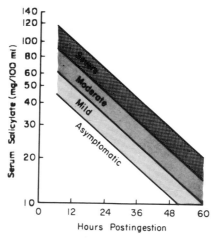

FIG 29–1.
Nomogram relating serum salicylate concentration and expected severity of intoxication at varying intervals following the ingestion of a single dose of salicylate. (From Done AK: Salicylate intoxication. *Pediatrics* 1960; 26:800. Used with permission.)

   b. In severe cases, IV fluids should be started. Elevation of the urine pH to above 7.5 is useful since the reabsorption of salicylate from urine is markedly reduced and excretion of salicylate is greatly enhanced at an alkaline pH. IV sodium bicarbonate, 20 to 50 mEq, is given over a period of 5 minutes. If after 10 minutes the urine is not alkaline, an additional 15 mEq is given and repeated every 10 minutes until the urine is alkaline. After the urine is alkaline, 10 mEq of sodium bicarbonate per 100 mL of 5% dextrose in half-normal saline is given as a drip at 1.5 to 3.0 mL/min. After a good urinary flow is obtained, serum potassium levels should be monitored and 30 mEq added as needed to each liter of IV fluid. The urine pH should be checked every 30 minutes, and if it is less than 7.5, another 15 to 25 mEq of sodium bicarbonate should be given over a 5-minute period. An indwelling catheter is useful if it is difficult to collect urine. After 2 to 5 hours of treatment, maintenance fluids may be started. In rare cases in which renal failure occurs, hemodialysis or peritoneal dialysis may be considered.

B. Lead poisoning.

   1. Lead poisoning occurs primarily among children 12 to 36 months old in urban areas. Housing in poor repair with peeling paint that has a high lead concentration is associated with lead poisoning. A history of pica generally can be elicited. There is a seasonal incidence of lead poisoning; most cases occur during the summer.

   2. Symptoms include vomiting, ataxia, change in personality, anorexia, constipation, anemia, incoordination, lethargy, apathy, convulsions, and stupor.

   3. The diagnosis may be difficult if there is no history of pica.

a. Roentgenograms of the abdomen often show radio-opaque material in the stomach. In chronic cases, films of the long bones reveal "lead lines"—areas of increased density at the metaphyses.

b. Anemia is usually present, and in some cases basophilic stippling may be seen in erythrocytes.

c. Coproporphyrin is found in the urine in most victims.

d. The best test for the diagnosis of lead poisoning is the whole blood lead level (not serum or plasma) done by an atomic absorption spectrophotometer. The erythrocyte protoporphyrin (EP) test is more sensitive but not as useful in the ED. A blood lead level higher than 50 μg/100 mL indicates significant exposure. A level above 60 μg/100 mL indicates lead poisoning.

4. Rapid deterioration may occur, and prompt treatment is therefore essential. Most children with lead poisoning should be hospitalized. Enemas should not be given.

a. Urine flow is established by the administration of 10% dextrose in water in a dose of 10 to 20 mL/kg over a period of 2 hours. Fluids are then continued on a maintenance basis so that the urine output ranges between 350 and 500 mL/day. Overhydration is dangerous in persons with lead poisoning and may induce seizures.

b. Shortly after the urinary flow is established, dimercaprol (BAL) is given intramuscularly (IM) in a dose of 4 mg/kg. Four hours later the dose of BAL is repeated, and calcium disodium edathamil (CaEDTA) in a dose of 12.5 mg/kg is also given IM. A small dose of procaine added to the EDTA will reduce local pain. BAL and EDTA are then administered every 4 hours for

5 days. If convulsions occur, anticonvulsants may be given (see Chapter 11).

c. If severe cerebral edema develops, IV mannitol, 20% solution, may be administered at an initial dose of 3 cc/kg, and dexamethazone (Decadron), 20 mg should be administered IV immediately and followed by 10 mg every 4 hours over a period of 24 hours.

d. Respiratory arrest is a constant threat, and preparations should be made for resuscitation and assisted respiration if they become necessary.

C. Iron poisoning

1. Iron poisoning is common in young children. Tablets that contain iron, particularly ferrous sulfate, are often mistaken for candy by children. Occasionally poisoning may occur from liquid preparations that contain iron.

2. The symptoms include vomiting, abdominal pain, pallor, diarrhea, and dehydration. Rarely does significant poisoning occur in the absence of these symptoms. Acidosis and shock may develop. A history of ingestion can usually be elicited.

3. The toxicity of iron poisoning is dependent on the amount of elemental iron ingested.

4. In the management of iron poisoning, the following measures are indicated.

a. Syrup of ipecac should be administered to induce vomiting, even if vomiting has occurred before admission, to empty the stomach further.

b. The stomach should be lavaged first with a 1% sodium bicarbonate solution by using a large-bore stomach tube. Follow with 200 to 500 cc of 2 to 3% solution and leave 50 to 100 cc in the stomach. Avoid phosphate lavage. It causes electrolyte imbalance.

c. Blood should be drawn on the patient's admission to the hospital for determining the serum iron content and the iron-binding capacity. Patients ingesting adult iron preparations need levels determined at least 4 to 6 hours after ingestion. For pediatric preparations, levels determined at 2 hours postingestion are adequate.

e. A "scout" film of the abdomen should be taken since iron-containing tablets are opaque and can often be seen in the roentgenogram.

e. Desferoxamine challenge.—Occasionally patients with less than 350 mg/dL exhibit significant toxicity. Thus the desferoxamine challenge test should be utilized in all patients with a strong possibility of iron ingestion, even in the absence of clinical evidence of toxicity. For adult patients, give desferoxamine, 2 gm, unless the patient is in shock. If shock is present, give IV at a maximum of 15 mg/kg/hr. For children, give 50 mg/kg up to a maximum of 2 gm. If shock is present, give IV as for adults. The absence of pink urine by 6 hours is a very reliable test for iron ingestion, i.e., a negative result. As soon as the urine turns pink, begin desferoxamine treatment.

f. Desferoxamine should be administered IV or IM for levels above 500 μg/dL and for levels above 350 μg/dL if there are clinical signs of toxicity. The dose is 20 mg/kg IM, or if the child is in shock, 40 mg/kg IV over a period of 4 hours. Give no more than 15 mg/kg in any single hour. The IM route is only appropriate if there is no evidence of acidosis or hypoperfusion. IV desferoxamine can cause hypotension, and careful monitoring is essential.

g. All urine should be collected, and any color change after administration of the drug should be noted. Red indicates a heavy excretion of iron and that additional desferoxamine should be given. If the urine does not change color or if it returns to a normal color, therapy may be discontinued.

h. Symptomatic therapy should be carried out as indicated. Occasionally treatment for shock is necessary. The chelation therapy with desferoxamine is effective only if there is good urinary output. If severe oliguria or anuria develops, dialysis should be considered to remove the iron chelate.

i. In rare cases when iron levels are greater than 1,000 µg/dL, the risk of massive liver damage necessitates the consideration of exchange transfusion and endoscopic or surgical removal of aggregated iron pills in the stomach.

D. Poisoning with kerosene and related hydrocarbons

1. Kerosene and other compounds that contain hydrocarbons are common causes of poisoning in young children. Products frequently involved are furniture polish, turpentine, lighter fluid, and benzene. A history of ingestion is usually elicited. These children may develop pneumonia, pneumonitis, and pulmonary edema. The hydrocarbon may be the vehicle for other drugs, e.g., organophosphates, and thus there may be additional symptoms.

2. Hydrocarbon ingestion signs and symptoms usually include choking and gagging, cough, nausea, characteristic breath odor, fever, weakness, and central nervous system depression. A chest roentgenogram may reveal pulmonary infiltration.

3. Treatment.

a. In this type of poisoning, decisions on emesis are based on the viscosity, surface tension, and volatility of the substance ingested. When the risks of toxicity outweigh those of aspiration, emesis is indicated (see Tables 30–2 and 30–3).

b. It may be necessary to use oxygen therapy, high humidity, and IV fluids.

c. Adrenocorticosteroids have been used in severe cases, but their value is questionable.

E. Caustic burns.

1. Lye is used in many households for cleaning drains and frequently is stored in a variety of receptacles including soda bottles. It may then be mistaken for the original edible material and ingested by small children. Most lye burns occur in children between 13 months and 5 years old. Many caustic or corrosive substances, including Clinitest tablets, that are found in the house are ingested accidentally.

2. Burns may be noted on the lips, in the mouth, and in the throat. Excessive salivation may be present. In such cases, the child should be hospitalized and observed. The great threat is the development of esophageal stenosis and stricture from an esophageal burn.

3. If an esophageal burn is suspected, parenteral corticosteroid treatment should be started.

4. Arrangement should be made for esophagoscopy to determine the presence and extent of the lye burn in the esophagus. If there is no esophageal burn, corticosteroid therapy may be discontinued. If a lye burn is present, prednisone, 2 mg/kg/day or the equivalent, is continued for 10 days, and arrangements are made for early bougienage.

5. Management of the ingestion of ammonium hydroxide and permanganate is essentially similar to that of lye. Household products such as bleach are frequently ingested by young children. However, such products almost never cause esophageal burns, and in most cases esophagoscopy is not indicated.

6. Battery ingestion can cause mechanical obstruction and electrical or chemical burn. Most pass uneventfully, and regular surveillance by x-ray is all that is required. A stuck or split battery requires removal by endoscopy, purging, or surgery.

7. Hydrofluoric acid burns require prompt specific treatment. Initial treatment with iced benzalkonium or 25% magnesium sulphate is useful. Then inject 10% calcium gluconate around and into the burned area by using a 30-gauge needle. Use the disappearance of pain as an indicator of the adequacy of treatment.

F. Organophosphate poisoning.

1. Organophosphates are commonly used as insecticides. These pesticides are a common and important source of poisoning in children and adults. Among the organophosphates are malathion, parathion, TEPP, and OMPA. These compounds may be ingested, inhaled, or absorbed through the skin or eye. They inactivate acetylcholinesterase and cause an accumulation of acetylcholine.

2. Symptoms include blurred vision, headache, profuse sweating, abdominal cramping, nausea, and vomiting. Respiratory distress, convulsions, cyanosis, shock, or coma may develop.

3. Physical examination.—Miosis is usually present, although mydriasis may develop terminally.

4. Mental confusion is frequently found, and muscular incoordination develops. Areflexia is usually present.

5. A history of exposure to an organophosphate pesticide 6 hours or less before the onset of symptoms can usually be elicited.

6. In the diagnosis of organophosphate poisoning, significant depression of cholinesterase activity in plasma and erythrocytes provides laboratory verification of the diagnosis. Heparinized blood (10 mL) should be sent to the laboratory. Treatment, however, should not await the result of laboratory tests.

7. Treatment.

a. Gastric lavage should be used, activated charcoal instilled, and a saline cathartic administered if the pesticide has been ingested.

   b. Skin and clothing should be decontaminated promptly. Use tincture of green soap if available.

   c. If there is respiratory difficulty, maintenance of an adequate airway is essential, and assisted respiration may become necessary.

   d. Anticonvulsants may be indicated (see Chapter 11).

8. A specific antidote for organophosphate poisoning is IV atropine. The dose is 0.05 mg/kg slowly every 10 to 30 minutes to ensure atropinization (decreased bronchial secretions). For adults, give 2 to 5 mg slowly, and repeat every 10 to 30 minutes to maintain atropinization (decreased bronchial secretions). Very large total doses may be required.

9. Pralidoxime (Protopam Chloride) is given after atropine. This drug reactivates cholinesterase. For adults, give 1 gm IV (500 mg/min). Repeat every 8 to 12 hours for three doses if muscle weakness persists. For children, give 25 to 50 mg/kg IV, and repeat every 8 to 12 hours for three doses if muscle weakness persists.

G. Poisoning with specific psychotropic drugs.—Psychotropic drug poisoning is particularly prevalent among adolescents and young adults. In general, the clinical manifestations are somewhat similar, and treatment is essentially the same, with some specific exceptions. The clinical picture and treatment of the more common psychotropic drug overdoses are discussed:

1. Barbiturates.

   a. A short-acting barbiturate (secobarbital, pentobarbital) overdose is most common, and single doses of 2 to 3 gm can be life-threatening or fatal. Long-acting barbiturates (phenobarbital) have a wider margin of safety; single doses of 5 gm or more are generally fatal (serum level higher than 120 μg/mL).

   b. The clinical presentation in mild cases includes drowsiness, nystagmus, ataxia, and dysarthria. In more severe cases, profound central nervous system depression may occur with deep coma, areflexia, hypotonia, apnea, hypotension, and hypothermia.

c. Treatment.

(1) The principles of management given in Section V should be followed, with special attention paid to the recognition of rapid deterioration in the level of consciousness and ventilation. Hypotension requires aggressive treatment with fluids first and then vasopressors if necessary.

(2) Short-acting barbiturates are poorly dialyzable, and forced diuresis is of little value. Supportive care is most important, with dialysis indicated if there is renal failure.

(3) Phenobarbital is well excreted in forced alkaline diuresis (see Tables 29–4 and 29–5). Hemodialysis is effective in long-acting barbiturate overdoses.

2. Glutethimide (Doriden).

a. The lipid solubility of this drug makes serum concentrations of almost no value.

b. The clinical presentation is similar to that of barbiturates, with the additional anticholinergic effects of tachycardia, paralytic ileus, and mydriasis.

c. Treatment.

(1) See Section V, and monitor for sudden changes in consciousness and ventilation.

(2) Hemodialysis is of little or no value.

3. Major tranquilizers.

a. Manifestations depend on the class of drug ingested. Chlorpromazine (Thorazine) abuse has diminished, and haloperidol (Haldol) abuse has increased lately.

b. Clinical presentation.

(1) Aliphatic and piperidine phenothiazines (Thorazine, Mellaril, Serentil) produce

central nervous system depression with coma and seizures after the ingestion of large amounts. Hypothermia or hyperthermia can result. Tachycardia, hypotension, paralytic ileus, urinary tract retention, and cardiac dysrhythmias including ventricular tachycardia can occur.

(2) Piperazine phenothiazines (Prolixin, Stelazine, Trilafon), haloperidol (Haldol), and thioxanthines (Navane) can produce central nervous system excitation with agitation, delirium, muscular rigidity, spasm, twitching, hyper-reflexia, tremor, and seizures. Other manifestations include impaired temperature regulation, autonomic nervous system dysfunction, and cardiac dysrhythmias. Frank extrapyramidal signs can occur with excessive intake or as a side effect with normal doses.

  c. Treatment.

(1) Emetics may not be effective because almost all phenothiazines have antiemetic properties. Gastric lavage should be instituted immediately and administer activated charcoal (see Section V).

(2) Patient surveillance must include cardiac monitoring for dysrhythmias.

(3) Hypotension should be treated with volume expansion and, if necessary, α-adrenergic stimulators (metaraminol, norepinephrine). The use of β-adrenergic drugs may cause further hypotension.

(4) Dystonic reactions are treated with IV diphenhydramine, up to 50 mg slowly, or IV benztropine (Cogentin), 2 mg.

(5) Forced diuresis and dialysis are of little value.

4. Lithium carbonate.

  a. Toxicity correlates with serum lithium levels; levels higher than 2 mEq/L are toxic. Toxicity

can follow an acute overdose or a maintenance dose due to poor monitoring of serum
levels, coadministration of diuretics, restricted
sodium intake, or dehydration.

b. Clinical presentation.
(1) Early signs are nausea, tremor, drowsiness, thirst, and muscle irritability.
(2) Severe poisoning produces muscle fasciculation, twitching, rigidity, clonus, hyper-
reflexia, seizures, hypothermia, obtundation, and coma. The electrocardiogram
(ECG) shows a prolonged QT interval and
inverted T waves.

c. Treatment.—Forced saline diuresis with alkalinization of the urine is the most effective
therapy in mild cases. If any serious clinical
signs, neuropsychiatric abnormality, or a
level of 4.0 mEq/L or more at 6 hours occurs, hemodialysis should be considered
very seriously, even if the patient is asymptomatic.

5. Tricyclic antidepressants (TCAs).

a. TCAs can present as an anticholinergic syndrome. Other causes include antihistaminics,
antiparkinsonian, antipsychotic and over-the-
counter (OTC) drugs. OTC drugs usually contain antihistamines and belladonna alkaloids.

b. After rapid oral absorption, TCAs are widely
distributed in body tissues and are highly protein bound, with less than 1% in the plasma
even after an overdose. Toxicity is due to the
blocked reuptake of norepinephrine, an atro-
pine-like anticholinergic effect, and a direct
myocardial depressant effect.

c. Clinical presentation.
(1) Cardiotoxicity is a major cause of mortality
and produces myocardial depression, prolongation of His-Purkinje conduction, and
dysrhythmias from anticholinergic activity.

    The latter includes supraventricular tachydysrhythmias.

  (2) The following can also occur: respiratory depression, grand mal seizures, hypotension, hypertension, shock, abnormal tendon reflexes, hypothermia, hyperthermia, choreoathetosis, myoclonus, coma, and death.

d. Treatment.

  (1) The half-life of TCAs in an overdose is greatly prolonged beyond 24 to 36 hours. Serum concentrations correlate with symptoms. Prolongation of the QRS interval beyond 0.12 seconds is associated with a TCA plasma level of 1,000 mg/mL, which correlates with severe symptoms.

  (2) Because of delayed gastrointestinal tract motility due to the anticholinergic effect, patients with a major ingestion can initially have relatively minor signs and symptoms of anticholinergic effects.

  (3) Emesis should be induced or gastric lavage instituted following tracheal intubation. Charcoal and a cathartic should be given every 4 hours for 24 hours in mild cases and every 2 hours via nasogastric tube in more severe cases.

  (4) Close surveillance for signs of cardiotoxicity, respiratory depression, and central nervous system toxicity is mandatory, with admission to the hospital if necessary. In a patient with dysrhythmia, monitoring should continue until he is free from dysrhythmia for 24 hours.

  (5) Physostigmine is indicated *only* for life-threatening dysrhythmias or coma, seizures, severe delirium and hallucinations, or severe hypotension. The adult dose is 1 to 2 mg slowly IV over a period

of 2 minutes; the pediatric dose is 0.5 mg slowly IV over a 2-minute period. If the symptoms reverse, the dose may be repeated every 30 minutes as necessary.

(6) Alkalinization of plasma may reverse dysrhythmias; use IV sodium bicarbonate, 1 to 2 mEq/kg, to raise the plasma pH to 7.50. Ventilated patients can be alkalinized by hyperventilation.

(7) Lidocaine is indicated when life-threatening ventricular dysrhythmias fail to respond to alkalinization. Use 1 mg/kg IV as a bolus, and a constant infusion at 3 to 4 mg/min is indicated.

(8) Phenytoin is indicated if lidocaine is ineffective. The adult dose is 1 gm IV at 50 mg/min and for children, 10 mg/kg.

(9) Propranolol is indicated for refractory ventricular dysrhythmias. The adult dose is 1 mg/min to a maximum of 5 mg. The pediatric dose is 0.01 mg/kg IV. Occasionally, this may aggravate conduction disturbances and depress myocardial contractility.

(10) Cardiac pacing may be necessary.

(11) Hypotension requires IV fluids and, if necessary, phenylephrine (Neo-Synephrine), 2 to 4 μg/min.

(12) Diazepam is indicated for seizures, including those that are resistant to physostigmine.

(13) Dialysis or hemoperfusion is not beneficial.

6. Phencyclidine (PCP).
   a. PCP, which is easily made in home laboratories, is one of the most dangerous street drugs available. It is sold under many names and in many forms, and it is often combined with other drugs. Like ketamine, PCP is a dissocia-

tive anesthetic with sympathomimetic and hallucinogenic properties. Its rapid onset of action, enteric recirculation, and affinity for adipose tissue make close surveillance and the availability of toxicological studies mandatory.

b. Clinical presentation.

(1) Low-dose intoxication is often an unpredictable state resembling drunkenness. Disorientation, agitation, and sudden rage are common. Mutism, ataxia, diminished response to painful stimuli, and intermittent horizontal, vertical, or rotatory nystagmus are characteristic. Catatonic rigidity or myoclonus with muscle rigidity on stimulation may occur, as can flushing, diaphoresis, facial grimacing, hypersalivation, and vomiting. Death in this setting is usually due to accidents, especially drowning, fire, automobile accidents, and police encounters with violent subjects.

(2) High-dose intoxication often induces coma lasting hours to days. The person is unresponsive to pain. Respiratory depression, hypertension, and tachycardia occur, occasionally producing cardiac failure, hypertensive encephalopathy, or intracerebral hemorrhage. Intense muscle rigidity, opisthotonos, and decerebrate rigidity can occur with myoclonus and generalized tonic-clonic seizures. Hyperthermia and rhabdomyolysis are also possible. As the plasma level falls, symptoms of low-dose toxicity appear.

c. Treatment.

(1) Low-dose intoxication.

a An atmosphere of minimal stimulation is ideal while the patient is observed for increasing toxicity.

      b A patient's stomach should be emptied only where a large overdose or mixed-drug ingestion is suspected.

      c Violent patients may require IV diazepam or IM haloperidol, 5 to 10 mg, if an antipsychotic agent is indicated.

      d A high fluid intake with cranberry juice and ascorbic acid should be encouraged.

  (2) High-dose intoxication.

      a If tracheal intubation is necessary, it should be done very carefully because of the high risk of laryngospasm, pharyngeal hypersecretion, and aspiration.

      b Fifty percent dextrose in water and naloxone, 0.8 mg, are given IV because of the possibility of hypoglycemia and mixed overdose in all unconscious patients.

      c Gastric lavage is followed by charcoal, 1 gm/kg, and cathartics given every 2 to 4 hours. Continuous nasogastric suction may be useful.

      d IV diazepam, 2 to 5 mg, is indicated to control excessive muscle activity and seizures.

      e Mannitol should be administered if myoglobinuria is detected, which signals rhabdomyolysis.

      f Neuromuscular blocking agents may be necessary if muscular relaxation cannot be induced with diazepam, phenytoin, or phenobarbital.

      g Cooling measures are indicated for hyperthermia.

      h Hypertensive crises respond to diazoxide, 100 to 150 mg by IV push, or nitroprusside, 3 µg/kg/min.

      i Brisk diuresis with IV furosemide, 40

mg, and acidification using ascorbic acid, 1 to 2 mg/L of IV fluid, promotes excretion but may worsen myoglobinuric damage (see Table 30–4).

j In massive overdoses, ammonium chloride (2.75 mEq/kg in a 1% to 2% solution of saline given IV every 6 hours) may be indicated. Blood gases, pH, serum electrolytes, and ammoniac levels must be monitored. An alternative regimen is to give 300 mEq of HCl in 1 L of sterile water over a period of 6 hours by *central venous line*. Both these treatments are controversial and may precipitate or aggravate myoglobinuria.

k PCP psychosis may mimic or reactivate classic schizophrenia (see Chapter 30). Hospitalization is usually required in a quiet room, and treatment with antipsychotic drugs including haloperidol or chlorpromazine may be indicated.

7. Opiates.
   a. An overdose is usually unintentional, either therapeutic or with drug abuse.
   b. Clinical presentation.
      (1) Altered levels of consciousness range from drowsiness to coma, shallow to absent respiration, cyanosis, and miosis. IV track marks may be visible.
      (2) Pulmonary edema with a normal-size heart on x-ray can occur, even in conscious patients.
   c. Treatment.
      (1) Institute airway management.
      (2) Administer 50 cc of 50% dextrose in water and naloxone immediately. If no respiratory depression is present, 0.8 mg IV is a satisfactory starting dose. Use 2.0 mg IV if

respiration is compromised in any way. This may be repeated up to 20 mg safely if clinically indicated. A continuous IV infusion may be needed (see below).

(3) If IV access is unavailable and hypotension is not present naloxone can be given IM or subcutaneously (SC). When hypotension is present, a blind sublingual injection may be very effective.

(4) Application of restraints prior to the administration of naloxone prevents an agitated patient emerging from an overdose from injuring himself or medical personnel.

(5) Pulmonary edema is treated with oxygen and positive-pressure ventilation. Digitalis, diuretics and phlebotomy are not usually indicated.

(6) Careful surveillance for clinical relapse is necessary since the duration of action of naloxone is about 45 minutes and opiate toxicity may reappear. For a continuous IV infusion, calculate the naloxone dose as follows: use two thirds of the dose needed initially to reverse respiratory depression, give it in 5% dextrose in water (D_5W) or normal saline hourly. Intermittent boluses or drip rate alterations may be necessary to maintain the effect.

H. Acetaminophen or paracetamol (Tylenol).

a. Abuse of this drug has become more common. It causes severe liver damage because it depletes the glutathione supply. It seldom causes significant symptoms prior to 24 hours after ingestion.

b. Clinical course.

(1) Evidence of hepatotoxicity including right upper quadrant pain, hepatomegaly, and bleeding over 2 to 3 days.

      (2) Uneventful recovery or progressive liver failure with coma, severe metabolic disturbances, and occasionally death.

   c. Treatment.

      (1) Induce emesis or perform gastric lavage. If it is a mixed overdose, give activated charcoal.

      (2) Obtain a serum acetaminophen level at least 4 hours after ingestion. If the ingestion time is unknown, determine the level immediately and 4 hours later.

      (3) If the level is above the diagonal line on the nomogram in Figure 29–2, start *N*-acetylcystine administration; load with 140 mg/kg, followed by 70 mg/kg every 4 hours for 18 doses given orally as a 5% solution.

      (4) If the serum level is not obtainable immediately, start administering *N*-acetylcystine until the level is available. The maximal effect is obtained if it is given within 10 hours of ingestion.

I. Mercury poisoning.

  1. Metallic mercury is not absorbed and does not cause mercury poisoning. Mercury salts, however, are extremely toxic. Poisoning may occur from mercury bichloride tablets or excessive amounts of calomel or ammoniated mercury.

  2. Symptoms.—Throat and esophageal lesions develop, and there may be abdominal pain, vomiting, bloody diarrhea, and signs of renal failure.

  3. Therapy includes copious lavage after a protein-containing food such as milk or raw egg has been introduced into the stomach.

   a. Fifteen to 30 mL of magnesium sulfate may be administered in 6 oz of milk. Activated charcoal (1gm/kg) should follow.

   b. The major therapy is dimercaprol (BAL), which is administered in a dose of 3 mg/kg

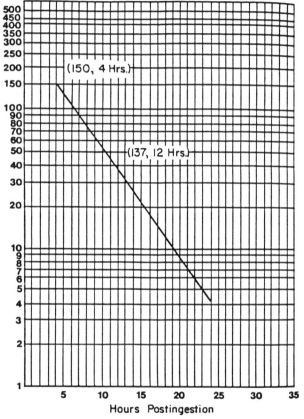

Plasma or Serum Acetaminophen Concentration μg/ml

(150, 4 Hrs.)

(137, 12 Hrs.)

Hours Postingestion

every 4 hours for six times for a 2-day period, then in a dose of 3 mg/kg every 6 hours for four times, and subsequently in a dose of 3 mg/kg every 12 hours for 2 days. In less severe cases, a smaller dose may be used.

    c. Urinalysis should be performed daily and the blood urea nitrogen (BUN) level monitored.

J. Noxious gases.

  1. Several noxious gases are toxic to humans. The major gases are carbon monoxide (CO), carbon disulfate, hydrogen sulfide, cyanide, and the products of fire damage to plastic and other synthetic materials.

  2. Hydrogen sulfide and carbon disulfide.

    a. These gases are found in petroleum refineries, tanneries, mines, and rayon factories.

    b. Clinical presentation.

      (1) Slight exposure causes skin and eye irritation, nausea and vomiting, headache, dysphagia, and stupor.

      (2) Extensive exposure causes nausea and vomiting, blurred vision, coma, pulmonary edema, and respiratory paralysis.

FIG 29–2.

Rumack-Matthew nomogram for acetaminophen poisoning. Semilogarithmic plot of plasma acetaminophen levels vs. time. *Cautions for use of the graph:* (1) the time coordinates refer to time of ingestion; (2) serum levels drawn before 4 hours may not represent peak levels; (3) the graph should be used only in relation to a single acute ingestion; (4) the *lower solid line* 25% below the standard nomogram is included to allow for possible errors in acetaminophen plasma assays and estimated time from ingestion of an overdose. (Adapted from Rumack BH, Matthew H: Acetaminophen poisoning and toxicity. *Pediatrics* 1975; 55:871. Used with permission.)

   c. Treatment.
- (1) Remove from the noxious atmosphere.
- (2) Follow the principles of management given in Section V.
- (3) Administer amyl nitrite and sodium nitrite as outlined below on cyanide poisoning.
- (4) Reduce the sensory input to the patient to avoid precipitating convulsions.

3. CO (see Chapter 5 on respiratory emergencies).
4. Cyanide.
   a. Cyanide is widespread in our environment, for example, in fertilizer, synthetic rubber, metal-cleaning solutions, fruit seeds, and medications. It appears to poison by inhibiting the cytochrome oxidase system for oxygen use in the cells.
   b. Clinical presentation.
- (1) Ingestion or inhalation of large amounts causes immediate unconsciousness, convulsions, and death within 1 to 15 minutes.
- (2) Ingestion, inhalation, or skin absorption of smaller amounts causes dizziness, tachypnea, drowsiness, hypotension, tachycardia, and unconsciousness.
- (3) Usually convulsions followed by death occur within 4 hours with all cyanide derivatives except sodium nitroprusside, which may cause death as late as 12 hours after ingestion.

   c. Treatment.
- (1) Remove from the contaminated area; administer 100% O_2.
- (2) Start amyl nitrate inhalation, 1 ampule every 5 minutes. Stop only if the patient is hypotensive.
- (3) Delay gastric lavage until an antidote is given.
- (4) Immediately give sodium nitrite, 3% solution IV at 2.5 to 5 ml/min, stopping only

for severe hypotension. *Read the cyanide kit package insert for dosage details.*

(5) After sodium nitrite, give sodium thiosulfate, 25% solution IV at 2.5 to 5 ml/min.

(6) Nitrite and nitrate administration produces methemoglobin, which combines with cyanide to form cyanmethemoglobin. Thiosulfate converts cyanide to thiocyanate.

5. Arsenic and arsine gas.

a. Arsenic is found in ant poisons, insecticides, weed killers, paint, and medicines. Arsine gas is formed when acid acts on metals in the presence of arsenic. It appears to cause toxicity by combining with sulfhydryl enzymes and interfering with cellular metabolism.

b. Clinical presentation.

(1) Massive ingestion causes violent gastroenteritis, with burning esophageal pain, vomiting, and watery or bloody diarrhea. Shock follows, with convulsions and coma as terminal signs. Smaller doses cause nausea and vomiting, cramps, and variable paralysis. Ventricular dysrhythmias can occur.

(2) Inhalation of arsenic dust causes acute pulmonary edema.

(3) Inhalation of arsine gas causes hemolysis.

c. Laboratory findings.

(1) In arsenic poisoning, proteinuria, hematuria, and cylindruria occur. In arsine gas inhalation, hemoglobinuria may be present.

(2) Arsenic compounds may appear as barium-like radio-opaque material in the gastrointestinal tract.

(3) Massive toxicity correlates with blood levels in a range of 0.1–1.5 mg/dL.

    d. Treatment.
      (1) Follow the principles of management given in Section V.
      (2) Give dimercaprol (BAL), 3 to 4 mg/kg every 4 hours for the first 2 days, then 3 mg/kg every 12 hours for a total of 10 days. If BAL causes severe nausea and sweating, use ephedrine or diphenhydramine.

  6. Combination of plastic and other synthetic materials (see Chapters 5 and 27).

K. Methanol and ethylene glycol.

  1. Methanol (methyl alcohol, wood alcohol) and ethylene glycol are found in antifreeze, paint remover, shellac, varnish, and denatured alcohol. For unexplained reasons, preparations with denatured methanol often cause toxicity greater than that expected from the methanol concentration.

  2. The toxicity of methanol is due to the metabolism of methyl alcohol to formic acid and formaldehyde, which are toxic to most major organs, especially retinal cells. Ethylene glycol toxicity is due to its metabolism to calcium oxalate formic acid, and other metabolites.

  3. Clinical presentations.

    a. Mild and moderate acute poisoning produces headache, nausea, vomiting, and blurred vision; the severity depends on the dose.

    b. Severe acute poisoning causes the progression of these symptoms to cyanosis, tachypnea, hypotension, and coma. Papilledema and mydriasis are present. Severe metabolic acidosis occurs and is often fatal. Urinalysis shows crystals and ketones.

    c. Evaluation of serum osmolality and electrolytes is very helpful when toxicity with these substances is suspected.

(1) Serum osmolality calculations.

    a Calculated serum osmolality $= 2 \times Na + \dfrac{BUN}{2.8} + \dfrac{Glucose}{18}$.

    b Osmolal gap = Measured osmolality − Calculated osmolality.

    c Normal = <10 mOsm/kg.

    d These solutes increase the osmolal gap, and their molecular weights (mol wts) can be used to estimate blood concentrations.

Alcohol	Mol Wt
Ethanol	46
Isopropanol	60
Ethylene glycol	62
Methanol	32

    e Estimated blood concentration in mg/dL
$$= \text{Osmol gap} \times \dfrac{\text{mol wt}}{10}.$$

(2) Electrolyte calculations.

    a Anion gap $= Na - (Cl + HCO_3)$.

    b Normal = <12 mEq/L.

    c An elevated anion gap is usually due to one of the following (A MUDPIE):

        A = Aspirin

        M = Methanol

        U = Uremia

        D = Diabetic ketoacidosis

        P = Paraldehyde or phenformin

        I = Idiopathic lactic acidosis, iron, or isoniazid

        E = Ethanol or ethylene glycol

4. Treatment.

  a. Immediately institute the principles of management given in Section V, and add sodium bicarbonate (20 gm/L) to the lavage fluid. Do

   not give activated charcoal if oral ethyl alcohol
   is to be used.
   b. Administer ethyl alcohol, 1 to 1.5 ml/kg orally
   (50%) or IV (10%) initially and 0.5 to 1 ml/kg
   every 2 hours for as long as 4 days. Ethyl alcohol reduces methanol toxicity by inhibiting
   the metabolism of methanol to formaldehyde
   and formic acid. Check the blood level often
   enough to keep the blood ethanol level between 100 and 200 mg/dL
   c. Aggressively treat the metabolic acidosis.
   d. Carefully monitor serum glucose levels in children because ethanol-induced hypoglycemia is
   much more common than in adults.
   e. Hemodialysis should be considered when the
   blood methanol level is higher than 50 mg/100
   mL.
L. Animal venoms.
   1. General considerations.
      a. Animal venoms are mixtures of many different
      substances that may produce several different
      toxic reactions in humans.
      b. Few venoms are specific to one organ; some
      have an effect on almost every organ. Occa-
      sionally, the patient may release pharmacolog-
      ical substances that increase the poison's se-
      verity.
      c. Venom composition depends on how the ani-
      mal uses the toxin. Mouth venoms are offen-
      sive and are intended to immobilize prey; they
      often contain lethal factors. Tail venoms are
      defensive and are intended to drive away pre-
      dators; the venom is less toxic and destroys
      less tissue.
   2. Snakebite.
      a. The majority of poisonous snakes are pit vi-
      pers, and in the United States they are rattle-
      snakes, copperheads, and cottonmouths. Coral
      snakes, a small but dangerous group, are

found mainly in the southern and southwestern states. See Figure 29–3.

b. Identification and clinical presentation.

(1) Pit vipers.

a Identification is made by noting the fa-

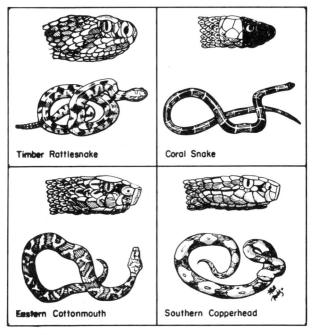

FIG 29–3.

Some venomous snakes found in the United States. (From *Emergency Management of Poisonous Snakes*. Chicago, American College of Surgeons, 1981. Used with permission.)

cial pit, the vertical elliptical pupils of the eye, a single row of subcaudal scales, and a triangular head.

b Clinical presentation.

   (i) Initial symptoms are one or more fang marks, burning, mild pain, and progressive local swelling. If paresthesia, perioral tingling and numbness, or facial muscle fasciculations occur, significant envenomation has occurred.

   (ii) Although swelling will progress very rapidly throughout the limb without treatment, it usually occurs slowly over 8 to 36 hours. Tissue destruction and tissue hemorrhage occur variably, depending on the species.

   (iii) Death is due to hypovolemic shock and pulmonary edema. Severe coagulopathy may occur within 6 hours. Occasionally neuromuscular toxins cause respiratory failure.

(2) Coral snakes.

a Identification is by the three-color ring pattern; snakes with red zones bordered by yellow or white are venomous, and those with red zones bordered by black are nonvenomous.

b Clinical presentation.

   (i) Early signs within 4 hours include tremors, drowsiness, euphoria, and marked salivation.

   (ii) After 5 to 10 hours, cranial nerve involvement leads to slurred speech, ocular muscle palsies, fixed miotic pupils, ptosis, dysphagia, and dyspnea. Survival past

24 hours is a favorable prognostic sign.

c Management.

(i) First aid, while important, should not delay transportation to a hospital. If medical care is available within a few hours, the only care in the field is patient immobilization and prompt transportation. If care is more than 3 to 4 hours away and if envenomation is certain, then reassurance, the application of a lymphatic tourniquet immediately and incision and suction within 30 minutes of the bite, immobilization, and rapid transportation, preferably on a stretcher, are the most useful measures. If possible, keep the limb level with the heart. Kill the snake, if possible to do so safely, for identification.

(ii) Perform a complete clinical evaluation and order baseline laboratory studies, complete blood cell count, a blood type and cross-match, prothrombin time, partial thromboplastin time, platelet count, urinalysis, and determinations of the levels of blood sugar, BUN, and electrolytes. For severe bites, also order tests for fibrinogen, red cell fragility, clotting time, and clot retraction time.

(iii) The degree of envenomation must be assessed, and 6 hours of observation is necessary to avoid underassessing severe envenomation.

- Minimal envenomation.—Local symptoms and signs, few systemic signs and symptoms, and minimally abnormal laboratory test results.
- Moderate envenomation.— Swelling progressing beyond the bite area, some systemic symptoms and signs, abnormal laboratory findings, especially abnormal clotting factors, falling hematocrit reading, and falling platelet count.
- Severe envenomation.—Marked local and severe systemic symptoms and signs with significant laboratory test abnormalities.

(iv) Start IV saline in all patients; give oxygen, and treat shock if present.

(v) Keep the limb level with the heart; remove the tourniquet *only* after shock is treated and antivenin is available.

(vi) Some sources recommend early surgical exploration to determine the depth and amount of tissue destruction.

(vii) For antivenin, *read the package insert carefully, and perform a skin test*. Antivenin should not be given to patients who have no signs and symptoms or even to those with local but no systemic symptoms and signs. Administer antivenin IV on the basis of a clinical grading of envenomation.

- Minimal.—0 to 4 vials.
- Moderate.—5 to 9 vials, especially in children and the elderly.

- Severe.—10 to 15 or *more* vials.
- The amount of antivenin is based on improvement of the clinical picture, not the patient's weight. Children may need more antivenin than adults do. Severe envenomation may require a rapid IV infusion of antivenin in large doses. Use polyvalent antivenin (Wyeth) for all bites with the exception of eastern coral snake bites, for which North American coral snake antivenin (Wyeth) is issued.

(viii) Hospitalize any patient who is receiving antivenin, and observe carefully for vascular insufficiency or compartment syndrome.

M. Arthropod bites.
  1. Arthropod venom is variable and complex. Some venoms, like that of the black widow, affect neuromuscular transmission, whereas other produce tissue necrosis only. Some digest food; others are for defense.
  2. Reactions to spider venom.
     a. Spider venom is more potent than is pit viper venom on a volume-for-volume basis, but the absolute amount of venom is less.
     b. Two major reactions occur: a neurotoxic reaction due to the black widow bite and local tissue necrosis due to most other spider bites.
  3. Black widow.
     a. The venom increases the amount of acetylcholine released from myoneural junctions, which exhausts end-plate activity and blocks synaptic transmission by depolarizing the postsynaptic membrane.
     b. Identification.—A shiny, coal-black spider with a red hourglass on the abdomen; the body is 1 to 5 cm long with up to a 5-cm leg span.

    c. Clinical presentation.

        (1) There is usually a history of a sharp pin-prick bite followed by a dull numbing pain in the affected extremity or body area.

        (2) Severe pain is followed by muscle rigidity of the limb or body area.

        (3) Other symptoms include headache, dizziness, ptosis, eyelid edema, conjunctivitis, skin rash and pruritus, nausea, vomiting, sweating, salivation, weakness, oliguria, and in severe cases hypotension and ECG abnormalities similar to those from a digitalis overdose.

        (4) The only local sign may be two fang marks with little local swelling. Multiple bites are rare.

    d. Treatment.

        (1) Give 2 to 10 cc of 10% calcium gluconate for immediate muscle relaxation. Methocarbamol (Robaxin), 1 gm, is given at 100 mg/min IV as an alternative.

        (2) For milder symptoms in adults and children over the age of 6, diazepam may be sufficient.

        (3) In severe cases, the elderly, and children under the age of 6, give antivenin (Lyovac *Latrodectus:* MSD), 1 ampule (2.5 cc) IV in 50 cc of saline. Perform a skin test first.

4. *Loxosceles* (brown recluse).

    a. Venom is a complex mixture of multiple enzymes that damage the endothelium of the arterioles and venules. Thrombosis, lysis of polymorphonuclear cells, and mast cell release of enzymes damage tissue.

    b. Identification.—The spider is fawn to dark brown. The body is 9 to 12 mm long. There are six white eyes in a semicircular head and a dark violin-shaped marking on the cephalothorax.

   c. Clinical presentation.
      (1) There is no significant pain initially but, later, localized pain and erythema.
      (2) In a few hours, a blister develops that is surrounded by an ischemic ring and further outlined by an erythematous ring—"bulls-eye lesion."
      (3) After several days, the area enlarges, necrosis occurs, and the center ruptures into an ulcer deep into the muscle layer.
      (4) At 7 to 8 days, an eschar develops, sloughs, and leaves a tissue defect.
   d. Treatment.
      (1) Steroids may delay the development of the lesion.
      (2) Some sources recommend excision of the bite.
N. Mushroom poisoning.
   1. Identifying mushroom species is very difficult and should be left to expert mycologists. Gastric contents should be examined microscopically to differentiate deadly toxic mushrooms from mildly toxic ones. High-power examination will show hyphae, and oil immersion examination will show spores the size of red blood cells. Staining the aspirate with Melzer's reagent will demonstrate the *Amanita* organisms as blue.
   2. Clinical presentation (see Table 29–1).
      a. While toxic and nontoxic cases show nausea, vomiting, cramps, and diarrhea, persons who ingested the lethal *Amanita* species may have a latent period of 6 hours before symptoms occur.
      b. Severe vomiting, watery diarrhea, elevated liver enzyme and bilirubin levels, and hypoglycemia suggest *Amanita* poisoning.
      c. Occasionally, hemoglobinuria, methemoglobinemia, and free hemoglobinemia indicate monomethylhydrazine poisoning (see Table 30–1).

        d. Symptoms that occur immediately or within 2 hours of ingestion make diagnosis more difficult. Treatment should shart and be accompanied by close surveillance. Identification using a reference source such as *Poisindex* is mandatory.

   3. Treatment.

      a. Specific treatment is based on the identification of the mushroom group and signs and symptoms.

      b. Induce emesis or perform gastric lavage, with tracheal intubation if necessary.

      c. Monitor blood sugar and liver enzyme levels and renal functions closely.

      d. Administer analgesics and occasionally opiates for pain.

      e. Chlorpromazine is used to treat anxiety or hallucinations.

      f. Severe seizures may occur (see Chapter 11).

O. Plant toxins.

   1. Although approximately 700 species of North American plants are considered poisonous, the number of related deaths is low given that plants are among the three most common substances ingested by children (Tables 29–8 and 29–9).

   2. Toxicity varies with region, plant maturity, quantity ingested, weight of the patient, degree of systemic absorption, and whether ingested seeds are cracked.

   3. Specific antidotes for plant poisons are rare; care is usually supportive (see Section V). The symptoms usually appear in 4 hours, and no treatment is necessary if they do not appear within 12 hours. Symptoms are related to the gastrointestinal tract in 75% of cases, but alkaloids produce systemic reactions as well. The toxic principles of commonly ingested plants are listed in Table 29–10. Actual plant identification is often difficult. Reference should be made to recent toxicology textbooks or *Poisindex* for assistance.

4. Major toxic principles.
   a. Alkaloids.
      (1) The major effect is on the nervous system, and the rate of onset varies with the mode of ingestion. Systemic effects vary with the chemical structure.

   a Atropine-containing plants produce an anticholinergic picture. Treatment is supportive, and in severe cases physostigmine, 1 to 2 mg IV, repeated as needed, is useful.

   b Colchicine produces severe dysphagia, nausea and vomiting, and profound fluid loss. Treatment is supportive, including fluid and electrolyte replacement.

   c Aconitine is rapidly absorbed and produces oral paresthesia, visual disturbances, respiratory difficulties, convulsions, and ventricular fibrillation. Treatment is rapid gastric lavage; for sensory or muscular disturbances, calcium chloride, 250-500 mg IV slowly, may be useful. Cardiac dysrhythmias should be treated as described in Chapter 3.

      (2) Polypeptides and amines.

   a The major sources are the akee plant, which is not found in the United States, and mistletoe.

   b Mistletoe is toxic in all forms, especially the berries, and causes hypertension, bradycardia, and smooth muscle contractions due to the toxins tyramine and β-phenylethylamine. Treatment is supportive and similar to that for digitalis intoxication.

      (3) Glycosides.

   a Cyanogenetic glycosides yield hydrocyanic acid (see Section J for the treatment of cyanide poisoning).

TABLE 29–8.
Mushroom Groups*

Chemical Groups	Onset of Symptoms	Treatment
I. Cyclopeptides	6 to 24 hr, typically 10 to 14 hr	Thioctic acid, 50–150 mg/kg q6h IV with glucose (questionable benefit) and penicillin G, 250 mg/kg/day in continuous IV infusion (controversial value as a displacer). Vitamin K, 40 mg IV daily. Massive doses of corticosteroids, e.g., dexamethasone 20–40 mg IV daily. Maintain fluid and electrolyte balance. Follow liver and renal parameters and blood sugar levels. Death may occur on the 4th–7th day, or recovery may take as long as 2 weeks
II. Ibotenic acid, muscimol (isoxazoles)	30 min to 2 hr	Physostigmine, 0.5–2 mg slowly IV, repeated hourly as needed for anticholinergic symptoms. Do *not* give atropine unless definite cholinergic symptoms are present. Recovery in 4 to 24 hrs

III. Gyromitrin, monomethylhydrazine (MMH)	6 to 12 hrs	Pyridoxine HCl, 2.5 mg/kg IV titrated with the patient's symptoms. Follow methemoglobin and free hemoglobin levels and hepatic parameters. Death may occur on the 5th–7th day. In mild poisonings, recovery may occur in 1 day
IV. Muscarine and other muscarinic compounds	30 min to 2 hr	Atropine, 1–2 mg IV, repeated as needed. Symptoms subside within 6 to 24 hr
V. Corpine (Antabuse-like)	About 30 min after drinking alcohol, as long as 5 days after eating mushrooms	Avoid elixirs and tinctures. Propranolol (Inderal) may be necessary to control arrhythmias. Recovery is usually spontaneous within 2–4 hr
VI. Psilocybin and psilocin (indoles)	30–60 (180) min†	Diazepam (Valium), 5–10 mg for seizures. Chlorpromazine (Thorazine), 50–100 mg IM for psychosis. Reassurance for apprehension. Recovery is usual within 6 hr
VII. Gastrointestinal irritants	½–2 hr	Death is rare; recovery varies according to species from 1 hr to several days or 1 wk

*From Rumack B, Peterson G: Diagnosis and treatment of mushroom poisoning. Aspen Systems Corp 1: 1979. Used with permission.
†Three hours is usually the latest onset.

TABLE 29–9.
The 11 Most Ingested Toxic Plants*

Plant	Toxic Part	Toxin	Symptoms	Treatment
Philodendron	All parts	Oxalates	See oxalates in text	See oxalates in text
Yew	All parts, especially seeds	Alkaloid taxine	See alkaloids in text	See alkaloids in text
Nightshade (includes bittersweet, eggplant, Jerusalem cherry, potato)	Green fruit and spoiled sprouts; ripe fruit is harmless	Alkaloid alkaloids	See alkaloids in text	See alkaloids in text
Holly	Berries	Ilicin, ilexanthin, and ilex acid; not identified as to structure and exact action	Nausea, vomiting, diarrhea, and stupor	Gastric lavage and symptomatic care
Poinsettia	White latex exuding from all parts of plant when broken	Not identified	Very similar to oxalates	See oxalates in text

Plant	Parts	Toxin	Symptoms	Treatment
Dieffenbachia	All parts	Oxalates	See oxalates in text	See oxalates in text
Black elder	All parts except berries	Cyanogenic glycoside sambunigrin	See cyanogenic glycoside in text	See cyanogenic glycoside in text
Oleander	All parts	Cardiac glycosides (nerioside and oleandroside)	See glycosides in text	See glycosides in text
Jerusalem cherry	Berries	Alkaloid solanine	See solanine in text	See solanine in text
Jimsonweed	Seed	Atropine alkaloids	See atropine alkaloid in text	See atropine alkaloid in text
Mistletoe	All parts, especially berries	Tyramine and β-phenylethylamine	Increased blood pressure, bradycardia, increased contractions of uterus and intestine	Gastric lavage, supportive care, potassium, procainamide, or quinidine

*From Burton D, Hanenson I (eds): *Plant Toxins in Quick Reference to Clinical Toxicology.* Philadelphia, JB Lippincott, 1980. Used with permission.

TABLE 29–10.
Commonly Ingested Plants*

Plant	Toxin
Aconitum (monkshood)	Aconitine alkaloid
Amaryllis	Lycorine alkaloid
Angel's trumpet	Atropine alkaloid
Apple (seed)	Cyanogenic glycoside
Apricot (seed)	Cyanogenic glycoside
Autumn croccus	Colchicine alkaloid
Azalea	Andromedotoxin alkaloid
Beet	Oxalates
Belladonna (deadly nightshade)	Atropine alkaloids
Bitter almond	Cyanogenic glycoside
Black locust	Phytotoxins
Buckeye	Saponins
Buttercup	Irritant oils
Caladium (elephant's ear)	Oxalates
Calla lilly	Oxalates
Castor bean	Phytotoxins
Cherry (seed)	Cyanogenic glycoside
Daffodil	Lycorine alkaloid
Delphinium	Aconitine alkaloid
Devil's ivy (pothos)	Oxalates
English ivy	Saponins
Foxglove	Cardiac glycosides
Glory lilly	Colchicine alkaloid
Hemlock, poison	Coniine alkaloid
Hyacinth	Lycorine alkaloid
Hydrangea	Cyanogenic glycoside
Hyoscyamus (henbane)	Atropine alkaloids
Iris	Resins
Jack-in-the-pulpit	Oxalates
Jonquil	Lycorine alkaloid
Larkspur	Aconitine alkaloid
Lilly-of-the-valley	Cardiac glycosides

Lima bean	Cyanogenic glycoside
Matrimony vine	Atropine alkaloids
Mayapple	Resins
Milkweed	Resins
Monkshood *(Aconitum)*	Aconitine alkaloid
Monstera species	Oxalates
Narcissus	Lycorine alkaloid
Peach (seed)	Cyanogenic glycoside
Plum (seed)	Cyanogenic glycoside
Pokeweed	Saponins and resins
Pothos (devil's ivy)	Oxalates
Privet	Andromedotoxin alkaloid
Rhododendron	Andromedotoxin alkaloid and resins
Rhubarb	Oxalates
Spider lily	Lycorine alkaloid
Syngonium (tri-leaf wonder)	Oxalates
Tuberose	Lycorine alkaloid
Wisteria	Resins

*From Burton D, Hanenson I (eds): *Plant Toxins in Quick Reference to Clinical Toxicology.* Philadelphia, JB Lippincott, 1980. Used with permission.

---

    b Cardiac glycosides produce gastrointestinal tract irritation and digitalis intoxication. Treatment is supportive, with dysrhythmia treatment based on the ECG and clinical presentation.

  (4) Oxalates.

    a Soluble oxalates are in high concentration in plants in the summer and fall. Rapid absorption leads to a decrease in the amount of blood-ionized calcium. While the kidneys can handle moderate amounts of soluble oxalates, large amounts precipitate oxalate crystals in tubules and cause proteinuria, hematuria, and crystaluria.

   b Symptoms include dysphagia, colic, dyspnea, and oropharyngeal edema, which can be severe.

   c Treatment is with 30 mL of aluminum magnesium hydroxide every 2 hours; gargle and swallow.

(5) Resins.

   a These act on nervous and muscle tissue and cause gastrointestinal tract distress.

   b Treatment is supportive and based on the symptoms.

(6) Phytotoxins or toxalbumins.

   a These are similar to bacterial toxins and elicit an antibody response and gastrointestinal tract distress, with hemorrhagic lesions of the gastrointestinal tract mucosa.

   b Treatment is supportive and based on the symptoms.

P. Rodenticides.—The most common rodenticide ingested is warfarin. This compound is not very toxic to humans and produces only hypoprothrombinemia after repeated administration. In most cases, therapy after ingestion is not necessary, although vitamin K can be administered.

30
Psychiatric Emergencies*

I. Introduction

A. Emergency management of psychiatric patients involves the following:
   1. Ensuring protection of the patient and the medical staff.
   2. Ruling out serious medical illness that is manifested psychiatrically (organic mental disorders).
      a. Acute (acute encephalopathy, often called *delirium*).
      b. Chronic or gradual intellectual deterioration (often called *dementia*).
   3. Ruling out life-threatening psychiatric conditions.
      a. Suicidal risk.
      b. Homicidal or assaultive risk.
      c. Grave mental disability.
   4. Formulating a working psychiatric diagnosis.
   5. Selecting the appropriate treatment and disposition.

*Chapter 30 contributed by Robert S. Hoffman, M.D., Assistant Clinical Professor of Psychiatry, University of California School of Medicine, San Francisco, and Clinical Instructor in Neurology, Stanford University School of Medicine, Stanford, California.

B. Decisions are made primarily on the basis of the history, physical and neurological examination and mental status examination (MSE). The latter is crucial; it will enable the examiner to distinguish between psychiatric presentations that require medical, neurological, or surgical treatment, and those that require only psychiatric treatment.

C. We will discuss the following areas:
1. Physical protection.
2. Mental status examination.
3. Specific psychiatric syndromes—diagnosis and treatment.
4. Differential diagnosis and disposition.

II. Physical Protection

A. Violent patients are seen frequently in the emergency department (ED). Ensuring physical protection of the medical staff as well as the patient is a high priority.

B. Early recognition of the violence-prone patient is essential.
1. Beware of the patient who is agitated, angry, suspicious, hostile, or delusional.
2. Have a high index of suspicion for the violence potential of patients taking alcohol, amphetamines, cocaine, or hallucinogens (especially phencyclidine [PCP]).
3. If you see this picture, have extra staff present during your examination, or ensure immediate access to them by leaving the door ajar.

C. Two principles of management are crucial.
1. Adopt a calm, reassuring, businesslike manner that communicates recognition of the patient's needs and a clear intent to help.
2. Ensure adequate physical controls.
   a. If the patient arrives accompanied by the police, ask them to remain until controls are

instituted or the patient is examined and found to be calm.

    b. If the patient arrives in restraints, *do not* remove them until a preliminary assessment is made. Ignoring this rule is the most frequent cause of injury.

D. If a patient unexpectedly becomes threatening or violent, *maximal force* should be deployed.

    1. Frequently a simple show of force (appearance of several burly staff members) will suffice by convincing the patient that any struggle is pointless.

    2. If a threat of force is unsuccessful, the maximum force is *applied* with the humane use of restraints. Ideally, four staff members should be used, one for each extremity.

E. Pharmacological intervention.

    1. If possible, avoid administering psychoactive drugs to a violent patient before full evaluation is performed and a diagnosis achieved. These agents may confuse an evolving neurological picture such as subdural hematoma and may increase organic confusion or obtundation.

    2. If necessary, agitated patients may be sedated.

       a. If the patient is nonpsychotic or intoxicated with central nervous system (CNS) stimulants, diazepam, 10 mg orally or intramuscularly, may be remarkably effective.

       b. If the patient is psychotic and agitated, haloperidol, 5 mg, or chlorpromazine, 50 mg, may be administered orally or intramuscularly and repeated every hour until the patient is calmer (*Only* haloperidol may be given intravenously, 3 to 5 mg over a period of 1 minute and repeated several times as needed at intervals of at least 20 minutes. This is reversed for severe agitation.) Monitor the patient for hypotensive response.

       c. In agitated patients with organic mental dis-

orders from any cause, particularly drug induced, sedatives are best avoided; the agitation will generally remit with time or
specific medical treatment of the underlying
condition.

III. Mental Status Examination

A. Before performing an MSE, it is essential to obtain
an adequate history from family and friends as
well as the patient. This should include the following:
1. Presenting symptoms, precipitating factors, and
chronology of events.
2. Associated symptoms (e.g., Is the patient depressed? Is there also anorexia, weight loss, insomnia, or suicidal ideation?).
3. Prior psychiatric history, medical history, and
medications (legal and otherwise).
4. Situational resources such as family, friends,
physicians, counselors, and living arrangements. Knowledge of these greatly simplifies
disposition.
B. A physical and neurological examination should
be done to rule out possible neuromedical disorders.
C. The MSE assesses the following (the first three of
which are usually evaluated automatically during
the initial conversation and history taking,
whereas cognitive function must be tested separately and specifically):
1. Behavior.
2. Mood.
3. Thought.
4. Cognition.
D. Behavior.—Note psychomotor agitation or retardation, restlessness, dishevelment, inattentiveness,
or unusual posturing.

E. Mood.—The patient's mood may be anxious, depressed, euphoric, hostile, withdrawn, suspicious, inappropriate, "speeding," or labile.

F. Thought.

1. Abnormal thought process.

   a. Looseness of associations, i.e., varying degrees of slippage in logical connections from mild rambling (tangential or circumstantial speech) to incoherence ("word salad"), as opposed to normal goal-directed conversation. (Note that apparent looseness may result from memory dysfunction in cases of organic mental disorders.)

   b. Looseness should be distinguished from the flight of ideas or pressured speech in mania (fast but understandable if one slows the patient down).

   c. Various types of faulty logic may also be seen.

2. Abnormal thought content.

   a. Delusions.—Fixed false beliefs that are not amenable to change via persuasion or evidence. Types are persecutory, grandiose, somatic, and depressive.

   b. Ideas of references.—Interpreting events falsely as related to oneself. ("The TV anchorman is sending me personal messages.")

   c. Feelings of influence.—Belief that one's thoughts or actions are controlled by other persons or uncanny forces.

   d. Thought broadcasting.—Belief that one's thoughts are audible to others or that one's mind can be read.

   e. Somatic preoccupations.—Unrealistic concern with one's body or fear of disease that is not responsive to facts or reassurance.

   f. Derealization.—Feeling that the world is unreal, as if in a dream.

g. Depersonalization.—Feeling that oneself is unreal, e.g., an inanimate object.

h. Suicidal thoughts.—Inquire about these in *every* depressed patient.

i. Homicidal thoughts.

3. Abnormal perception.

a. Illusions.—False interpretations of actual perceptions, e.g., belief that a passing cloud represents a radioactive vapor (compare with delusions).

b. Hallucinations.—False perceptions in the absence of external stimuli.

(1) Auditory.—Most common in schizophrenia.

(2) Visual, gustatory, olfactory, or tactile.—Most common in organic mental disorders including drug intoxications. *If present, assume an organic cause until proved otherwise.*

G. Cognition.

1. Testing cognitive (intellectual) function is perhaps the most crucial factor in evaluating psychiatric patients. *Impairment of cognition is pathognomonic of organic mental disorders,* many of which are due to medical, neurological, pharmacological, or surgical pathology. It is thus extremely important to evaluate cognitive function in order to accurately diagnose and treat the illness. Many people have died because treatable medical or surgical illnesses were not considered because of psychiatric symptoms.

2. Cognitive function testing includes evaluation of the following:

a. Level of consciousness.

b. Orientation.

c. Attention.

d. Memory.

e. Fund of information.

3. The level of consciousness may vary from full

alertness, through various levels of obtundation, to frank coma.

4. Orientation.
   a. The patient should be "oriented × 4," i.e., to situation, time, place, and person.
   b. Impaired orientation indicates severe cognitive dysfunction. However, the presence of orientation × 4 does *not* rule out organic mental disorder.

5. Attention.
   a. When grossly impaired, wandering attention and distractibility are obvious.
   b. Subtle degrees of impairment are tested by asking the patient to repeat a series of numbers. (A normal person can repeat six digits in the same order as spoken by the examiner and four in reverse order.) Simple two-digit arithmetic calculations can also be tested.

6. Memory.
   a. Immediate memory is evaluated by the examiner mentioning three words or objects; the patient should be able to remember these at 1- and 5-minute intervals.
   b. Recent memory is tested by asking the patient about events of the last few hours or days. Confabulation is ruled out by asking the same question more than once.
   c. Remote memory is reflected in the capacity to give a past medical history. The examiner should be sure that failure is due to the inability to remember as opposed to a lack of interest or cooperation.

7. Fund of information.
   a. The patient should have a knowledge appropriate to his age and social situation.
   b. Information can include current events, political figures or others in the news, or local geography.

IV. Diagnostic Categories of Psychiatric Syndromes

A. Psychiatric presentations are broadly divided between psychotic and nonpsychotic disorders (Fig 30–1).

B. Psychotic disorders are further divided into two general categories: organic and nonorganic (sometimes called functional). This division is made on the basis of the MSE.

1. Organic disorders cause abnormal cognitive function.

   a. Organicity may be acute (delirium) or chronic (dementia).

   b. Medical, surgical, neurological, or pharmacological causes underlie many organic disorders. A correct diagnosis is therefore crucial.

2. Nonorganic (functional) psychoses do not generally cause abnormal cognitive function, although other parts of the MSE may show substantial impairment. The nonorganic psychoses include the following:

   a. Schizophrenia.

   b. Mood disorders (major depression and bipolar disorders).

3. Nonpsychotic disorders.

   a. The MSE findings are normal. The patient is neither confused nor psychotic.

   b. ED visits are often due to acute anxiety reactions.

V. Organic Mental Disorders

Organic mental disorders may be either acute (delirium) or chronic (dementia) and are characterized by *impaired cognitive function* on MSE.

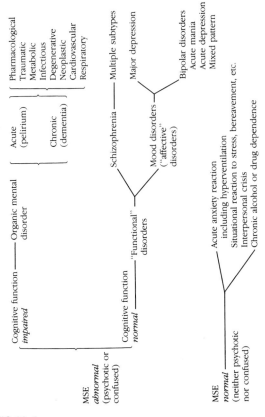

FIG 30–1.

Diagnostic flowchart. Note that testing of cognitive function part of the mental status examination (MSE) is crucial to the differential diagnosis.

A. General considerations.
   1. Cause.—Medical illness presenting psychiatrically (Table 30–1).
      a. Medications or abused drugs.
      b. Endocrine or metabolic disorders.
      c. Infections: systemic or CNS.
      d. Neurological degenerative diseases.
      e. Seizure disorders, especially postictal states.
      f. Chronic subdural hematoma.
      g. Oncological diseases including cerebral metastases or hormone-producing tumors.
      h. Autoimmune disorders.
      i. Vascular occlusion.
   2. Early recognition of the underlying medical or surgical cause is essential.
   3. A frequent error is to neglect an adequate medical workup in patients who already carry a psychiatric diagnosis and now have new symptoms, particularly impaired cognitive function.
   4. Clues to an underlying medical or surgical cause are the following:
      a. Personality change after the age of 40.
      b. Onset of psychiatric symptoms related in time to the onset or exacerbation of medical illness or trauma or to a change in medications.
      c. Prominent cognitive dysfunction (disorientation, inattention, memory loss).
      d. Hallucinations other than auditory.
      e. Brief or transient behavioral aberrations lasting minutes or hours (rule out especially psychomotor seizures or postictal states following major motor seizures).
B. Acute organic mental disorders (delirium or acute encephalopathy).
   1. Definition.—An *acute* global impairment of brain function, usually transient and/or treatable. Although delirium can mimic any major

TABLE 30–1.
Common Medical Illnesses Presenting as "Psychiatric" Disorders*

Metabolic disorders.—Glucose, sodium, calcium, or magnesium imbalance, acid/base imbalance, acute hypoxia or posthypoxic encephalopathy, renal failure, hepatic failure, anemia, copper disorders (Wilson's disease)

Endocrine disorders.—Thyroid disease, parathyroid disease, adrenal hormone imbalance (corticosteroids, mineralocorticoids, catecholamines [pheochromocytoma]), other catecholamine disorder (carcinoid), insulinoma

Infectious diseases.—Encephalitis, meningitis, brain abscess, tertiary syphilis, generalized sepsis or any severe systemic infection

Trauma.—Concussion or postconcussive syndrome, intracranial hematoma (especially occult subdural hematoma)

Cardiovascular disorders.—Cardiac dysrhythmia, hypotension, TIA,† CVA, migraine, vasculitis (temporal arteritis, lupus, periarteritis nodosa), hypertensive encephalopathy, multi-infarct dementia

Neoplastic diseases.—CNS tumors or metastases, remote tumors with hormonal secretion (insulin, ADH, ACTH)

Degenerative diseases.—Senile or presenile dementia of the Alzheimer type

Drug abuse.—Alcohol, barbiturates, sedative hypnotics, amphetamines and other stimulants, hallucinogens

Drug reactions.—L-Dopa, steroids, β-adrenergic blockers, antihypertensives (reserpine, α-methyldopa, hydralazine), cardiac drugs (digoxin, quinidine, procainamide, lidocaine), bronchodilators (methylxanthines [aminophylline], β-adrenergic agonists [ephedrine, terbutaline]), anticonvulsants, thyroid preparations, cimetidine, isoniazid, rifampin

*From Callham M, Bresler MJ, Hoffman RS: Behavioral emergencies, in Callaham M (ed): *Current Therapy in Emergency Medicine.* Philadelphia, BC Decker, 1987. Used with permission.
†TIA = transient ischemic attack; CVA = cerebrovascular accident; ADH = antidiuretic hormone; ACTH = adrenocorticotropic hormone.

psychiatric disorder, the hallmark is that *cognitive* (intellectual) functioning is acutely impaired over a period of several hours to days.

2. Characteristics.

a. Impaired cognition is demonstrated on MSE (disorientation, memory dysfunction, decreased level of consciousness, or reduced fund of information).

b. Sudden or recent onset in the context of medical illness, trauma, or drugs. However, these factors may not be apparent initially.

c. Fluctuation of signs, even minute to minute, which tend to increase at night.

d. Disorders of any of the following: behavior (psychomotor agitation, apathy), mood (excited, apathetic, labile), thought process (disordered speech), thought content (delusions), or perception (hallucinations).

3. Cause.—Often lies outside the CNS. Causes include systemic infections, metabolic disorders, hepatic or renal disease, thiamine deficiency, drug intoxication or withdrawal, hypertensive encephalopathy, hypotension, hypoxia, encephalitis, postictal state, and subdural hematoma.

4. Differential diagnosis.—Nonorganic (functional) disorders such as schizophrenia, mania, or major depression.

5. Management.

a. An immediate medical workup is mandatory. The patient should be admitted to a medical or surgical service. A toxicology screen of urine and blood should be obtained as soon as possible when appropriate.

b. The major danger is to misdiagnose acute organic disorders as nonorganic psychosis. *Testing of cognition on MSE will avoid this pitfall.*

c. Another error is to misdiagnose an acute, potentially treatable delirium as chronic dementia. Taking an accurate history is crucial. Remember that dementia proceeds very slowly; if a known demented patient *acutely* becomes worse, a superimposed delirium is usually present, and the cause must be found.

C. Chronic organic mental disorders (dementia).

1. Definition.—A progressive impairment of *cognitive* function, usually of insidious onset and *gradual* course.

2. Characteristics.

a. Impaired cognition (especially memory).

b. Subtle or major personality change, impaired judgment, and occasionally frankly psychotic symptoms (*nonauditory* hallucinations, delusions).

c. Fluctuation of symptoms, worse at night.

3. Cause.

a. Most common are primary degenerative dementia of the Alzheimer type and multi-infarct dementia.

b. Other causes—many of which are treatable—may be CNS or non-CNS related.

(1) CNS.—Hemorrhage (especially chronic subdural hematoma), infarct, low-pressure hydrocephalus, tumors.

(2) Non-CNS.—Neoplasm, nutrition (vitamin B_{12}, folate), endocrine, toxic, metabolic.

4. Differential diagnosis.

a. Major depression.—Depressed patients may perform poorly on cognitive tests owing to a lack of motivation (pseudodementia).

b. Delirium.—Elderly patients, even with a clear history of progressive dementia, may have a rapid onset of confusion, clouded consciousness, delusions, hallucinations, or agitation; this most often represents a superimposed delirium related to underlying medical illness.

    c. Chronic schizophrenia.—In late stages of schizophrenia, apathy may lead to poor performance on cognitive testing.

  5. Management.—Admission as indicated to a psychiatry or neurology service for a definitive workup.

D. *DSM-III-R.*

  1. *The Diagnostic and Statistical Manual of Mental Disorders,* third edition, revised (American Psychiatric Association: *Diagnostic and Statistical Manual of Mental Disorders,* ed 3, revised. Washington, DC, American Psychiatric Association, 1987.), is the official psychiatric classification system of the American Psychiatric Association. It is frequently revised in accordance with the continuing evolution of our understanding of mental disorders. The actual definitions of the various psychiatric terms thus have changed over the years and continue to do so.

  2. Because the emphasis in emergency medicine is somewhat different from that in general psychiatry, we have elected in this book to use a slightly different classification scheme (see Fig 30–1). This emergency medicine classification system stresses the difference between acute vs. chronic organic mental disorders because immediate treatment and disposition in the ED are largely a function of the degree of acuity.

  3. Organic mental disorders—*DSM-III-R.*
DSM-III-R considers organic mental disorders in three broad categories.

    a. Dementias arising in the senium and presenium.—Primary degenerative dementia of the Alzheimer type and multi-infarct dementia.

    b. Psychoactive substance–induced organic mental disorders.—Acute intoxication and withdrawal syndromes of the various drugs.

c. Organic mental disorders associated with specific physical disorders or whose etiology is unknown.

4. Delirium and dementia—*DSM-III-R.*—The current use of these words roughly corresponds with the acute-vs.-chronic implications implied earlier in this chapter. However, the *DSM-III-R* further defines each of these words with characteristics not specifically relating to the level of acuity.

VI. Nonorganic Psychoses

Previously called "functional" psychoses, schizophrenia and the mood disorders are distinguished by abnormal findings on the MSE but *normal cognitive function.*

A. Schizophrenia.
1. Definition.—A psychotic disorder that may be acute or chronic, often relapsing or remitting, with impaired behavior, mood, thought process, thought content, perception, and judgment, but *without* clouding of consciousness or cognitive dysfunction. If the latter is present, the diagnosis is much more likely to be dementia or delirium.
2. Characteristics.
   a. Onset in adolescence or early adulthood (nobody gets it after 45).
   b. Poor premorbid history, e.g., a long history of social withdrawal, eccentricity, and impaired educational/vocational function.
   c. Family history of schizophrenia often positive.
   d. Psychotic symptoms.—Bizarre delusions (usually persecutory); *auditory* hallucinations; loose associations or incoherence; blunted, flat, or inappropriate affect; bizarre motor mannerisms, e.g., catatonic posturing or unresponsiveness.

      e. *No* clouding of consciousness, disorientation, confusion, or cognitive impairment as in delirium or dementia.

   3. Management.

      a. Decide whether psychiatric hospitalization, urgent or elective, is indicated. If not, provide for psychiatriac follow-up.

      b. For psychotic agitation, give haloperidol (Haldol), 5 mg, or chlorpromazine (Thorazine), 50 mg, orally or intramuscularly; this may be repeated every hour until the patient is calm.

         (1) Postural hypotension may occur with these drugs, especially with chlorpromazine. Monitoring of the blood pressure is therefore important.

         (2) Dystonic (extrapyramidol) side effects may also occur, especially with haloperidol. These may be controlled with benztropine mesylate (cogentin), 2 mg, or diphenhydramine (Benadryl), 50 mg, either orally or intramuscularly.

      c. Treatment will eventually include an antipsychotic agent; haloperidol or chlorpromazine may be started on a two- or three-times-a-day schedule pending referral.

B. Mood disorders, (previously called affective disorders).

   1. There are two types: bipolar disorder, consisting of recurrent episodes of mania and depression, and unipolar depressive disorder, consisting of depressions alone. At a given time, a patient is said to be suffering a manic episode or a depressive episode, depending on the direction of the mood swing.

   2. Characteristics of manic episodes.

      a. Euphoric or irritable mood.

      b. Pressure of speech, flight, of ideas, racing thoughts.

    c. Inflated self-esteem, often to point of grandiose delusions.

    d. Restlessness, increased activity, decreased need for sleep.

    e. Self-destructive activities, e.g., spending sprees, hypersexuality, foolish investments or projects, reckless driving, all inconsistent with previous behavior.

    f. With severe impairment, bizarre delusions, hallucinations, and incoherence.

    g. A useful point to remember is that manic patients can be humorous, whereas schizophrenic patients generally cannot.

3. Characteristics of major depressive episodes.

    a. A depressed mood with a loss of interest in usual activities; must be prominent, persistent (not momentary mood shifts from day to day), and severe enough to impair daily functioning.

    b. Poor appetite and weight loss or increased appetite and weight gain.

    c. Insomnia or hypersomnia.

    d. Psychomotor retardation or agitation.

    e. Fatigue, loss of energy, and multiple somatic complaints.

    f. Feelings of worthlessness, self-reproach, or guilt. These may be of delusional proportions but are consistent with depression, and not bizarre as in schizophrenia.

    g. Suicidal ideation.

    h. *No* cognitive dysfunction suggesting delirium or dementia (distinguish depressive refusal to answer test questions from actual cognitive inpairment).

4. Management.

    a. Psychiatric hospitalization is usually indicated.

    b. Always assess for suicidal intent in patients with any level of depression.

        c. Definitive treatment includes lithium for mania and antidepressants or electroconvulsive therapy (ECT) for major depression. However, the initial use of antipsychotic agents may be helpful, especially in emergency situations involving agitation, e.g., chlorpromazine or haloperidol in the same doses as for schizophrenia (see Section A,3).

        d. Be sure to rule out organic causes, especially in patients over 40.

    5. *Note:* Patients with major mood (affective) disorders usually function normally between acute episodes of mania or depression. By contrast, schizophrenic patients often appear abnormal or eccentric and function poorly between acute exacerbations of their illness. Such history greatly assists in the diagnosis.

VII. Nonpsychotic Disorders

The hallmark of nonpsychotic disorders is MSE findings that are essentially normal (neither confused nor psychotic). Nonpsychotic behavioral problems are common in the ED.

    A. Chronic alcohol or drug dependence.—Acute intoxication and withdrawal are discussed in Section VIII. These may impair cognitive function and result in abnormal MSE findings.

    B. Acute anxiety reactions.

        1. The MSE reveals signs of anxiety but not those of psychosis or cognitive dysfunction.

        2. Acute anxiety frequently is related to certain physical symptoms. In addition to feelings of tension, restlessness, or dread, prominent symptoms may include tremulousness, abdominal cramps, diarrhea, headache, and the hyperventilation syndrome (panic, dyspnea, paresthesias, dizziness, carpopedal spasm, and sometimes chest discomfort or syncope).

3. After appropriate medical workup as indicated (e.g., electrocardiogram [ECG] and a blood gas determination), the principal treatment is reassurance, with an explanation of how stress or anxiety can produce real physical symptoms. Bag rebreathing may be helpful in treating hyperventilation. During acute panic states, a one-time dose or a short course of benzodiazepines may be useful. Psychiatric follow-up is important in preventing a recurrence.

VIII. Drug Abuse

A. General considerations.
   1. While patients with chronic drug abuse present frequently to the ED with a variety of related medical and emotional problems, the emergencies directly caused by drugs are generally due to either acute intoxication or acute withdrawal.
   2. Medical management of intoxication and withdrawal is discussed more fully in Chapter 29. The following section deals primarily with the behavioral manifestations, many of which cause acute encephalopathy (delirium).
B. Specific drug syndromes.
   1. Alcohol.
      a. Simple intoxication.—No specific treatment is necessary unless the following occur:
         (1) Deep coma with aspiration or impairment of ventilation.
         (2) Descending level of consciousness. Suspect a mixture with other drugs or associated medical condition, e.g., trauma.
         (3) Suicidal or assaultive risk. This generally clears as the alcohol is metabolized.
         (4) Gross disorientation, confusion, agitation, or bizarre psychotic thinking. This

requires hospitalization on a psychiatric or medical unit for protection and diagnosis.

b. Intoxication with medical complications of alcohol abuse (head trauma, gastrointestinal tract bleeding, pancreatitis).

c. Wernicke-Korsakoff syndrome.—In a chronic drinker after a binge: confusion, memory deficit, ataxia, nystagmus, ocular palsies. Treat with intravenous thiamine after determining a serum level to confirm the diagnosis.

d. Alcohol withdrawal (see Chapter 17, p 125).—Escalating tremulousness, weakness, ataxia, confusion, agitation, delusions, visual or tactile hallucinations, seizures.

(1) In early stages of tremulousness, give chlordiazepoxide, 50 to 100 mg, or diazepam, 10 to 20 mg, orally every 2 hours until a response occurs. Oral absorption is faster than intramuscular. One half the oral dosage may be used intravenously.

(2) Full-blown delirium tremens has more than a 15% mortality. Admit the patient to an inpatient service that can provide full medical treatment including benzodiazepines and electrolyte and fluid management.

2. Opiates.

a. Intoxication.—Naloxone and supportive care as indicated (see Chapter 29, p 475).

b. Withdrawal.—Uncomfortable but not dangerous; rarely requires admission; refer to methadone maintenance program for specialized treatment.

3. Barbiturates and other sedative hypnotics (see Chapter 29, p. 467).

a. Intoxication.—Usual supportive care.

b. Withdrawal.—Resembles alcohol withdrawal

with restlessness, diaphoresis, vomiting, tremors, hypotension, fever, potentially fatal seizures, and/or toxic psychosis.

   c. Hospitalize for reintoxication and gradual withdrawal.

4. CNS stimulants (amphetamines, cocaine).

   a. Intoxication.—Insomnia, euphoria or irritability, belligerence, panic reactions, paranoid ideation, hallucinations (especially visual and tactile), tachycardia, hypertension; eventually arrhythmias, fever, seizures, coma. Coronary spasm with or without myocardial infarction may also occur (see Chapter 3).

     (1) The toxic psychosis may be indistinguishable from paranoid schizophrenia.

     (2) Immediate treatment is often required: diazepam, 10 mg, chlorpromazine, 50 to 75 mg, or haloperidol, 5 to 10 mg, all orally or intramuscularly. Fever is an ominous sign; if the patient is physically deteriorating, antipsychotic agents (haloperidol or phenothiazines) have a specific neutralizing effect because of their dopamine-blocking properties.

     (3) Respiratory support if indicated.

   b. Withdrawal.—Fatigue, weakness, hypersomnia. Severe depression can be a complication, but it is treatable with tricyclic antidepressants.

5. Hallucinogens (LSD, PCP, marijuana) (see Chapter 29, p 472).

   a. Medical complications are relatively benign (see Chapter 29), but psychiatric ones can be severe and lethal, e.g., falls or accidents.

   b. Mild "bad trip".—Extended period of intoxication, panic reactions.

   c. Severe intoxication.—Toxic delirium with agitation, thought disorder, delusions, hallucinations. PCP produces a virulent picture of extreme agitation and violence plus neurological findings. Death can result from violence or suicide (acute renal failure from rhabdomyolysis has been reported).

d. Management.—For mild bad trips, "talking down" often suffices. For severe reactions, admit to psychiatry service. Withhold antipsychotic agents for at least 24 hours if possible to permit an accurate diagnosis (rule out schizophrenia), but sedation is acceptable with agents such as diazepam or diphenhydramine. If the symptoms are very severe or continue beyond 24 to 48 hours, antipsychotic agents may be used.

IX. Life-Threatening Psychiatric Conditions

Patients may require hospitalization involuntarily if their condition appears to be life-threatening. Such risk generally falls within three categories.

A. Suicide risk.—The following factors are associated with higher risk:
1. Detailed plan or recent attempt.
2. Previous serious attempt.
3. Advanced age, living alone, unemployed, with no money or other resources.
4. Major depressive illness, schizophrenia, chronic alcoholism, or delirium.
5. Immobilization and feeling of life impasse without solutions persisting after interview; no response to helpful advice, interventions, and referrals.

B. Homicidal risk.—Factors associated with high risk are as follows:
1. Concrete plans and preparations.
2. Past history of violence—the best predictor.
3. Persecutory delusions, with the potential victim seen as the main persecutor.

4. Intoxication or chronic use of drugs thought to stimulate or release violent behavior: alcohol, amphetamines, cocaine, or hallucinogens (especially PCP).

5. A provocative victim (e.g., spouse who goads patient with "You'd never have the guts" or repeatedly starts violent arguments).

6. Postpartum depression, which is associated with the risk of injury to the newborn.

7. Factors associated with a loss of control: constant preoccupation with the homicidal ideas, no concern about expected legal consequences, state of agitation or rage objectively evident, no response to the interview in terms of relaxation and increased control.

C. Grave mental disability (defined as a state of impaired judgment such that the patient is unable to provide for basic needs such as food, clothing, and shelter).

1. Many patients with a functional psychosis or organic mental disorder are gravely disabled, but many are not and function quite well.

2. In contrast, persons without psychiatric illness who are under severe stress may occasionally develop acute panic reactions that disable them as much as would a psychosis.

3. Assessment is carried out by attention to three sources of information.

   a. MSE evidence of gross impairment in thought processes (looseness, incoherence), thought content (extensive delusions), perception (hallucinations), and especially cognitive function (disorientation, confusion, memory loss).

   b. Questions posed to the patient to test judgment. Inquire in detail about the patient's immediate plans: destination after leaving the ED; method of transportation; arrangements for meals, sleeping, income; etc. If the answers are unintelligible or unconvincing, a grave disability is presumed.

c. Information from family, friends, and other professionals who know the patient. Some seriously impaired patients may converse normally, whereas such collateral information may reveal severe deterioration in life functioning.

X. Differential Diagnosis and Disposition

A. Differential diagnosis (see Fig 30–1).

1. The essential distinctions are between the following:

   a. Psychotic and nonpsychotic.

   b. If psychotic or confused, the differential diagnosis is between an organic mental disorder and a "functional" psychosis (schizophrenia or mood disorder).

   c. If organic, the differential diagnosis is between delirium and dementia.

2. The distinction between psychotic and nonpsychotic is frequently made immediately and intuitively when the patient is severely disturbed. The psychotic patient is recognized by thought disorder, gross confusion, or inappropriate, bizarre, or unexpected behavior. In questionable cases, the best way to elicit psychotic material is to permit the patient to speak freely and encourage him with broad-focus questions.

3. Once a patient is determined to be psychotic, the distinction must be made between organic (delirium or dementia) and functional (schizophrenia or affective) disorders. This distinction rests *solely* on the findings of cognitive dysfunction (consciousness, orientation, attention, memory, fund of information, and abstraction).

Accordingly, the MSE with these test questions should *never* be omitted with any seriously disturbed patient. Misdiagnosis in either direction may result in grossly inappropriate treatment.

4. If cognitive testing reveals the patient to have an organic mental disorder (impaired cognitive function), the distinction between acute (delirium) and chronic (dementia) is made by history. This may require collateral history from others.

5. If the patient is found to have a functional psychosis, further distinction is made among schizophrenia, mania, and major depression with the help of a history and the MSE.

   a. If the disturbance recurs as discrete episodes lasting weeks to months with excellent function between, it is probably an affective disorder (mania or depression).

   b. If the patient has residual symptoms or signs and poor functioning between acute episodes, the disturbance is probably schizophrenia.

   c. A number of medical illnesses and drugs produce "secondary" depression, mania, or psychosis, rather than the strictly "functional" type, and these should always be considered.

6. In a nonpsychotic patient, further diagnostic distinctions are made by history; the categories in Figure 31–1 are self-explanatory. Except for the highly agitated patient who will require some verbal management and possibly a few doses of sedative medication, the major goal with such patients is correct triage and referral for psychotherapy, special treatment programs, social services, or psychiatric hospitalization in the case of suicidal or homicidal ideation.

7. As a final note on diagnosis in the elderly: one should always maintain a high index of suspi-

cion of organic mental disorders. The major pitfall with the elderly is failing to distinguish major depression, which may be treatable, from dementia, which is often less amenable to treatment. Although affective symptoms such as depression or anxiety may occur in patients with dementia, elderly patients with major depression may be too inert and unmotivated to make any effort to answer cognitive test questions and thus be mistakenly diagnosed as demented. Such patients with "pseudodementia" may then be denied effective antidepressant drugs or ECT—and worse, be consigned to a nursing home or a state hospital. These facts again emphasize the importance of adequate cognitive testing in the elderly.

B. Disposition.

   1. Indications for *medical* hospitalization.

      a. Delirium due to medical illness, trauma, or unknown cause.

      b. Serious drug intoxication.

      c. Withdrawal syndrome from alcohol (delirium tremens), barbiturates, or other sedative hypnotics.

      d. Certain medical illnesses manifesting themselves psychiatrically (even if not delirium), e.g., endocrine or metabolic encephalopathies or temporal lobe epilepsy.

   2. Indications for urgent (involuntary if necessary) *psychiatric* hospitalization.

      a. Suicidal risk.

      b. Homicidal or assaultive risk.

      c. Grave mental disability.

      d. Initial presentation of acute behavioral changes in an elderly patient.

   3. Indications for elective psychiatric hospitalization depend on the individual's medical, emotional, and social situation.

4. If hospitalization is not indicated, decide on immediate treatment (reassurance or medication) and arrange for appropriate follow-up (psychiatric referral, medical referral, drug or alcohol treatment program, or social service involvement).

Index

A

Abdominal aortic aneurysm,
238–239
Abdominal emergencies,
167–184
acute inflammatory disease
and, 172–175
anorectal conditions and,
181–184
constipation and, 175–176
diarrhea and, 176
intestinal obstruction and,
167–172
massive gastrointestinal
hemorrhage and,
179–181
traumatic wounds and,
176–179
Abdominal irradiation effects,
340
Abdominal reflex in spine
injuries, 161
Abdominal x-ray
aortic aneurysm and, 239
intestinal obstruction and,
168, 169, 172
peptic ulcer and, 173
poisoning and overdose and,
444
arsenic, 481
iron, 463

lead, 461
Abductor pollicis longus, 262,
264
Abortion
rape and, 212
spontaneous, 201–202
Abrasion of cornea, 319–320
Abruptio placenta, 208–209
Abscess, 221–228
axillary, 228
Bartholinian, 207
definition of, 213
dental emergencies and, 311
perirectal, 181–182, 228
peritonsillar, 305
Absorption spectrophotometer
in lead poisoning, 461
Accidental tattoo, 284
Acetaminophen
chemotherapy side effects
and, 343
head injuries and, 158
overdose of, 476–477
antidote for, 447
determining level of, 444,
477, 478–479
pediatrics and
fever in, 358
seizures in, 360
tonsillitis and pharyngitis
in, 370
Acetanilid, 348

529

Acetazolamide
  angle-closure glaucoma and,
    318
  central retinal artery
    occlusion and, 318
Acetone, 128
Acetylcholine
  black widow spider and, 489
  organophosphate poisoning
    and, 466
Acetylcholinesterase, 466
N-Acetylcysteine,
    acetaminophen
    overdose and, 447, 477
Acetylsalicylic acid (*see*
    Aspirin)
Acid-base balance in
    hyperglycemia,
    128–129
Acid-base disorders, 51–56
    (*see also* Acidosis;
    Alkalosis)
Acid diuresis, 455
Acidosis
  adrenal crisis and, 133
  ventricular tachycardia and,
    38
Acids
  burns of conjunctiva and
    cornea and, 314
  caustic ingestion and, 296
ACLS termination (*see*
    Advanced cardiac life
    support termination)
Aconitine, 493, 498, 499
Acoustic neuroma, 146
Acquired immunodeficiency
    syndrome, 325–331
Acromioclavicular separation,
    244
Activated charcoal, 450–451,
    477
  ethyl alcohol and, 484
  mercury and, 477
  organophosphates and, 466

phencyclidine and, 474
  tranquilizers and, 469
  tricyclic antidepressants and,
    471
Acute myocardial infarction,
    17–24 (*see also*
    Myocardial
    infarction)
Acute respiratory failure,
    83–86
Acyclovir
  herpes genitalis and, 206
  herpes simplex and, 399
  herpes zoster and, 399
  stomatitis and, 312
Addisonian crisis in cancer,
    338
ADH (*see* Antidiuretic
    hormone)
Adnexal mass
  ectopic pregnancy and, 201
  ovarian cyst and, 204
  pelvic inflammatory disease
    and, 203
Adrenal crisis, 132–133
Adrenal insufficiency in cancer,
    338
α-Adrenergics, tranquilizer
    overdose and, 469
β-Adrenergics
  cardiogenic pulmonary
    edema and, 24
  psychiatric disorders and,
    511
  tranquilizer overdose and,
    469
Adrenocorticosteroids
  hydrocarbon overdose and,
    465
  septic shock and, 10
Adult respiratory distress
    syndrome
  acute respiratory failure and,
    84
  lung contusion and, 111

thermal burns and, 409
viral pneumonia and, 82, 83
Advanced cardiac life support
termination, 41–42
Adynamic ileus, 168–169
Aeromonas, 329
Affective disorders, 516–518
Aged, psychiatric emergencies
in, 525–526
AHF (*see* Antihemophilic
factor)
AIDS (*see* Acquired
immunodeficiency
syndrome)
AIDS-related complex, 326
Airway management
anaphylactic shock and, 384
cardiac arrest and, 42–47
head injuries and, 155
neurological emergencies
and, 117, 124
regional anesthesia toxicity
and, 435
spine injuries and, 163
thermal burns and, 408
thoracic injuries and, 97–99
trauma and, 11
Airway obstruction, 293–294
foreign body and, 294–296
Akee plant, 493
Albumin, false calcium levels
and, 73
Alcohol (*see also* Ethanol)
atrial fibrillation and, 31
atrial flutter and, 30
dialysis and, 456
diuresis and, 456
facial injuries and, 276
multifocal atrial tachycardia
and, 30
neurological emergencies
and, 125–127
nonpsychotic disorders and,
518
nystagmus and, 157

overdose of, 519–520
premature ventricular
contractions and, 36
psychiatric disorders and,
511
violence and, 502, 523
Aldomet (*see* Methyldopa)
Alkaline diuresis, 455
Alkalis
in burns of conjunctiva and
cornea, 314
ingestion of, 296
Alkaloids in plants, 493, 496
Alkalosis
bronchial asthma and, 378
false calcium levels and, 73
Allen test, 265
Allergic emergencies, 377–388
anaphylactic shock and,
384–387
angioedema and, 387
bronchial asthma and,
377–383
chemotherapy reactions and,
343
serum sickness and,
387–388
urticaria and, 387
Allergic shock, 384–387
Alpha-adrenergics, tranquilizer
overdose and, 469
Aluminum magnesium
hydroxide, 500
Alveolar partial pressure of
oxygen, 85
Amanita poisoning, 491–492
hemoperfusion and, 457
Amantadine, 83
American Psychiatric
Association, 514
Amines in plants, 493
Aminoglycosides
meningitis and, 335
pyelonephritis and,
192

Aminophylline
  anaphylactic shock and, 385
  bronchial asthma and, 380,
    382
  cardiogenic pulmonary
    edema and, 24
  pediatrics and
    asthma in, 364
    dosage in, 371–372
  psychiatric disorders and,
    511
Amitriptyline, 143
Ammonia
  caustic ingestion and, 296
  gastric lavage and, 450
Ammonium chloride
  acid diuresis and, 455
  phencyclidine overdose and,
    475
Ammonium hydroxide
    ingestion, 465
Amniotic fluid embolism, 208
Amobarbital, 153
Amoxicillin
  bites and, 218, 219
  cystitis and, 191
  gonococcal dermatitis and,
    394
  otitis media and, 307
  sinusitis and, 309
Amoxicillin/clavulanic acid
  bites and, 218, 219
  otitis media and, 307
Amphetamine overdose
  cardiac effects of, 443
  dialysis and, 456
  diuresis and, 456
  psychiatric emergencies and,
    511, 521
  violence and, 502, 523
Ampicillin
  bacterial vaginosis and, 206
  bronchial asthma and,
    382

gonococcal dermatitis and,
    394
  Haemophilus pneumonia
    and, 80, 370–371
  meningitis and, 335, 368,
    369
  otitis media and, 307, 370
  paranasal sinus fracture and,
    291
  pediatrics and
    epiglottitis in, 363–364
    Haemophilus influenzae
      pneumonia in, 370–371
    meningitis in, 368, 369
    otitis media in, 370
    pneumonia in, 370
  pyelonephritis and, 192
  septic shock and, 9
  sinusitis and, 309
Amputation
  frostbite and, 414
  hand and, 273
A MUDPIE, 483
Amylase
  pancreatitis and, 175
  septic shock and, 9
Amyl nitrate, 480
Amyl nitrite, 480
Amytal, 153
Anal fissure, 375
Anaphylactic shock, 1,
    384–387
  causes of, 1
  clinical findings in, 2
Anatomy of hand, 260–263
Andromedotoxin alkaloid, 498,
    499
Anemia
  emergent, 345–346
  hemolytic, 346, 347, 348
  lead poisoning and, 461
  red cell destruction,
    346–348
  syncope and, 139

Anesthesia, 419–439
  muscular paralysis and,
    438–439
  regional, 419–436
    complications of, 433–436
    local infiltration block
      and, 419–420
    nerve block and, 420–433
      (*see also* Regional
      nerve blocks)
  sedation and, 436–438
Anesthetic spray for airway
  obstruction, 294
Aneurysm
  aortic, 237–239
  false, 230
Angioedema, 387
Angle-closure glaucoma,
  318–319
Aniline overdose, 453
Animal venoms, 484–489
Anion gap
  metabolic acidosis and, 54
  respiratory acidosis and, 53
Ankle injuries, 254–255
Ankle stretch reflex in spine
  injuries, 160
Anorectal conditions, 181–184
Anorexia in appendicitis, 173
Anoscopy, 182
Anterior tibial muscle, spinal
  cord levels and, 161
Anthracyclines, 341–343
Antiarrhythmics, 38
Antibiotics (*see also specific
    antibiotic*)
  abdominal gunshot wounds
    and, 179
  bacterial conjunctivitis and,
    323
  bites and, 218
  caustic ingestion and,
    297

central nervous system
    infection and, 130–132
  corneal abrasion and,
    319–320
  dialysis and, 456
  epiglottitis and, 363
  felon and, 226
  foreign bodies in eye and,
    317
  hand fractures and, 272
  herpes genitalis and, 206
  infective endocarditis and,
    216
  meningitis and, 335, 336
  olecranon bursitis and,
    228
  open fracture and, 15
  paronychium and, 227
  pulmonary aspiration and,
    90
  pyelonephritis and, 192
  rape and, 211
  septic shock and, 9
  soft-tissue infections and,
    213–214
  thermal burns and, 408
  wound infections and, 215
Anticholinergics
  cystitis and, 192
  overdose of
    antidote for, 447
    dialysis and, 457
    symptoms of, 442
  pupils and, 123
Anticoagulants in
    gastrointestinal
    hemorrhage, 180 (*see
    also specific
    anticoagulant*)
Anticonvulsants, 149–153
  head injuries and, 158
  psychiatric disorders and,
    511

Antidepressants
  cardiac arrest and, 39
  mood disorders and, 518
  premature ventricular
    contractions and, 36
  syndrome of inappropriate
    secretion of antidiuretic
    hormone and, 339
  torsade de pointes and, 38
Antidiarrheal medication in
  fecal impaction, 181
Antidiuretic hormone
  hyponatremia and, 63
  syndrome of inappropriate
    secretion of, 338–339
Antidotes for poisoning and
  overdose, 446, 447–449
Antiemetics in chemotherapy,
  341
Antifreeze (*see* Ethylene
  glycol)
Antihemophilic factor, 353,
  355
Antihistamines
  anaphylactic shock and, 385,
    386
  angioedema and, 387
  atopic dermatitis and, 389
  bronchial asthma and, 381
  chemotherapy and, 343
  dialysis and, 457
  drug eruption and, 393
  rabies and, 221
  serum sickness and, 388
  urticaria and, 387, 403
  vertigo and, 147
Antihypertensives
  atrioventricular block and,
    34
  psychiatric disorders and,
    511
  syncope and, 139
Antimalarials in hemolytic
  anemia, 348

Antineoplastic drugs, 339,
  340–343
Antipruritics in urticaria, 403
Antipyretics in hemolytic
  anemia, 348 (*see also*
  specific antipyretic)
Antiseptics in facial injuries,
  276
Antivenin
  black widow spider and, 490
  coral snake bite and,
    488–489
Anxiety reactions, 518–519
  to regional nerve block, 436
Aortic aneurysm, 237–239
Aortic injuries, 112–113
Aortic insufficiency, 237, 238
Aortic valve disease, 138
Aortography
  aorta and great vessel
    injuries and, 112
  rib fracture and, 100
Apnea
  hypokalemia and, 68
  neurological emergencies
    and, 124
  spine injuries and, 163
Appendicitis, 173
  in child, 375–376
Apresoline (*see* Hydralazine)
Aqueous epinephrine (*see*
  Epinephrine)
Aramine (*see* Metaraminol)
ARC (*see* AIDS-related
  complex)
ARDS (*see* Adult respiratory
  distress syndrome)
Aristocort (*see* Fluocinonide)
Arm
  injuries of, 242–250
  regional nerve blocks and,
    423–430
Arrest
  cardiac (*see* Cardiac arrest)

cardiopulmonary (*see*
Cardiopulmonary
arrest)
Arrhythmias
carbon monoxide poisoning
and, 91
hypokalemia and, 68
syncope and, 138
ARS (*see* Equine Antirabies
Serum)
Arsenic poisoning, 481–482
Arsine gas poisoning, 481–482
Arterial blood gases (*see also*
Partial pressure)
acid-base balance and, 51
acquired immunodeficiency
syndrome and, 327, 330
acute respiratory failure and,
85
bronchial asthma and, 378,
379
cardiogenic pulmonary
edema and, 23
formulas for, 85
hypovolemic shock and, 5
metabolic acidosis and,
53–54
metabolic alkalosis and, 56
pulmonary aspiration and,
89
pulmonary embolus and, 75
respiratory acidosis and, 52
respiratory alkalosis and, 55
toxic inhalation and, 92
Arterial contusion, 230
Arterial diseases, syncope and,
139
Arterial embolization, 233
Arterial ischemia, 229–230
Arteriography
allergic reaction to,
386–387
aortic aneurysm and,
238

arterial embolization and,
233
arteriosclerosis obliterans
and, 234
femoral shaft fracture and,
251
humerus and, 246
pulmonary embolus and,
76–77
vessel injuries and, 233
Arteriosclerosis obliterans, 234
Arteriosclerotic cardiovascular
disease, 29 (*see also*
Atherosclerotic disease)
Arteriovenous fistula, 230
Arthrocentesis, 252
Arthropod bites, 489–491
Ascorbic acid
acid diuresis and, 455
phencyclidine overdose and,
474, 475
ASCVD (*see* Arteriosclerotic
cardiovascular disease)
Aspiration
needle (*see* Needle
aspiration)
peritonsillar abscess and,
305
pulmonary, 89–90
Aspirin
bronchial asthma and, 377,
381
head injuries and, 158
hemolytic anemia and, 348
metabolic acidosis and, 53
overdose of, 450
rib fracture and, 100
scarlet fever and, 397
urticaria and, 403
Asthma, 377–383
in child, 364
Asystole, ventricular (*see*
Ventricular asystole)
Atarax (*see* Hydroxyzine)

Ataxic breathing in
  neurological
  emergencies, 124
Atherosclerotic disease, 29
  aortic aneurysm and, 238
  vertigo and, 146
Atmospheric pressure injuries,
  416–417
Atomic absorption
  spectrophotometer in
  lead poisoning, 461
Atopic dermatitis, 389–391
Atracurium, 439
Atrial fibrillation, 31–32
Atrial flutter, 30–31
Atrial thrombi, 138
Atrioventricular block, 33–35
Atropine
  allergic reaction to contrast
    material and, 386–387
  as antidote, 447
  atrioventricular block and,
    34
  cardiac arrest and, 47
    pediatric, 366
  cardiogenic pulmonary
    edema and, 24
  electromechanical
    dissociation and, 49
  mushroom poisoning and,
    494, 495
  organophosphate poisoning
    and, 467
  pancuronium and, 439
  in plants, 493, 497, 498, 499
  premature ventricular
    contractions and, 36
  pupils and, 123
  regional anesthesia toxicity
    and, 435
  sinus bradycardia and, 33
  sinus tachycardia and, 26
  tubocurarine and, 438
  uveitis and, 323
    ventricular asystole and, 49
    ventricular fibrillation and,
      48
Atropine sulfate as antidote,
  449
Attention in cognition
  assessment, 507
Augmentin (*see* Amoxicillin/
  clavulanic acid)
Auricular nerve block, 423
Autoamputation in frostbite,
  414
Avulsion
  hand, 273
  tooth, 310
Axillary abscess, 228
Axillary block, 428–430
Axillary nerve injury, 243

B

Babinski reflex, 123–124, 157
Bacitracin
  bacterial conjunctivitis and,
    323
  corneal abrasion and, 320
Bacterial conjunctivitis,
  322–323
Bacterial meningitis, 131
Bacterial pneumonia, 369
Bacterial septic shock, 8
Bacterial vaginosis, 205–206
Bactrim (*see* Trimethoprim/
  sulfamethoxazole)
Bag-valve mask
  cardiac arrest resuscitation
    and, 44
  thoracic injuries and, 99
Ballet fracture, 255–256
Balloon, epistaxis, 302
Barbiturates
  convulsive disorders and,
    150
  dialysis and, 456

hemoperfusion and, 457
hydroxyzine and, 436
overdose of, 467–468
psychiatric emergencies and, 511, 520–521
regional anesthesia toxicity and, 434
Barium swallow, 295
Barotrauma, 416–417
Bartholinian abscess, 207
Battered child, 371
Battery ingestion, 465
Baxter formula, 410
Beclomethasone, 383
Beevor's sign, 162
Behavior assessment in mental status examination, 504
Belladonna compounds overdose, 457
Benadryl (*see* Diphenhydramine)
Bends in decompression illness, 417
Benign positional vertigo, 146
Benzalkonium, 466
Benzathine penicillin
    impetigo and, 400
    pediatrics and
        pharyngitis in, 370
        tonsillitis in, 370
    pharyngitis and, 304, 370
    scarlet fever and, 397
    syphilis and, 402
Benzene poisoning, 452, 454
Benzine poisoning, 453, 454
Benzocaine
    foreign body in air or food passages and, 295
    overdose of, 443
Benzodiazepines
    abscess and, 221
    alcohol withdrawal and, 126, 520
    anxiety reactions and, 519

delirium tremens and, 126
dialysis and, 457
sedation and, 437–438
Benztropine
    schizophrenia and, 516
    tranquilizer overdose and, 469
Beta-adrenergics (*see* β-Adrenergics)
Beta-hydroxybutyric acid in hyperglycemia, 128
Beta-lactamase–resistant agent, 215–216
Betamethasone
    bronchial asthma and, 382
    dermatologic disorders and, 391
Bethanechol overdose, 448
Bicarbonate value in acid-base balance, 51 (*see also* Sodium bicarbonate)
Biceps muscle, spinal cord levels and, 161
Biceps stretch reflex in spine injuries, 161
Bicillin, 304
Bier block, 430–431
    wrist and hand injuries and, 248
Bilirubin in cholecystitis, 173
Bipolar mood disorders, 516
Bismuth subsalicylate, 176
Bites, 217–219 (*see also* Rabies)
    antibiotics and, 215
Black widow spider, 489–490
Bladder infections, 193
Bladder injuries, 178, 188–189
Blakemore-Sengstaken tube, 89
Bleeding (*see* Hemorrhage)
Bleomycin sulfate, 342
Blisters in thermal burns, 408
Blood gases (*see* Arterial blood gases)

Bloodless field in hand injuries, 270, 271

Blood pressure
  hypovolemic shock and, 4, 5
  syncope and, 137

Blood transfusion in hypovolemic shock, 6

Blood urea nitrogen, 54

Blowout fracture, 322

Bone trauma, 241–257
  hip and, 250–251
  lower extremity and, 251–256
  pelvis and, 256–257
  upper extremity and, 242–250

Boxer's fracture, 249–250

Brachial plexus injury, 243

Bradycardia
  in cardiogenic pulmonary edema, 24
  fear of regional nerve blocks and, 436
  regional anesthesia toxicity and, 435
  spinal shock and, 10
  vagal reaction and, 386

Brain abscess in cancer, 335

Brain cancer, antidiuretic hormone and, 339

Brain herniation, pupils and, 156

Breast cancer
  spinal cord compression and, 333
  thrombosis and, 344

Breathing (*see also* Airway management)
  thoracic injuries and, 99
  trauma and, 11–12

Bretylium
  pediatric dosage of, 372
  premature ventricular contractions and, 36

torsade de pointes and, 39
  ventricular fibrillation and, 48
  ventricular tachycardia and, 38

Bromide overdose, 456

Bronchial asthma, 377–383
  in child, 364

Bronchial rupture, 111

Bronchiolitis, 364–365

Bronchitis, 382

Bronchodilators
  bronchial asthma and, 379–381
  multifocal atrial tachycardia and, 30
  psychiatric disorders and, 511

Bronchopneumonia in Legionnaire's disease, 82

Bronchoscopy
  pulmonary aspiration and, 90
  tracheal or bronchial rupture and, 111

Bronchospasm in cardiogenic pulmonary edema, 23, 24

Bronkosol (*see* Isoetharine)

Brown recluse spider, 490–491

Bullous impetigo, 400

BUN (*see* Blood urea nitrogen)

Bupivacaine
  local infiltration block and, 419
  rib fracture and, 101
  thrombosed hemorrhoids and, 183

Burn center, 407, 410

Burns
  caustic, 465–466

chemical
  airway, 408–409
  conjunctival and corneal, 314–315
  electrical, 410–411
    mouth and, 309–310
  respiratory, 93, 408–409
  thermal, 405–410
Burow's solution
  contact dermatitis and, 392
  herpes genitalis and, 206
  stasis dermatitis and, 392
Bursitis
  olecranon, 227–228
  trochanteric, 250–251
Busulfan, 342
Butyrophenones, 341

C

CaEDTA (*see* Calcium disodium edathamil)
Cafergot, 143
Caffeine
  headache and, 143
  premature ventricular contractions and, 36
  sinus tachycardia and, 26
Caisson disease, 416
Calamine, 393
Calcaneal fracture, 255
Calcium
  falsely elevated, 73
  hypercalcemia and, 71–73
  hypocalcemia and, 69–71
Calcium chloride
  aconitine and, 493
  cardiac arrest in child and, 366
  magnesium sulfate and, 209
  verapamil reversal and, 27–28
Calcium disodium edathamil, 461

Calcium gluconate
  black widow spider and, 490
  cardiac arrest in child and, 366
  hydrofluoric acid burns and, 466
  hyperkalemia and, 66
  hypocalcemia and, 71
  magnesium sulfate and, 209
Calomel, 477
Campylobacter
  acquired immunodeficiency syndrome and, 329
  diarrhea and, 176
Cancer emergencies (*see* Oncological emergencies)
Candida, 200
  in acquired immunodeficiency syndrome, 328
  vaginitis and, 200, 205
Carbenicillin
  gram-negative pneumonia and, 81
  meningitis and, 335
  septic shock and, 10
Carbocaine, nerve block and (*see* Mepivacaine, nerve block and)
Carbon dioxide
  partial pressure of (*see* Partial pressure of carbon dioxide)
  in respiratory acidosis, 51–52
Carbon disulfide poisoning, 479–480
Carbon monoxide
  acquired immunodeficiency syndrome and, 327, 330
  neurological emergencies and, 124

Carbon monoxide *(cont.)*
  poisoning from, 91–92
    determining level of, 444
Carbon tetrachloride overdose,
  452, 454
Carboxyhemoglobin
  carbon monoxide poisoning
    and, 91
  toxic inhalation and, 92
Carcinoma
  gastrointestinal hemorrhage
    and, 180
  herpes genitalis and, 207
Cardiac arrest, 39–49 *(see also*
    Cardiopulmonary arrest)
  airway establishment in,
    42–45
  closed cardiac compression
    in, 40–41
  defibrillation in, 47–49
  evaluation and treatment in,
    42–49
  IV line and, 45–47
  resuscitation in, 40
    termination of, 41–42
  treatment plan in, 39–40
Cardiac compression
  in child, 365
  closed, 40–41
Cardiac disorders
  anaphylactic shock and, 384
  chemotherapy and, 343
  presenting as psychiatric
    disorders, 511
  regional anesthesia toxicity
    and, 434, 435
  sickle cell disease and, 349
  syncope and, 138
Cardiac emergencies, 17–49
  acute myocardial infarction
    and, 17–24 *(see also*
    Myocardial infarction)
  cardiac arrest and, 39–49
    (see also Cardiac
    arrest)

  dysrhythmias and, 24–38
    (see also Dysrhythmias)
  torsade de pointes and,
    38–39
Cardiac failure
  cancer and, 343
  in child, 365–366
Cardiac glycosides in plants,
  498, 499
Cardiac massage, internal
  for cardiac arrest, 41
  in thoracotomy, 116
Cardiac rate in resuscitation
  monitoring, 12
Cardiac rhythm
  myocardial infarction and,
    19
  resuscitation monitoring
    and, 12, 47–49
Cardiac tamponade, 113–115
  aorta injuries and, 112
  aortic aneurysm and, 237,
    238
  obstructive shock and, 1, 3
Cardiac toxicity in
    chemotherapy, 341–343
Cardiogenic pulmonary edema
    in myocardial infarction,
    22–24
Cardiogenic shock
  causes of, 1
  clinical findings in, 2
  myocardial infarction and,
    21–22
Cardiopulmonary arrest *(see
    also* Cardiac arrest)
  cancer and, 343
  in child, 365–366
Cardiopulmonary resuscitation
    in hypothermia, 416
Cardiovascular disorders *(see*
    Cardiac disorders)
Cardioversion *(see also*
    Defibrillation)
  atrial fibrillation and, 32

atrial flutter and, 30–31
cardiogenic pulmonary
  edema and, 24
ventricular tachycardia and,
  37
Caries, 311
Carmustine, 342
Carotid sinus massage
  atrial flutter and, 30
  paroxysmal supraventricular
    tachycardia and, 27
Carotid sinus syndrome, 138
Carpal tunnel, 260, 262
Cartilage injury, 252
Cast
  ankle injuries and, 255
  bone and joint trauma and,
    242
  humerus and, 245
  metatarsal fracture and, 256
  navicular fracture and, 249
  patellar fracture and, 251
  wrist and hand injuries and,
    248
Cat bites and scratches, 217,
  218
  rabies prophylaxis and, 222
Catecholamines
  epistaxis and, 302
  premature ventricular
    contractions and, 36
Catgut
  eyelid lacerations and, 284
  suture techniques and, 278
Cathartics, poisoning and, 451
  organophosphate, 466
  phencyclidine, 474
  tricyclic antidepressant, 471
CAT scan (*see* Computed axial
  tomography scan)
Caustic burns, 296–297,
  465–466
  activated charcoal and, 451
  gastric lavage and, 450
Cautery in epistaxis, 302

CDC (*see* Centers for Disease
  Control)
Cecal volvulus, 172
Ceclor (*see* Cefaclor)
Cefaclor
  otitis media and, 307, 371
  pyelonephritis and, 192
  sinusitis and, 309
Cefazolin, 216
Cefotaxime
  central nervous system
    infection and, 132
  gonococcal dermatitis and,
    394
  meningitis and, 335
Cefoxitin
  abdominal gunshot wounds
    and, 179
  gonococcal dermatitis and,
    394
  pelvic inflammatory disease
    and, 203
  septic shock and, 9
Ceftriaxone
  epididymitis and, 195
  gonococcal dermatitis and,
    394
  gonococcal urethritis in men
    and, 193
  pelvic inflammatory disease
    and, 203
  pharyngitis and, 304
Celestone (*see* Betamethasone)
Cellulitis
  definition of, 213
  dental emergencies and,
    311
Centers for Disease Control
  acquired immunodeficiency
    syndrome and, 330–331
  rabies and, 221
Central herniation of brain,
  122 (*see also*
  Cerebral herniation
  syndromes)

Central nervous system
  acute respiratory failure and,
    83
  infection of, 130–132
    cancer and, 334–337
  regional anesthesia toxicity
    and, 434
  sickle cell disease and,
    349
Central venous pressure
  cardiogenic shock and,
    21–22
  hypovolemic shock and, 5
  pulmonary aspiration and,
    89
  resuscitation monitoring
    and, 12–13
Cephalexin
  bites and, 218
  hand fractures and, 272
  infective endocarditis and,
    216
  wound infections and, 216
Cephalosporin
  bites and, 218
  infective endocarditis and,
    216
  meningitis and, 335
  olecranon bursitis and, 228
  wound infections and, 216
Cephalothin
  eye injuries and, 320
  gram-negative pneumonia
    and, 81
Cephazolin, 272
Cerebral edema
  head injuries and, 159
  hypernatremia and, 59
  lead poisoning and, 462
Cerebral embolism, 136
Cerebral hemorrhage in
  epistaxis, 301
Cerebral herniation syndrome,
  cancer and, 332–333

Cerebral herniation
    syndromes, 121, 122
Cerebrospinal fluid (*see also*
    Spinal tap)
  head injuries and, 157
  meningitis and, 131
Cerebrovascular accident,
    136
  myocardial infarction and,
    19
Cervical adenopathy in
    mononucleosis, 304
Cervical carcinoma, herpes
    genitalis and, 207
Cervical collar, 160, 165
Cervical plexus block,
    422–423
Cervical spine
  injuries to, 160–165
  metastases to, 333
  x-ray of
    head injuries and, 159
    spine injuries and, 163
Cesarean section
  herpes genitalis and, 207
  placenta previa and, 208
Cetacaine (*see* Benzocaine)
Chalazion, 324
Chancre in syphilis, 401–402
Charcoal (*see* Activated
    charcoal)
Cheek
  infraorbital nerve block and,
    422
  injuries to, 283
Chemical burns
  of airway, 408–409
  of conjunctiva and cornea,
    314–315
Chemical cautery in epistaxis,
    302
Chemical pneumonitis, 92
Chemotherapy
  effects of, 340–343

syndrome of inappropriate
  secretion of antidiuretic
  hormone and, 339
Chest
  in shock, 2–3
  superficial cervical plexus
    block and, 423
Chest escharotomy in thermal
  burns, 409
Chest pain in myocardial
  infarction, 18
Chest x-ray
  acquired immunodeficiency
    syndrome and, 330
  aortic aneurysm and, 238
  bronchial asthma and, 381
  cardiogenic pulmonary
    edema and, 23
  caustic ingestion and, 297
  diaphragmatic rupture and,
    112
  fever in child and, 358
  hemothorax and, 110
  hydrocarbon overdose and,
    464
  Legionnaire's disease and, 82
  noncardiogenic pulmonary
    edema and, 88
  pneumonia and, 78
    gram-negative, 80–81
    Haemophilus, 80
    Mycoplasma, 81
    pneumococcal, 78
    staphylococcal, 79
    streptococcal, 79
    viral, 82
  pneumothorax and, 107
  pulmonary aspiration and,
    89–90
  pulmonary embolus and, 76
  rib fracture and, 100
  toxic inhalation and, 92
Cheyne-Stokes breathing, 124

Chickenpox, 398
Child (*see* Pediatric
  emergencies)
Child abuse, 371
Chin, mental nerve block and,
  422
CHIPES, 444–445
Chlamydia
  acquired immunodeficiency
    syndrome and, 329
  cystitis and, 191
  nongonococcal urethritis in
    men and, 194
  pelvic inflammatory disease
    and, 202, 203
  rape and, 211
  urethritis in men and, 193
Chloral hydrate
  convulsive disorders and,
    153
  dialysis and, 456
Chlorambucil, 342
Chloramphenicol
  central nervous system
    infection and, 132
  Haemophilus pneumonia
    and, 80
  meningitis in child and, 368,
    369
  meningococcemia and, 396
  septic shock and, 9
Chlordiazepoxide
  alcohol withdrawal and, 126,
    520
  delirium tremens and, 126
Chloride in metabolic alkalosis,
  56
Chlorine poisoning, 92
Chloroquine overdose, 450
Chlorpromazine
  antidote for, 448
  chemotherapy and, 341
  heat stroke and, 413

Chlorpromazine *(cont.)*
  mood disorders and, 518
  mushroom poisoning and,
    492, 495
  overdose of, 468
  phencyclidine overdose and,
    475
  schizophrenia and, 516
  stimulant overdose and, 521
  violence and, 503
Cholecystitis, 173
Cholinergic overdose, 442
  antidote for, 447
Chondromalacia of patella, 254
Christmas disease, 355
Chromic catgut *(see* Catgut)
Chronic obstructive
    pulmonary disease, 86
Chvostek's sign, 70
Ciliary margin, 283–284
Cimetidine, 511
Circulation
  thoracic injuries and, 99
  trauma and, 12, 14
Circumstantial speech, 505
Cirrhosis, gastrointestinal
    hemorrhage and, 180
CK in myocardial infarction
    (see Creatine phos-
    phokinase in
    myocardial infarction)
Clavicle injuries, 242
Clavulanic acid
  bites and, 218, 219
  otitis media and, 307
Clindamycin
  abdominal gunshot wounds
    and, 179
  bites and, 218
  septic shock and, 9
Clinitest tablets, 465
Clothing of trauma patients, 13
Clotrimazole
  dermatologic disorders and,
    390

  fungal infections and, 398
  vaginitis and, 205
Cloxacillin, 403
Cluster headaches, 142
CO *(see* Carbon monoxide)
Coagulation emergencies,
    348–355
Coagulation pathway, 350
  disorders of, 351–353
Coagulopathy in hypovolemic
    shock, 6
Cocaine
  epistaxis and, 301
  overdose of, 443
  psychiatric emergencies and,
    521
  violence and, 502, 523
Codeine
  headache and, 143
  herpes zoster and, 399
  rib fracture and, 100
Cogentin *(see* Benztropine)
Cognition
  assessment of, 506–507
  in dementia, 513
  in nonorganic psychoses,
    515
  in organic mental disorders,
    508, 512
  psychiatric emergencies and,
    524–525
  in schizophrenia, 515–516
COHg *(see*
    Carboxyhemoglobin)
Coins in airway obstruction,
    294
Colchicine in plants, 493, 498
Cold injury, 413–416
Cold water
  heat stroke and, 412–413
  thermal burns and, 407–408
Cold water caloric test,
    syncope and, 139
Collateral ligament injuries,
    253

Colles' fracture, 248–249
Coma
  alcohol abuse and, 125–127
  causes of, 121–123
  central nervous system
    infection and, 130–132
  cerebrovascular accident
    and, 136
  endocrine dysfunction and,
    132–134
  evaluation of, 117, 120
  hepatic failure and, 130
  hyperglycemia and,
    127–129
  hypertensive
    encephalopathy and,
    134–135
  hypoglycemia and, 129
    pediatric, 366
  uremia and, 129
Compazine (*see*
  Prochlorperazine)
Complete blood cell count,
  fever in newborn and,
  357
Computed axial tomography
  scan (*see also*
  Computed tomography)
  central nervous system
    infection and, 130
  neurological emergencies
    and, 124
Computed tomography (*see
  also* Computed axial
  tomography scan)
  acquired immunodeficiency
    syndrome and, 327
  allergic reaction to,
    386–387
  cerebrovascular accident
    and, 136
  convulsive disorders and,
    150
  encephalitis and, 337
  headache and, 143

injuries and
  abdominal, 178
  bladder, 189
  eye, 320
  head, 159
  renal, 187, 188
  spine, 163
  ureteral, 188
  meningitis and, 335
Confabulation, 507
Congenital heart disease,
  syncope and, 138
Congestive heart failure,
  aminophylline and, 380
Coniine alkaloid in plants, 498
Conjunctiva
  chemical burn of, 314–315
  foreign bodies in, 316
Conjunctivitis
  bacterial, 322–323
  viral, 322
Consciousness
  altered levels of, 117–136
    (*see also* Neurological
    emergencies)
  cognition assessment and,
    506–507
  head injuries and, 155–156
  myocardial infarction and,
    19
  syncope and, 137–139
Constipation, 175–176
Contact dermatitis, 392
Contagious diseases of eyes,
  322–323
Contrast studies
  allergic reaction to,
    386–387
  caustic ingestion and, 297
  foreign body in air or food
    passages and, 295
  shock and, 187
Contusion
  arterial, 230
  of lung, 111

Contusion *(cont.)*
of myocardium, 113
of penis, 189
Convulsions (*see* Seizures)
Copperheads, 484, 485
Coproporphyrin
lead poisoning and, 461
poisoning and overdose and, 445
Coracoclavicular ligament injuries, 244
Coral snakes, 484–485, 486–489
Cornea
abrasion of, 319–320
chemical burn of, 314–315
foreign bodies in, 316–317
Corpine in mushrooms, 495
Corpora cavernosa rupture, 190
Cortef (*see* Hydrocortisone)
Corticosteroids (*see* Steroids)
Cortisporin, 308
Corynebacterium vaginale, 200, 205
Costovertebral angle tenderness
pyelonephritis and, 192
renal colic and, 195
Cottonmouths, 484, 485
Cough in acquired immunodeficiency syndrome, 330
Coumadin, 77
Coxsackievirus
hand-foot-and-mouth disease and, 394
stomatitis and, 311
Cramps, heat, 412
Cranberry juice in phencyclidine overdose, 474

Creatine phosphokinase in myocardial infarction, 18
Creatinine in pancreatitis, 175
Cremasteric reflex, 161
Cricothyroidotomy in head injuries, 155
Cricothyrotomy
airway obstruction and, 294
anaphylactic shock and, 384
cardiac arrest resuscitation and, 43
laryngeal trauma and, 299
thoracic injuries and, 98–99
Cromolyn, 383
Crotamiton, 401
Croup, 362–363
Cruciate ligament injuries, 253
Cryoprecipitate, 352, 353
Cryptococcus
acquired immunodeficiency syndrome and, 326
meningitis and, 336
Cryptosporidium in acquired immunodeficiency syndrome, 329
Crystalline penicillin (*see* Penicillin)
CSM (*see* Carotid sinus massage)
CT (*see* Computed tomography)
Culdocentesis, 201
Cyanide poisoning, 480–481
antidote for, 448
Cyanmethemoglobin, 481
Cyanogenic glycosides in plants, 497, 498, 499
Cyclizine, 147
Cyclopeptides in mushrooms, 494
Cyclophosphamide chemotherapy and, 342, 343

syndrome of inappropriate secretion of antidiuretic hormone and, 339
Cycloplegics
  foreign bodies in eye and, 317
  uveitis and, 323
Cystitis, 191–192
Cystospaz (*see* Hyoscyamine)
Cystostomy in urinary retention, 196
Cystourethrography in bladder injuries, 178
Cytoxan (*see* Cyclophosphamide)

D

Darvon (*see* Propoxyphene)
Daunorubicin, 341–343
Debridement
  abscess and, 221
  bites and, 217
  hand fractures and, 272
  inground foreign material and, 284
  olecranon bursitis and, 228
  perirectal abscess and, 228
  thermal burns and, 408
  wound infections and, 215
Decadron (*see* Dexamethasone)
Decompression illness, 416–417
Decongestants
  otitis and
    external, 308
    middle ear, 306
    serous, 306
  sinusitis and, 309
Deep-tendon reflex in head injuries, 157
Deferoxamine as antidote, 448

Defibrillation (*see also* Cardioversion)
  in thoracotomy, 116
  ventricular fibrillation in cardiac arrest and, 47–48
Degenerative diseases presenting as psychiatric disorders, 511
Dehydration
  in child, 358–360
  hyponatremia and, 60
Delirium, 501, 508, 510–513 (*see also* Encephalopathy)
  dementia and, 513
  The Diagnostic and Statistical Manual of Mental Disorders and, 515
  drug abuse and, 519
Delirium tremens, 126, 520
Delta-Cortef (*see* Prednisolone)
Deltasone (*see* Prednisone)
Delusions, 505
Demeclocycline, 63
Dementia, 501, 508, 513–514
  The Diagnostic and Statistical Manual of Mental Disorders and, 514, 515
Demerol (*see* Meperidine)
Dental emergencies, 309–312
Dentures in airway obstruction, 294
Depersonalization, 506
Depo-Provera (*see* Medroxyprogesterone)
Depression, 517
  dementia and, 513
  differential diagnosis of, 525

Depression *(cont.)*
  in elderly, 526
Derealization, 505
Dermatitis
  atopic, 389–391
  contact, 392
  stasis, 392
Dermatologic disorders,
    389–403
  dermatitis and
    atopic, 389–391
    contact, 392
    stasis, 392
  drug eruption and, 393
  erythema multiforme and,
    393–394
  febrile illness with rash and,
    394–398
  fungal infection and, 398
  herpes virus infection and,
    398–400
  impetigo and, 400
  infestations and, 400–401
  pemphigus vulgaris and, 401
  syphilis and, 401–402
  toxic epidermal necrolysis
    and, 402–403
  urticaria and, 403
Dermatophytoses, 398
Desferoxamine challenge in
    iron poisoning, 463
Desonide, 391
Desoximetasone, 391
DEV (*see* Duck Embryo
    Vaccine)
Dexamethasone
  bronchial asthma and, 382
  caustic ingestion and, 297
  cerebral herniation and, 333
  chemotherapy and, 341
  croup and, 362
  head injuries and, 159
  poisoning and
    lead, 462
    mushroom, 494

Dextroamphetamine overdose,
    450
Dextrose, hypoglycemia in
    child and, 366
Dextrostix, 129
Diabetes
  abscess and, 225
  in child, 366–368
  diarrhea and, 176
  hyperglycemia and, 127–129
  hypoglycemia and, 129
  myocardial infarction and,
    19
  vitreous hemorrhage of eye
    and, 323
Diabetic ketoacidosis, 367–368
*The Diagnostic and Statistical
    Manual of Mental
    Disorders*, 514–515
Dialysis, poisoning or overdose
    and, 451, 456–457 (*see
    also* Hemodialysis)
  lithium, 470
  methanol, 484
Diamox (*see* Acetazolamide)
Diaphragmatic rupture, 112
Diaphyseal fracture, 251
Diarrhea, 176
  acquired immunodeficiency
    syndrome and, 327, 329
Diastolic filling in cardiac
    tamponade, 113
Diazepam
  abscess and, 221
  alcohol abuse and, 126
  black widow spider and, 490
  in cardioversion, 31, 32, 37
  convulsive disorders and,
    151
  eclampsia and, 209
  head injuries and, 158
  mushroom poisoning and,
    495
  overdose and
    hallucinogen, 522

phencyclidine, 474
  stimulant, 521
  tricyclic antidepressant,
    472
pediatric dosage of, 372
regional anesthesia toxicity
  and, 434
respiratory alkalosis and, 56
seizures in child and, 361
shoulder dislocation and,
  243
violence and, 503
Diazoxide
  hypertensive
    encephalopathy and,
    135
  pediatric dosage of, 372
  phencyclidine overdose and,
    474
DIC (*see* Disseminated
    intravascular
    coagulation)
Dicloxacillin
  bites and, 218
  dermatologic disorders and,
    390
  hand fractures and, 272
  impetigo and, 400
  infective endocarditis and,
    216
  olecranon bursitis and, 228
  wound infections and, 216
Digitalis
  atrial fibrillation and, 32
  atrial flutter and, 30
  atrioventricular block and,
    34
  hypokalemia and, 68
  overdose of
    determining level of, 444
    dialysis and, 457
  paroxysmal atrial
    tachycardia and, 29
  premature ventricular
    contractions and, 36

syncope and, 138
Digital nerve block, 423–425
Digoxin
  atrial fibrillation and, 32
  atrial flutter and, 31
  paroxysmal supraventricular
    tachycardia and, 28
  pediatric dosage of, 372
  psychiatric disorders and,
    511
  sinus bradycardia and, 33
Dihydroergotamine, 143
Dilantin (*see* Phenytoin)
Dilation and evacuation in
    spontaneous abortion,
    202
Dilutional coagulopathy in
    hypovolemic shock, 6
Dimenhydrinate, 147
Dimercaprol, poisoning and
  arsenic, 482
  lead, 461
  mercury, 477–479
Diphenhydramine, 353
  anaphylactic shock and, 385,
    386
  angioedema and, 387
  as antidote, 448
  arsenic poisoning and, 482
  bronchial asthma and, 381
  clotting studies and, 20
  overdose and
    hallucinogen, 522
    tranquilizer, 469
  schizophrenia and, 516
  urticaria and, 387
  vertigo and, 147
Diphenoxylate overdose
  antidote for, 449
  dialysis and, 457
Diphtheria-tetanus toxoid, 214
Diplococcus pneumoniae, 336
Dislocation
  of cervical spine, 163
  of elbow, 246–247

Dislocation *(cont.)*
  of hip, 250
  of mandible, 288–289, 291
  patellar, 252
  septal, 291
  of shoulder, 243–244
Disopyramide
  atrial fibrillation and, 32
  torsade de pointes and, 38, 39
  Wolff-Parkinson-White syndrome and, 29
Disseminated intravascular coagulation, 354, 355
  abruptio placenta and, 208
  in cancer, 337
  septic shock and, 8–9
Distal radius fracture, 248–249
Distension in intestinal obstruction, 167, 168
Diuresis, overdose and, 451, 455–456
  lithium, 470
  phencyclidine, 474–475
  phenobarbital, 468
Diuretics
  cardiogenic pulmonary edema and, 23–24
  electric shock and, 411
  hypercalcemia and, 72
  hyperkalemia and, 65, 66
  hypertensive encephalopathy and, 135
  hyponatremia and, 60–64
  metabolic alkalosis and, 56
  noncardiogenic pulmonary edema and, 89
Diverticulitis, 173
Diverticulum, 375
Dizziness, 145–147
Dobutamine, 22
Dog bites, 217, 218
  rabies prophylaxis and, 222

Doll's eyes
  head injuries and, 156
  neurological emergencies and, 123
Domeboro *(see* Burow's solution*)*
L-Dopa, 511
Dopamine
  anaphylactic shock and, 385
  cardiac arrest in child and, 366
  cardiogenic shock and, 22
  regional anesthesia toxicity and, 435
Doppler stethoscope
  arterial ischemia and, 229
  in extremity trauma, 14
Doppler ultrasound in torsion of spermatic cord, 197
Doriden *(see* Glutethimide*)*
Double-cuffed tourniquet, 431
Doxorubicin, 341
Doxycycline
  Bartholinian abscess and, 207
  cystitis and, 191
  epididymitis and, 195
  gonococcal dermatitis and, 394
  pelvic inflammatory disease and, 203
  prostatitis and, 195
  urethritis in men and, 194
Draping for facial injuries, 276–277
Droperidol, 341
Drowning, 87, 88–89
Drug abuse *(see also* Poisoning and overdose*)*
  abscess and, 221
  nonpsychotic disorders and, 518

presenting as psychiatric disorder, 511
psychiatric emergencies and, 519–522
Drug dosages for children, 371–373
Drug eruption, 393
Drug overdose (*see* Poisoning and overdose)
DSM-III-R (*see The Diagnostic and Statistical Manual of Mental Disorders*)
Duck embryo vaccine, 223
dosages for, 224
Duodenal ulcer, 375
Dysequilibrium, 145
Dysphagia in acquired immunodeficiency syndrome, 330
Dyspnea in cardiogenic pulmonary edema, 22–23
Dysrhythmias, 24–38
atrial fibrillation, 31–32
atrial flutter, 30–31
atrioventricular block and, 33–35
cancer and, 343
cardiogenic pulmonary edema and, 24
hypothermia and, 415
multifocal atrial tachycardia, 29–30
myocardial contusion and, 113
paroxysmal atrial tachycardia, 29
paroxysmal supraventricular tachycardia, 27–29
premature ventricular contraction, 35–37
sinus bradycardia, 32–33
sinus tachycardia, 26

syncope and, 138
ventricular tachycardia, 37–38

E

Ear
bleeding from, 157
foreign body in, 296
great auricular nerve block and, 423
infections of, 305–308
Eardrum perforation, 300–301
Ecchymotic orbit, 285
ECG (*see* Electrocardiogram)
Eclampsia, 209
Econazole, 391
ECT (*see* Electroconvulsive therapy)
Ectopic pregnancy, 200–201
Edema
in hyponatremia, 60
pulmonary (*see* Pulmonary edema)
window, 20
Edrophonium, 28
EDTA (*see* Ethylenediamine tetraacetic acid)
Effusion, 94–95
Elbow
injuries to, 246–248
olecranon bursitis and, 227
Elderly, psychiatric emergencies in, 525–526
Electrical burns of mouth, 309–310
Electric shock, 410–411
internal cardiac massage and, 41
Electrocardiogram
atrial fibrillation and, 31
atrial flutter and, 30

Electrocardiogram *(cont.)*
  atrioventricular block and,
    33–34
  cardiac arrest resuscitation
    and, 45, 47
  electromechanical
    dissociation and, 49
  hypercalcemia and, 72
  hypocalcemia and, 70
  hypokalemia and, 68
  hypothermia and, 414, 415
  lithium overdose and, 470
  multifocal atrial tachycardia
    and, 29
  myocardial contusion and,
    113
  myocardial infarction and,
    18
  pacemaker malfunction and,
    25
  paroxysmal atrial
    tachycardia and, 29
  paroxysmal supraventricular
    tachycardia and, 27
  phenytoin and, 152
  premature ventricular
    contractions and, 35
  pulmonary embolus and,
    75–76
  sinus bradycardia and,
    32–33
  sinus tachycardia and, 26
  torsade de pointes and, 38
  ventricular tachycardia and,
    37
Electrocautery
  epistaxis and, 302
  facial injuries and, 275
Electroconvulsive therapy, 518
Electrolyte disorders, 57–73
  hypercalcemia and, 71–73
  hyperkalemia and, 64–67
  hypernatremia and, 57–59
  hypocalcemia and, 69–71

  hypokalemia and, 67–69
  hyponatremia and, 60–64
Electrolytes *(see also*
    Electrolyte disorders*)*
  heat cramps and, 412
  hypothermia and, 415
  metabolic acidosis and, 54
  metabolic alkalosis and, 56
  methanol poisoning and,
    482, 483
  respiratory acidosis and,
    52–53
Electromechanical dissociation
    in cardiac arrest, 49
Embolectomy, pulmonary,
    77–78
Embolization, arterial, 233
Embolus, pulmonary *(see*
    Pulmonary embolus*)*
EMD in cardiac arrest *(see*
    Electromechanical
    dissociation in cardiac
    arrest*)*
Emergent anemia, 345–346
Emesis
  overdose and, 446–450
    acetaminophen, 477
    hydrocarbon, 452–453,
      464
    tricyclic antidepressant,
      471
  poisoning and, 446–450
    iron, 462
    mushroom, 492
Empyema, 94–95
  pneumonia and, 79
Encephalitis, 130–132
  cancer and, 337
Encephalopathy, 510–513
  drug abuse and, 519
  hepatic, 127
  hypertensive, 134–135
  Wernicke's, 127
Endocarditis, cancer and, 337

Endocrine disorders
  neurological emergencies
    and, 132–134
  presenting as psychiatric
    disorders, 511
Endoscopy
  caustic ingestion and, 297
  foreign body in air or food
    passages and, 295
  gastrointestinal hemorrhage
    and, 180
Endotracheal drug
  administration in
  cardiac arrest, 47
Endotracheal intubation
  (*see also* Nasotracheal
    intubation; Tracheal
    intubation)
  acute respiratory failure and,
    86
  bronchial asthma and, 381
  epiglottitis and, 363
  flail chest and, 102
  lung contusion and, 111
  pulmonary aspiration and,
    90
  respiratory burns and, 93
  thoracic injuries and, 97
  toxic inhalation and, 93
Enterobacter in septic shock, 8
Envenomation (*see* Venoms)
Environmental trauma,
    405–417
  decompression illness and,
    416–417
  electric shock and, 410–411
  hyperthermic states and,
    411–413
  hypothermic states and,
    413–416
  thermal burns and, 405–410
Eosinophil count, total,
    378–379, 383

Ephedrine
  arsenic poisoning and, 482
  psychiatric disorders and,
    511
Epidemic keratoconjunctivitis,
    322
Epidermal necrolysis, toxic,
    402–403
Epididymitis, 194–195
  torsion of spermatic cord
    and, 197
Epidural metastases, 333
Epiglottitis, 363–364
Epileptic seizures, 149–153
    (*see also* Seizures)
Epinephrine
  anaphylactic shock and, 384
  angioedema and, 387
  asthma and, 364, 379
  bronchiolitis and, 365
  cardiac arrest and, 47
    pediatric, 366
  croup and, 362
  digital nerve block and, 423
  electromechanical
    dissociation and, 49
  facial injuries and, 275
  local infiltration block and,
    419
  oral soft-tissue trauma and,
    309
  perirectal abscess and, 182
  rabies and, 221
  reaction to, 435–436
  sinus tachycardia and, 26
  trigeminal nerve block and,
    420
  urticaria and, 387
  ventricular asystole and, 49
  ventricular fibrillation and,
    47–48
Epistaxis, 301–303
Epistaxis balloon, 302

Equine antirabies serum, 223
  dosages for, 224
Ergot, 143
Ergotamine, 143
Erythema in perirectal abscess, 182
Erythema multiforme, 393–394
Erythrocyte protoporphyrin test, 461
Erythrocytes
  excessive destruction of, 346–348
  in sickle cell disease, 349
Erythrocytosis, cancer and, 344
Erythromycin
  bites and, 218
  dermatologic problems and, 390
  impetigo and, 400
  Legionnaire's disease and, 82
  Mycoplasma pneumonia and, 81
  nongonococcal urethritis and, 194
  otitis media and, 307
    pediatric, 370
  pharyngitis and, 304
    pediatric, 370
  scarlet fever and, 397
  tonsillitis and, 370
  wound infections and, 216
Erythromycin/sulfisoxazole, 307
Escharotomy in thermal burns, 409
Escherichia coli
  central nervous system infection and, 132
  meningitis in child and, 368
  septic shock and, 8

Escherichia histolytica in acquired immunodeficiency syndrome, 329
Esmarch bandage, 430, 431
Esophageal varices, 180
Esophagus
  caustic burns and, 465
  foreign body in, 294–295
    child and, 376
Estrogen, rape and, 212
ET (*see* Endotracheal intubation)
Ethanol (*see also* Alcohol)
  as antidote, 448, 449
  methanol poisoning and, 484
  overdose of, 443, 451
    determining level of, 444
Ethchlorvynol overdose, 457
Ethinyl estradiol, 212
Ethyl alcohol (*see* Ethanol)
Ethylenediamine tetraacetic acid, 73
Ethylene glycol
  metabolic acidosis and, 53
  overdose of, 443, 482–484
    antidote for, 448
    determining level of, 444
    dialysis and, 456
Eucerin, 389
Eurax (*see* Crotamiton)
Evacuation of stomach, 446–450, 452–453
Extensor carpi radialis brevis or longus, 262–263, 264
Extensor pollicis longus, 269
Extensor tendons of hand, 260–261, 263
  injuries of, 272
External otitis, 307–308
  foreign body in ear canal and, 296

Extraperitoneal rupture, 188–189
Extremity trauma, 14–15 (*see also* Lower extremity; Upper extremity)
Eyebrows in facial injuries, 276
Eyelid
  infraorbital nerve block and, 422
  injuries to, 321–322
  laceration of, 283–284
Eyes, 313–324 (*see also* Ophthalmologic emergencies)
  movement of, head injuries and, 156–157
  sickle cell disease and, 349

F

Facial injuries, 275–292
  eyelid lacerations and, 283–284
  fractures and, 285–292
  inground foreign material and, 284–285
  oral mucosa and, 281–283
  respiratory burn and, 93
  suture techniques and, 278–279, 281
  tongue and, 281–283
  untidy wound and, 278
  wound care and, 276–277
  wound types in, 280–281
  x-ray in, 285
Factor VII deficiency, 351
Factor VIII$_{AHF}$, 353, 355
Factor VIII deficiency, 352–355
Factor IX, 355
Faintness, 137–139, 145
False aneurysm, 230

False labor, 209–210
Fascial compartment syndrome, 7
Fat cells in decompression illness, 417
Fava beans, 348
Fear (*See* Anxiety reactions)
Fecal impaction, 181
Federal Hazardous Substance Act, 443
Feelings of influence, 505
Felon, 225–226
Femoral cutaneous nerve block, 432, 433
Femoral nerve block, 431–432
Femoral shaft injuries, 251
Ferric chloride test, 458
Ferrous gluconate overdose, 448
Ferrous sulfate
  antidote for, 448
  iron poisoning and, 462
Fever
  acquired immunodeficiency syndrome and, 326–327, 328
  cancer and, 345
  in child, 357–358
  rash and, 394–398
Fiberoptic bronchoscopy in pulmonary aspiration, 90
Fiberoptic laryngoscopy
  foreign body in air or food passages and, 295
  laryngeal trauma and, 298
Fibrillation, ventricular (*see* Ventricular fibrillation)
Fibrinogen in septic shock, 9
Fibrinogen scanning in thrombophlebitis, 236
Finger
  abscess of, 226

Finger *(cont.)*
  infection of, 225, 226
  regional nerve blocks and, 423–430
First-degree burns, 407, 408
Fishbones in airway obstruction, 294
Fissure in ano, 182–183
Flagyl *(see* Metronidazole)
Flail chest, 101–103
  rib fracture and, 100
  symptoms of, 99
Flexor carpi radialis, 260, 261
Flexor carpi ulnaris, 260, 261
Flexor digitorum profundus, 267
Flexor digitorum superficialis, 267, 268
Flexor pollicis longus, 260, 262
Flexor tendon injuries of hand, 272
Florinef *(see* Fludrocortisone)
Fludrocortisone, 382
Fluids *(see also* Hydration)
  anaphylactic shock and, 385
  aorta and great vessel injuries and, 112
  cardiogenic shock and, 21–22
  diabetic ketoacidosis in child and, 367
  hyperglycemia and, 128
  hypovolemic shock and, 5–7
  pulmonary aspiration and, 90
  septic shock and, 9
  thermal burns and, 407, 409–410
Fluocinolone acetonide, 391
Fluocinonide, 391
Fluonid *(see* Fluocinolone acetonide)

Fluorescein in corneal abrasion, 319
Fluphenazine, overdose of, 448, 469
Focal motor status, 149
Foley catheter in resuscitation monitoring, 12
Food, headaches and, 142
Food passage, foreign body in, 294–296
Foot
  femoral nerve block and, 431
  injuries to, 255–256
  posterior tibial nerve block and, 433
  regional nerve blocks and, 431–433
  sciatic nerve block and, 431
Foramen magnum herniation, 122
Forearm
  injuries to, 248
  regional nerve blocks and, 423–430
Forehead, nerve blocks and, 422
Foreign bodies
  in air or food passages, 294–296
  airway obstruction and, 293
  cardiac arrest and, 42
  in ear canal, 296
  in eye, 316–317
  in gastrointestinal tract, 376
  in nose, 296
  wound infections and, 216–217
Foreign material in facial injuries, 284–285
Fracture
  ankle, 255
  antibiotics and, 15

arterial contusion and, 230, 231, 233
ballet, 255–256
boxer's, 249–250
calcaneal, 255
cervical spine, 163
of clavicle, 242
Colles', 248–249
diaphyseal, 251
electric shock and, 410
extremity trauma and, 14
of facial bones, 285–292
foot, 256
hand, 272
hip, 250–251
of humerus, 244–246
hyoid bone, 298
malar bone, 285, 286, 322
of mandible, 285, 288–289, 291
of maxilla, 285, 289–292
metacarpal bone, 249–250
metatarsal bone, 255–256
nasal bone, 289–291
navicular, 249
olecranon, 247
orbital bone, 322
orbital floor, 285–287, 322
paranasal sinus, 291
patellar, 251–252
pelvic, 256
of penis, 190
radial head, 247
of radius, 248, 248–249
rib, 100–101 (*see also* Rib fracture)
of scapula, 242–243
of symphysis, 289
tibial shaft, 254
tooth, 311
of ulna, 248
zygomatic arch, 287–288
Free water calculation, 360

Frenulum, 309
Frostbite, 413–414
Full-thickness burns, 407, 408
Functional psychoses, 515–518
definition of, 508
differential diagnosis of, 524, 525
Funduscopic examination, 313
Fungal infection
dermatologic disorders and, 398
meningitis and, 131
septic shock and, 8
Furosemide
cardiogenic pulmonary edema and, 23–24
hypercalcemia and, 72
hyperkalemia and, 66
hypertensive encephalopathy and, 135
hyponatremia and, 63–64, 340
pediatric dosage of, 372
phencyclidine overdose and, 474–475

G

Gallbladder
cholecystitis and, 173
sickle cell disease and, 349
Gallium scan in acquired immunodeficiency syndrome, 327, 330
Gamma benzene hexachloride
pediculosis and, 400
scabies and, 401
Gangrene in frostbite, 414
Gantrisin (*see* Sulfisoxazole)
Gardnerella vaginalis, 200, 205
Gardner-Wells tongs, 164–165

Gas, intestinal obstruction and, 168, 169–170

Gastric aspiration in pulmonary aspiration, 89–90

Gastric carcinoma, 180

Gastric lavage
overdose and, 446, 450, 452–453
acetaminophen, 477
aconitine, 493
phencyclidine, 474
tranquilizer, 469
tricyclic antidepressant, 471
poisoning and, 446, 450, 452–453
cyanide, 480
iron, 462
mercury, 477
mushroom, 492
organophosphate, 466

Gastrocnemius muscle, spinal cord levels and, 161

Gastrointestinal cancer, 344

Gastrointestinal hemorrhage, 179–181
in child, 375

Gastrointestinal system
anaphylactic shock and, 384
chemotherapy and, 341
foreign bodies in, 376
radiation and, 340

General anesthesia for convulsive disorders, 153

Genitourinary tract, 185–198
disorders of external genitalia in, 196–198
external genitalia disorders and, 196–198
herpes simplex and, 398–399
infections of, 191–195

injuries to, 185–190
sickle cell disease and, 349
syphilis and, 402
urinary tract obstruction and, 195–196

Gentamicin
abdominal gunshot wounds and, 179
bacterial conjunctivitis and, 323
gram-negative pneumonia and, 81
meningitis in child and, 368
pulmonary aspiration and, 90
pyelonephritis and, 192
septic shock and, 9

German measles, 395, 397

Giardia lamblia in acquired immunodeficiency syndrome, 329

Glasgow Coma Scale, 14, 117, 120

Glass in eye, 316

Glaucoma, angle-closure, 318–319

Globulin, false calcium levels and, 73

Glomerulonephritis
impetigo and, 400
pharyngitis and, 303

Glucagon
foreign body in air or food passages and, 295
hypoglycemia and, 129
neurological emergencies and, 124

Glucocorticoids
effect of, 383
in hypercalcemia, 72

Glucose
cancer and, 338
cerebrovascular accident and, 136

hypoglycemia and, 129
    pediatric, 366
hyponatremia and, 61
neurological emergencies
    and, 117, 124
pediatric dosage of, 372
Glucosuria, 128
Glutamic oxaloacetic
    transaminase, 9
Glutethimide
    overdose of, 468
        activated charcoal and,
            451
        dialysis and, 457
        pupils and, 123
Glycerin in angle-closure
    glaucoma, 318
Glycosides in plants, 493–499
Gonococcal dermatitis, 394
Gonococcal urethritis,
    193–194
Gonorrhea
    noncardiogenic pulmonary
        edema and, 87
    pelvic inflammatory disease
        and, 203
    pharyngitis and, 303, 304
    rape and, 211
G-6–PD deficiency, 348
Gram-negative bacteria (*see
    also* Gram stain)
    central nervous system
        infection and, 132
    meningitis and, 335, 336
        pediatric, 368
    pneumonia and, 80–81
    septic shock and, 8
    urinary tract infections and,
        193
Gram-positive bacteria in
    septic shock, 8
Gram stain (*see also* Gram-
    negative bacteria)
    acquired immunodeficiency
        syndrome and, 330

bronchial asthma and, 382
Legionnaire's disease and, 82
meningitis and, 335, 336
Mycoplasma pneumonia
    and, 81
olecranon bursitis and, 228
pneumococcal pneumonia
    and, 78
septic shock and, 8
urinary tract infections in
    men and, 193
viral conjunctivitis and, 322
Grease gun injuries of hand,
    273
Great auricular nerve block,
    423
Great vessel injuries, 112–113
Gums
    mandibular nerve block and,
        420
    mental nerve block and, 422
Gunshot wounds to abdomen,
    179
Gynecologic disorders,
    199–212 (*see also*
    Obstetric disorders)
    Bartholinian abscess and,
        207
    herpes genitalis and,
        206–207
    ovarian cyst and, 204
    pelvic inflammatory disease
        and, 202–204
    rape and, 210–212
    symptoms of, 199–200
    vaginitis and, 204–206
Gyne-Lotrimin (*see
    Clotrimazole*)
Gyromitrin in mushrooms, 495

H

Haemophilus influenzae
    central nervous system
        infection and, 132

Haemophilus influenzae
(*cont.*)
epiglottitis and, 363
meningitis and, 368, 369
otitis media and, 307, 370
pneumonia and, 80, 369
sickle cell disease and, 348
sinusitis and, 309
Haemophilus vaginalis
vaginitis and, 200
vaginosis and, 205
Haldol (*see* Haloperidol)
Haldrone (*see* Paramethasone)
Hallucinations, mental status
examination and, 506
Hallucinogens
overdose of, 521–522
dialysis and, 457
psychiatric disorders and,
511
violence and, 502, 523
Haloperidol
antidote for, 448
chemotherapy and, 341
mood disorders and, 518
overdose of, 468, 469
phencyclidine overdose and,
474, 475
schizophrenia and, 516
stimulant overdose and, 521
violence and, 503
Haloprogin, 398
Hand
anatomy of, 260–263
infections of, 227
injuries of, 259–273
bone and joint and,
248–250
diagnosis of, 263–269
treatment for, 269–273
regional nerve blocks and,
423–430
Hand-foot-and-mouth disease,
394–396

HCG in ectopic pregnancy
(*see* Human chorionic
gonadotropin in ectopic
pregnancy)
HCO₃ value in acid-base
balance (*see*
Bicarbonate value in
acid-base balance)
HDCV (*see* Human diploid cell
rabies vaccine)
Headache, 141–143
acquired immunodeficiency
syndrome and, 327
Head cancer
central nervous system
infection and, 334
meningitis and, 336
Head injuries, 155–160
neurological monitoring and,
13
regional nerve blocks and,
420–423
vertigo and, 146
Head tilt–chin lift maneuver,
42, 44
Head tilt–neck lift maneuver,
42, 46
Heart block, complete, 34
(*see also*
Atrioventricular block)
Heart failure
cancer and, 343
in child, 365–366
Heart rate in hypovolemic
shock, 5
Heat cramps, 412
Heat exhaustion, 412
Heat stroke, 412–413
Heimlich maneuver, 293
Hematemesis in aortic
aneurysm, 237
Hematocele, 190
Hematocrit test in poisoning
and overdose, 445

Hematologic emergencies,
    345–348
  cancer and, 344
Hematoma
  septal, 300
  vessel injuries and, 230
Hematuria
  radiation and, 340
  renal injuries and, 187
Hemodialysis (*see also*
    Dialysis, poisoning or
    overdose and)
  lithium overdose and, 470
  methanol poisoning and,
    484
Hemoglobin test in poisoning
    and overdose, 445
Hemolysis, false potassium
    levels and, 66
Hemolytic anemia, 346, 347,
    348
Hemoperfusion in poisoning
    and overdose, 451, 457
Hemopericardium, 115, 116
Hemophilia A, 352–353
Hemophilia B, 355
Hemoptysis, 93–94
  aortic aneurysm and, 237
  differential diagnosis for,
    93–94
Hemorrhage
  control of, 12
  gastrointestinal, 179–181
    pediatric, 375
  in third-trimester pregnancy,
    207–209
Hemorrhoids, thrombosed,
    183
Hemostatic ligature materials,
    278
Hemothorax, 94–95, 110–111
  aorta injuries and, 112
  differential diagnosis for,
    94–95

Heparin
  arterial embolization and,
    233
  cardiac arrest and, 40
  disseminated intravascular
    coagulation and, 355
  pulmonary embolus and, 77
  thrombophlebitis and, 237
Hepatic encephalopathy, 127
Hepatic failure in neurological
    emergencies, 130
Hepatotoxicity of
    acetaminophen, 476
Hernia, incarcerated, 374
Herniated bowel, 112
Herniation of brain, 121, 122
  cancer and, 335
  pupils and, 156
Herpes genitalis, 206–207
Herpes simplex, 398–399
  stomatitis and, 311, 312
Herpes simplex keratitis, 323
Herpes virus in dermatologic
    disorders, 398–400
Herpes zoster, 399–400
  encephalitis and, 337
Hexadrol (*see*
    Dexamethasone)
Hidradenitis, 228
Hippocrates method, 243
Hip trauma, 250–251
HIV (*see* Human
    immunodeficiency
    virus)
Hives, 403
Hodgkin's lymphoma, 399
Hollow viscus rupture,
    176–179
Homans' sign, 236
Homatropine, 317
Homicidal thoughts, 522–524
  mental status examination
    and, 506
Hordeolum, 324

HRIG (*see* Human rabies immune globulin)
Human bites, 217, 218
Human chorionic gonadotropin in ectopic pregnancy, 201
Human diploid cell rabies vaccine, 220
  dosages for, 224
Human immunodeficiency virus, 325, 326 (*see also* Acquired immunodeficiency syndrome)
Human rabies immune globulin, 220
  dosages for, 224
Human tetanus antitoxin, 214, 215
Humerus, injuries to, 244–246
Humidity
  bronchiolitis and, 365
  croup and, 362
Hydralazine
  eclampsia and, 209
  hypertensive encephalopathy and, 135
  pediatric dosage of, 372
  psychiatric disorders and, 511
Hydration (*see also* Fluids)
  bronchial asthma and, 379
  erythema multiforme and, 394
Hydrocarbons, overdose of, 464–465
  emesis and, 446, 452–453
Hydrocortisone
  adrenal crisis and, 133
  anaphylactic shock and, 385
  bronchial asthma and, 381, 382
  fissure in ano and, 183

hypercalcemia and, 72
myxedema coma and, 133
tennis elbow and, 247
thyroid storm and, 134
Hydrocyanic acid overdose, 448
Hydrofluoric acid burns, 466
Hydrogen chloride poisoning, 92
Hydrogen peroxide
  abscess and, 225
  mouth injuries and, 283
Hydrogen sulfide poisoning, 479–480
β-Hydroxybutyric acid in hyperglycemia, 128
Hydroxyurea, 342
Hydroxyzine
  anaphylactic shock and, 385
  angioedema and, 387
  headache and, 143
  sedation and, 436
  urticaria and, 387, 403
Hymenoptera sting, 384
Hyoid bone fracture, 298
Hyoscyamine, 192
Hyperaeration, foreign body in air or food passages and, 295
Hyperbaric chamber
  carbon monoxide poisoning and, 92
  decompression illness and, 417
Hypercalcemia, 71–73
  cancer and, 338
Hypercarbia
  acute respiratory failure and, 83, 84
  cardiogenic pulmonary edema and, 23
  endotracheal intubation and mechanical ventilation and, 86

Hypercoagulability, cancer and, 337
Hyperglycemia, 127–129
  hyponatremia and, 61
Hyperkalemia, 64–67
  adrenal crisis and, 133
  uremia and, 129
Hypernatremia, 57–59
  dehydration and, 359–360
Hypernephroma, 344
Hypersensitivity to regional anesthesia, 435
Hyperstat (*see* Diazoxide)
Hypertension
  aortic aneurysm and, 238
  epinephrine and, 379
  vitreous hemorrhage and, 323
Hypertensive cerebral hemorrhage in epistaxis, 301
Hypertensive encephalopathy, 134–135
Hyperthermic states, 411–413
  heat stroke and, 412–413
Hyperthyroidism, 133–134
Hypertonic dehydration, 359
Hypertonic saline in hyponatremia, 63
Hypertrophic aortic stenosis, 138
Hyperventilation, 518
  respiratory alkalosis and, 55
  syncope and, 139
Hyphema, 321
Hypnotics
  overdose of, 443
  psychiatric emergencies and, 511, 520–521
Hypoaeration, foreign body in air or food passages and, 295
Hypoalbuminemia, 69

Hypocalcemia, 69–71
  torsade de pointes and, 38
Hypocapnia, cancer and, 343
Hypocarbia
  bronchial asthma and, 378
  cardiogenic pulmonary edema and, 23
Hypofibrinogenemia, 9
Hypoglycemia, 129
  cancer and, 338
  in child, 366
Hypokalemia, 67–69
  atrial fibrillation and, 31
  paroxysmal atrial tachycardia and, 29
  premature ventricular contractions and, 36
  sinus bradycardia and, 33
  torsade de pointes and, 38
  ventricular tachycardia and, 38
Hypomagnesemia
  torsade de pointes and, 38
  ventricular tachycardia and, 38
Hyponatremia, 60–64
  adrenal crisis and, 133
  cancer and, 339–340
  dehydration and, 359
Hypotension
  anaphylactic shock and, 385
  barbiturate overdose and, 468
  bretylium side effects and, 38
  ectopic pregnancy and, 201
  fear of regional nerve blocks and, 436
  hypernatremia and, 59
  narcotics and, 437
  orthostatic (*see* Orthostatic hypotension)
  regional anesthesia toxicity and, 435

Hypotension *(cont.)*
  septic shock and, 8
  tranquilizer overdose and,
    469
Hypothermia, 413–416
  cardiac arrest and, 40
  hypovolemic shock and, 6
  internal cardiac massage
    and, 41
  myocardial infarction and,
    18
  myxedema coma and, 133
  sinus bradycardia and, 33
Hypothyroidism, 33
Hypotonic dehydration, 359
Hypoventilation
  cervical spine injury and, 14
  respiratory acidosis and,
    51–53
Hypovolemia
  ovarian cyst and, 204
  splenic injury and, 178
  ventricular fibrillation and,
    48
  ventricular tachycardia and,
    38
Hypovolemic shock, 4–7
  causes of, 1
  clinical findings in, 2
  hemothorax and, 110
  pit vipers and, 486
Hypoxemia
  acute respiratory failure and,
    83, 84
  arterial blood gases and, 85
  cardiogenic pulmonary
    edema and, 23
  noncardiogenic pulmonary
    edema and, 88
  pulmonary aspiration and,
    89
  toxic inhalation and, 93
Hypoxia
  correction of, 85

  hemothorax and, 110
  nasal pack and, 303
  noncardiogenic pulmonary
    edema and, 88
  premature ventricular
    contractions and, 36
  respiratory alkalosis and, 55
  tension pneumothorax and,
    104
  ventricular fibrillation and,
    48
  ventricular tachycardia and,
    38
Hysterical syncope, 139

I

Ibotenic acid in mushrooms,
    494
Ice
  heat stroke and, 412
  oral soft-tissue trauma and,
    309
ICP *(see* Intracranial pressure *)*
Ideas of references, 505
Ilex acid in plants, 496
Ilexanthin in plants, 496
Ilicin in plants, 496
Iliofemoral thrombophlebitis,
    236
Iliopsoas muscle, spinal cord
    levels and, 161
Illusions, 506
Immobilization
  hand injuries and, 270
  scapula injuries and, 243
  shoulder dislocation and,
    243–244
Immunoassay in ectopic
    pregnancy, 201
Impedance plethysmography,
    236
Impetigo, 400
Inapsine *(see* Droperidol *)*

Incarcerated hernia, 374
Incoherence, 505
Inderal (*see* Propranolol)
Indoles in mushrooms, 495
Indomethacin
  bronchial asthma and, 377
  epididymitis and, 194
  headache and, 143
  olecranon bursitis and, 228
Infant (*see* Newborn; Pediatric
    emergencies)
Infections
  acquired immunodeficiency
    syndrome and, 326
  bronchial asthma and,
    381–382
  cancer and, 343, 345
  childhood diseases and,
    368–371
  dental emergencies and,
    311–312
  fungal, 398
  of genitourinary tract,
    191–195
  otolaryngologic emergencies
    and, 303–309
  presenting as psychiatric
    disorders, 511
  soft-tissue, 213–228 (*see
    also* Soft-tissue
    infections)
Infectious enterocolitis, 329
Infective endocarditis, 216
Infestations, 400–401
Infiltration block, local,
    419–420
Inflammatory bowel disease,
    329
Inflammatory disease, acute,
    172–175
Information, fund of, 507
Infraorbital nerve block, 421,
    422

Inhalation injury, 408–409
Inhalation therapy in bronchial
    asthma, 380
Insecticide poisoning,
    466–467
  antidote for, 449
  noncardiogenic pulmonary
    edema and, 87
Insect sting, anaphylactic
    shock and, 384
Insulin
  diabetic ketoacidosis in
    child and, 367
  hyperglycemia and, 128
  hyperkalemia and, 66
Intellectual function (*see*
    Cognition)
Intercostal nerve block
  flail chest and, 103
  pneumothorax and, 433
  rib fracture and, 101
Intermittent positive-pressure
    breathing, 380
Internal fixation
  hip fracture and, 250
  radius-ulna fracture and, 248
Interosseous muscle, spinal
    cord levels and, 161
Intestinal obstruction,
    167–172
Intoxication (*See* Alcohol;
    Drug abuse)
Intracranial hemorrhage,
    155–156
Intracranial pressure, 332
Intraocular pressure, normal,
    314
Intraperitoneal rupture,
    188–189
Intrauterine device, 203
Intravenous drug
    administration in
    cardiac arrest, 45–47

Intravenous pyelography
    allergic reaction to,
        386–387
    bladder injuries and, 189
    renal colic and, 196
    renal injuries and, 187–188
Intravenous regional
    anesthesia, 430–431
Intubation
    airway obstruction and, 293
    trauma and, 13
Intussusception, 374
Iodine
    abscess and, 225
    facial injuries and, 276
    impetigo and, 400
    thyroid storm and, 134
Ipecac syrup (*see* Syrup of
        ipecac)
IPPB (*see* Intermittent
        positive-pressure
        breathing)
Iridocyclitis, 323
Iritis, 323
Iron poisoning, 462–464
    activated charcoal and, 451
    antidote for, 448
    determining level of, 444
Irrigation
    abscess and, 221, 225
    bites and, 217
    facial injuries and, 276
    hand fractures and, 272
    inground foreign material
        and, 284
    olecranon bursitis and, 228
    ophthalmologic emergencies
        and, 314–315
    perirectal abscess and, 228
Irritant oils in plants, 498
Ischemia
    arterial, 229–230
    arterial embolization and,
        233

arteriosclerosis obliterans
        and, 234
    carbon monoxide poisoning
        and, 91
    syncope and, 138
Isoetharine, 380, 383
Isoetharine in asthma
    in child, 364
Isoniazid overdose, 443
    dialysis and, 456
    diuresis and, 456
    psychiatric disorders and,
        511
Isoproterenol
    atrioventricular block and,
        34
    bradycardia from regional
        anesthesia toxicity and,
        435
    cardiac arrest in child and,
        366
    cardiogenic pulmonary
        edema and, 24
    paroxysmal atrial
        tachycardia and, 29
    premature ventricular
        contractions and, 36
    sinus bradycardia and, 33
    sinus tachycardia and, 26
Isospora belli, 329
Isotonic dehydration, 359
Isotonic saline in
    hyponatremia, 63
Isoxazoles in mushrooms,
    494
IUD (*see* Intrauterine device)
IVP (*see* Intravenous
    pyelography)

J

Jaw thrust maneuver, 42, 45
Joint trauma, 241–257
    hip and, 250–251

lower extremity and,
251–256
pelvis and, 256–257
upper extremity and,
242–250
J wave in hypothermia, 414,
415

K

Kaposi's sarcoma, 330
Kayexalate (*see* Polystyrene
sulfonate)
Kenalog (*see* Fluocinonide)
Keratitis, herpes simplex, 323
Keratoconjunctivitis, 322
Kerosene ingestion, 464–465
Ketoacidosis
in child, 367–368
hyperglycemia and, 127–129
Ketonemia, 128
Ketonuria, 128
Kidney injuries, 185–188
Kidney stone, 195–196
Klebsiella
pneumonia and, 80–81
septic shock and, 8
Knee injuries, 251–254
Knee stretch reflex, 160, 161
Koplik's spots, 396
Kwell (*see* Gamma benzene
hexachloride)
Kyphoscoliosis, 41

L

Labetalol, 135
Labor, true versus false,
209–210
Laboratory studies
bronchial asthma and,
378–379
septic shock and, 9

Labyrinthine dysfunction, 145
Lacrimal canaliculus laceration,
322
β-Lactamase–resistant agent,
215–216
Lactic acidosis, 53
convulsive disorders and,
151
Laetrile overdose, 448
Lagomorphs, rabies
prophylaxis and, 219,
223
Laparoscopy in tubo-ovarian
abscess, 204
Laparotomy
abdominal injuries and, 177,
178, 179
appendicitis and, 173
renal injuries and, 187
Large bowel obstruction,
167–172
Laryngeal edema in allergic
emergencies, 387
Laryngeal trauma, 297–299
Laryngoscopy
airway obstruction and, 293
epiglottitis and, 363
foreign body in air or food
passages and, 295
laryngeal trauma and, 298
thoracic injuries and, 98
Laryngospasm in airway
obstruction, 294
Lasix (*see* Furosemide)
Lateral femoral cutaneous
nerve block, 432, 433
Lavage (*see* Gastric lavage)
Laxatives
activated charcoal and, 451
fecal impaction and, 181
fissure in ano and, 183
L-Dopa, 511
Lead lines, 461

Lead poisoning, 460–462

LeFort maxillary fracture, 289–292

Leg
  injuries to, 251–256
  nerve block and
    femoral, 431
    regional, 431–433
    sciatic, 431

Legionnaire's disease, 81–82

Leukemia
  central nervous system
    infection and, 334
  meningitis and, 336

Leukeran (*see* Chlorambucil)

Leukocytes in sickle cell
  disease, 349

Leukocytosis
  cancer and, 344
  false potassium levels and,
    67
  pelvic inflammatory disease
    and, 203
  septic shock and, 9

Leukopenia in septic shock, 9

Levarterenol
  anaphylactic shock and, 385
  regional anesthesia toxicity
    and, 435

Level of consciousness (*see*
    Consciousness;
    Neurological
    emergencies)

Levodopa, 511

Librium (*see*
    Chlordiazepoxide)

Lice, 400

Lidex (*see* Fluocinonide)

Lidocaine
  abscess and, 221
  airway obstruction and, 294
  axillary block and, 429, 430
  cardiac arrest and, 47
    pediatric, 366

cardiogenic pulmonary
    edema and, 24
convulsive disorders and,
    152–153
epinephrine and, 435–436
epistaxis and, 302
facial injuries and, 275
foreign body in air or food
    passages and, 295
inground foreign material
    and, 284
intracranial pressure and,
    332
intravenous regional
    anesthesia and,
    430–431
metacarpal fracture and,
    249
multifocal atrial tachycardia
    and, 30
myocardial infarction and,
    20
nerve block and
    digital, 423
    local infiltration, 419, 420
    median, 425
    posterior tibial, 433
    trigeminal, 420
    ulnar, 425
oral soft-tissue trauma and,
    309
perirectal abscess and, 182
premature ventricular
    contractions and, 36
psychiatric disorders and,
    511
rectal prolapse and, 184
septal hematoma and, 300
stomatitis and, 311
thrombosed hemorrhoids
    and, 183
torsade de pointes and, 39
tricyclic antidepressant
    overdose and, 472

trochanteric bursitis and, 251

tube thoracostomy and, 108

ventricular fibrillation and, 48

ventricular tachycardia and, 37

Wolff-Parkinson-White syndrome and, 28

Ligament tears of knee, 252

Lightning, 411

Lip

  injuries of, 281–283

  nerve block and

    infraorbital, 422

    mandibular, 420

    mental, 422

Listeria monocytogenes, 335, 336

Lithium

  mood disorders and, 518

  overdose of, 469–470

    activated charcoal and, 451

    determining level of, 444

Liver disease

  aminophylline and, 380

  sickle cell disease and, 349

Liver failure in neurological emergencies, 130

Local infiltration block, 419–420

Loculations, 225

Lomotil overdose (*see* Diphenoxylate overdose)

Lomustine, 342

Looseness of associations, 505

Lotrimin (*see* Clotrimazole)

Louse, 400

Lower extremity

  injuries of, 251–256

  regional nerve blocks and, 431–433

Loxapine succinate, overdose of, 448

Loxitane, overdose of (*see* Loxapine succinate,overdose of)

Loxosceles, 490–491

LSD (*see* Lysergic acid diethylamide)

Lumbar puncture (*see* Spinal tap)

Lumbrical muscle, spinal cord levels and, 161

Lung cancer

  antidiuretic hormone and, 339

  spinal cord compression and, 333

Lung cells in decompression illness, 417

Lung contusion, 111

Lycorine alkaloid in plants, 498, 499

Lye burns, 465

  caustic ingestion and, 296

  conjunctiva and cornea and, 314

Lymphadenopathy

  acquired immunodeficiency syndrome and, 327–330

  definition of, 213

Lymphangitis, 213

Lymphoma

  central nervous system infection and, 334

  meningitis and, 336

  spinal cord compression and, 333

Lyovac *Latrodectus:* MSD, 490

Lysergic acid diethylamide, 123

Lysergic acid diethylamide overdose, 521–522

M

Macrodantin (*see*
  Nitrofurantoin)
Magnesium sulfate
  eclampsia and, 209
  hydrofluoric acid burns and,
    466
  hypocalcemia and, 69, 70,
    71
  mercury poisoning and, 477
  poisoning and overdose and,
    451, 477
Magnetic resonance imaging in
  acquired
  immunodeficiency
  syndrome, 327
Magnet rate, 26
Malar bone fracture, 285, 286,
  292, 322
Malathion overdose, antidote
  for, 449
Malathion poisoning, 466
Mallet finger deformity, 269
Malocclusion in facial bone
  fractures, 285
Mandibular dislocation,
  288–289, 291
Mandibular fracture, 285,
  288–289, 291
Mandibular nerve block, 420,
  421
Mania, 525
Manic episode, 516–517
Mannitol
  angle-closure glaucoma and,
    318
  cerebral herniation and, 333
  head injuries and, 159
  hyponatremia and, 61,
    63–64
  lead poisoning and, 462
  phencyclidine overdose and,
    474

Marcaine (*see* Bupivacaine)
Marijuana abuse, 521–522
MAST (*see* Military antishock
  trousers)
MAT (*see* Multifocal atrial
  tachycardia)
Maxillary fracture, 285,
  289–292
Measles, 395, 396
Meat in esophagus, 295
Meat tenderizer, 295
Mechanical ventilation
  acute respiratory failure and,
    86
  bronchial asthma and, 381
  lung contusion and, 111
  noncardiogenic pulmonary
    edema and, 88
Meckel's diverticulum, 375
Meclizine, 147
Median nerve, 260, 262
  anatomy of, 260
  sensation and, 265
Median nerve block, 425, 426
Medrol (*see*
  Methylprednisolone)
Medroxyprogesterone, 212
Medullary lesions, 123
Meibomian gland infection,
  324
Mellaril, overdose of (*see*
  Thioridazine, overdose
  of)
Melzer's reagent, 491
Memory in cognition
  assessment, 507
Meniere's disease, 145–146
Meningitis, 130–132
  cancer and, 334–335, 336
  cerebrospinal fluid in, 131
  in child, 368–369
  convulsive disorders and,
    150
Meningococcemia, 396

Meningococcus
central nervous system
infection and, 132
meningitis in child and, 368,
369
Meniscus, injuries of, 252, 253
Mental disability, grave,
523–524
Mental disorders (*see*
Psychiatric
emergencies)
Mental nerve block, 421, 422
Mental status examination
grave mental disability and,
523
hypovolemic shock and, 4
neurological emergencies
and, 117, 118–119
nonpsychotic disorders and,
518
organic mental disorders
and, 512
psychiatric emergencies and,
504–507
septic shock and, 8
Meperidine
abscess and, 221
headache and, 143
sedation and, 437
shoulder dislocation and,
243
Mepivacaine, nerve block and
local infiltration, 419, 420
posterior tibial, 433
trigeminal, 420
Meprobamate overdose, 456
Mercury poisoning, 477–479
Metabolic acidosis, 53–55
hyperglycemia and, 128–129
respiratory acidosis and, 52
respiratory alkalosis and, 55
Metabolic alkalosis, 56
respiratory acidosis and, 52

Metabolic disorders
cancer and, 338–340
presenting as psychiatric
disorders, 511
Metacarpal fracture, 249–250
Metacortelone (*see*
Prednisolone)
Metal in eye, 316
Metallic mercury ingestion,
477
Metaproterenol, 380
bronchial asthma and, 383
Metaraminol
hypovolemic shock and, 7
paroxysmal supraventricular
tachycardia and, 28
tranquilizer overdose and,
469
Metatarsal fracture, 255–256
Methacholine overdose, 448
Methanol
metabolic acidosis and, 53
overdose of, 443, 482–484
activated charcoal and,
451
antidote for, 449
determining level of, 444
dialysis and, 456
Methaqualone overdose, 457
Methemoglobinemia, 445
Methemoglobin overdose, 444
Methicillin
meningitis in child and, 369
pulmonary aspiration and,
90
Methocarbamol, 490
Methotrexate, 342
Methsuccimide overdose, 457
Methyl alcohol (*see* Methanol)
Methyldopa
hypertensive
encephalopathy and,
135

Methyldopa *(cont.)*
  pediatric dosage of, 372
  psychiatric disorders and, 511
Methylene blue
  as antidote, 449
  hemolytic anemia and, 348
Methylene chloride overdose, 452
Methylprednisolone
  bronchial asthma and, 382
  pulmonary aspiration and, 90
Methylxanthine, 511
Methyprylon overdose, 457
Methysergide, 143
Metoclopramide
  chemotherapy and, 341
  headache and, 143
Metronidazole
  bacterial vaginosis and, 206
  vaginitis and, 205
Miconazole
  fungal infections and, 398
  vaginitis and, 205
Micturition syncope, 138 (*see also* Urinary output; Urinary tract)
Midazolam
  abscess and, 221
  in cardioversion, 31, 32, 37
  sedation and, 437–438
Midbrain lesion, 123
  pupils and, 156
Migraines, 141, 142
Miliary tuberculosis, 87
Military antishock trousers
  anaphylactic shock and, 385
  aorta and great vessel injuries and, 112
  aortic aneurysm and, 239
  ectopic pregnancy and, 201
  hypovolemic shock and, 7

neurological emergencies and, 124–125
Mineral acid overdose, 451
Mineralocorticoid effect, 383
Mini-mental state, 118–119
Miotics, 318
Mistletoe, 493
Mithramycin, 72
Mitomycin C, 342
Mitral myxoma, 138
Mitral valve disease, 138
MMH poisoning (*see* Monomethylhydrazine poisoning)
Moban, overdose of (*see* Molindone, overdose of)
Mobitz I atrioventricular block, 33–34
Mobitz II atrioventricular block, 34
Molindone, overdose of, 448
Monilia (*see Candida*)
Monistat (*see* Miconazole)
Monofilament nylon sutures (*see* Nylon sutures)
Monomethylhydrazine poisoning, 491
  mushrooms and, 495
Mononucleosis, pharyngitis and, 304
Mood disorders, 516–518
  differential diagnosis of, 525
  mental status examination and, 505
Morphine
  abscess and, 221
  cardiogenic pulmonary edema and, 23
  myocardial infarction and, 19–20
  noncardiogenic pulmonary edema and, 89

pediatric dosage of, 372
sedation and, 437
shoulder dislocation and, 243
sinus bradycardia and, 33
Mouth (*see* Oral lesions)
MSE (*see* Mental status examination)
Mucosa, suture materials for, 278
Mucous membrane burn, 93
Multifocal atrial tachycardia, 29–30
Muscarine, 495
Muscimol, 494
Muscle
  neurological emergencies and, 123
  spinal cord levels and, 161
  suture materials for, 278
  suture techniques for, 279
Muscular paralysis anesthesia, 438–439
Mushroom poisoning, 491–492, 494–495
Mycobacterium, acquired immunodeficiency syndrome and, 328, 330
Mycolog (*see* Nystatin)
Mycoplasma pneumonia, 81
Mycostatin (*see* Nystatin)
Myleran (*see* Busulfan)
Myocardial contusion, 113
Myocardial infarction
  cardiogenic pulmonary edema and, 22–24
  cardiogenic shock and, 21–22
  definition of, 17
  diagnosis of, 18–19
  incidence of, 17
  risk factors for, 17
  syncope and, 138

treatment of, 19–20
  thrombolytics in, 20
Myoglobin, 445
Myoglobinuria
  convulsive disorders and, 151
  electric shock and, 411
Myonecrosis in electric shock, 411
Myringotomy in otitis media, 307
Myxedema coma, 133
Myxoma, 138

N

Nafcillin
  staphylococcal pneumonia and, 79
  staphylococcal scalded skin syndrome and, 403
  toxic shock syndrome and, 10
Nail abscess, 226
Nalidixic acid
  cystitis and, 192
  hemolytic anemia and, 348
Naloxone
  as antidote, 449
  cancer and, 338
  cardiac arrest and, 39
  cerebrovascular accident and, 136
  hypoglycemia and, 129
  narcotics and, 437
  neurological emergencies and, 117, 124
  overdose and, 446
    opiate, 475–476, 520
    phencyclidine, 474
  pediatric dosage of, 372
  reversal of morphine and, 20
Naphazoline, 322

Napthalene, 348
Narcan (*see* Naloxone)
Narcotics (*see also* Opiates;
    specific narcotic)
  abscess and, 221
  hydroxyzine and, 436
  noncardiogenic pulmonary
      edema and, 87
  oncological emergencies
      and, 338
  overdose of, 442
    antidote for, 449
    dialysis and, 457
  regional anesthesia toxicity
      and, 434
  renal colic and, 196
  sedation and, 436–437
  sickle cell disease and, 348
  syndrome of inappropriate
      secretion of antidiuretic
      hormone and, 339
Nasal fractures, 289–291
Nasal pack, 302–303
Nasal trauma, 299–300
Nasogastric tube insertion, 13
Nasotracheal intubation
    (*see also* Endotracheal
    intubation; Tracheal
    intubation)
  spine injuries and, 163
  thoracic injuries and, 98
Navane, overdose of (*see*
    Thioxanthines, overdose
    of)
Navicular fracture, 249
Near drowning, 87, 88–89
Nebs (*see* Acetaminophen)
Neck
  cancer of, central nervous
      system infection and,
      334
  regional nerve blocks and,
      420–423

superficial cervical plexus
    block and, 423
Neck veins in shock, 2–3
Necrolysis, toxic epidermal,
    402–403
Needle aspiration
  cardiac tamponade and,
      113–115
  olecranon bursitis and,
      228
NegGram (*see* Nalidixic acid)
Neisseria gonorrhoeae
  acquired immunodeficiency
      syndrome and, 329
  pelvic inflammatory disease
      and, 202
Neomycin
  bacterial conjunctivitis and,
      323
  corneal abrasion and, 320
  hepatic encephalopathy and,
      127
Neonate (*see* Newborn)
Neoplasms (*see also*
    Oncological
    emergencies)
  acquired immunodeficiency
      syndrome and, 326
  presenting as psychiatric
      disorders, 511
Neostigmine
  antidote for, 447
  pancuronium and, 439
  paroxysmal supraventricular
      tachycardia and, 28
  tubocurarine and, 438
Neo-Synephrine (*see*
    Phenylephrine)
Nerve blocks, 420–433 (*see
    also* Regional nerve
    blocks)
Nerve injuries of hand,
    271–272

Neurological emergencies,
117–136, 155–165
alcohol abuse and, 125–127
cancer and, 332–337
central nervous system
infection and, 130–132
cerebrovascular accident
and, 136
endocrine conditions and,
132–134
headache and, 142, 143
head injuries and, 155–160
hepatic failure and, 130
hyperglycemia and, 127–129
hypertensive
encephalopathy and,
134–135
hypoglycemia and, 129
spinal injuries and, 160–165
syncope and, 138
uremia and, 129
Neurological monitoring in
trauma, 13–14
Neuromuscular blocking
agents, 438–439
in convulsive disorders,
153
phencyclidine overdose and,
474
Neuromuscular dysfunction in
acute respiratory failure,
84
Neurotoxicity of
chemotherapy, 343
Neutropenia, 345
Newborn
fever in, 357
gastrointestinal tract
bleeding in, 375
herpes genitalis and, 207
hypoglycemia in, 366
meningitis in, 368
pyloric stenosis in, 373–374

Nicotine, sinus tachycardia
and, 26
Nifedipine, 135
Nitrates
cyanide poisoning and, 480
overdose of, 442
antidote for, 449
Nitrites
antidote for, 448, 449
cyanide poisoning and,
480–481
noxious gas poisoning and,
480
overdose of, 442–443
Nitrobenzene overdose, 443,
453, 454
Nitrofurans, 348
Nitrofurantoin, 191–192
Nitrogen in decompression
illness, 416–417
Nitrogen oxide poisoning, 92
Nitroglycerine
cardiogenic pulmonary
edema and, 23
myocardial infarction and,
19
Nitrophenol overdose, 443
Nitroprusside
antidote for, 448
aortic aneurysm and, 238
hypertensive
encephalopathy and,
134–135
overdose of, 480
pediatric dosage of, 372
phencyclidine overdose and,
474
Nitrosoureas, 342
Nitrous oxide, abscess and,
221
Nocturnal dyspnea in
cardiogenic pulmonary
edema, 22–23

Nonbony injury of knee, 252–253
Noncardiogenic pulmonary edema, 87–89
  pulmonary aspiration and, 89
  toxic inhalation and, 92
Nondepolarizing agents in muscular paralysis, 438–439
Nongonococcal urethritis, 193, 194
Non-Hodgkin's lymphoma, 330
Nonorganic psychoses, 515–518
  definition of, 508
  differential diagnosis of, 524, 525
Nonpsychotic behavioral disorders, 518–519
  definition of, 508
  differential diagnosis of, 524
Nonsteroidal anti-inflammatory drugs
  bronchial asthma and, 377
  olecranon bursitis and, 228
  temporomandibular joint disorders and, 312
Norepinephrine
  cardiac arrest in child and, 366
  hypovolemic shock and, 7
  overdose and
    tranquilizer, 469
    tricyclic antidepressant, 470
Norgestrel, 212
Nose
  bleeding from, 301–303
    head injuries and, 157
  foreign body in, 296
  fracture of, 289–291
  infraorbital nerve block and, 422

injuries of, 299–300
Noxious gas poisoning, 479–482
Nursemaid's elbow, 246
Nuts, airway obstruction from, 294
Nylen-Barany test, 146–147
Nylon sutures
  eyelid and, 284
  facial injuries and, 275
  skin and, 278
Nystagmus
  eardrum perforation and, 300
  head injuries and, 157
  Nylen-Barany test and, 147
Nystatin
  dermatologic disorders and, 391
  vaginitis and, 205

O

Oat cell carcinoma, 339
Obesity, cardiac arrest resuscitation and, 42
Obstetric disorders, 199–212
  (*see also* Gynecologic disorders; Pregnancy)
  abruptio placenta and, 208–209
  eclampsia and, 209
  ectopic pregnancy and, 200–201
  herpes genitalis and, 206–207
  labor and, 209–210
  placenta previa and, 207–208
  rape and, 210–212
  spontaneous abortion and, 201–202
  symptoms of, 199–200
  vaginitis and, 204–206

Obstipation in intestinal
obstruction, 167, 169
Obstructive disease, acute
respiratory failure and,
84
Obstructive shock
causes of, 1
clinical findings in, 3
Oculocephalic reflex, 156
Olecranon bursitis, 227–228
Olecranon fracture, 247
OMPA poisoning, 466
Oncological emergencies,
331–345
cardiopulmonary conditions
and, 343–344
hematologic disorders and,
344
infections and, 345
neurological disorders in,
332–337
radiation and chemotherapy
and, 340–343
toxic and metabolic
abnormalities in,
338–340
vascular disorders in,
337–338
Open pneumothorax (*see*
Pneumothorax, open)
Ophthalmologic emergencies,
313–324
angle-closure glaucoma and,
318–319
central retinal artery
occlusion and, 317–318
chemical burns and,
314–315
contagious diseases and,
322–323
corneal abrasion and,
319–320
eye injuries and, 320–321
eyelid injuries and, 321–322

foreign bodies and, 316–317
Opiates (*see also* Narcotics)
cardiac arrest and, 39
diarrhea and, 176
headache and, 143
mushroom poisoning and,
492
overdose of, 475–476
psychiatric emergencies and,
520
Oral lesions
in acquired
immunodeficiency
syndrome, 330
injuries and, 281–283
electrical burns in,
309–310
mucosal, 281–283
soft-tissue, 309–310
Orbital bone fracture, 322
Orbital floor fracture,
285–287, 322
Orbital x-rays
eye injuries and, 320
foreign bodies and, 316
Orchiopexy, 197, 374
Organic mental disorders,
508–515
*The Diagnostic and
Statistical Manual of
Mental Disorders* and,
514–515
differential diagnosis of, 524,
525
Organophosphates, 466–467
activated charcoal and, 451
antidote for, 449
noncardiogenic pulmonary
edema and, 87
Orientation in cognition
assessment, 507
Orotracheal intubation
spine injuries and, 163
thoracic injuries and, 97–98

Orthopnea in cardiogenic
  pulmonary edema,
  22–23
Orthostatic hypotension, 139
Osborne wave in hypothermia,
  414, 415
Osmolal gap
  metabolic acidosis and, 54
  methanol poisoning and,
    483
  respiratory acidosis and, 53
Osmolality (*see* Serum
    osmolality)
Osmotics, 318–319
Osteochondral fracture of
    knee, 252
Otalgia, 306
Otitis, external, 307–308
Otitis media, 306–307
  in child, 370–371
  foreign body in ear canal
    and, 296
  serous, 305–306
Otolaryngologic emergencies,
  293–312
  airway obstruction and,
    293–294
  caustic ingestion and,
    296–297
  dental emergencies and,
    309–312
  epistaxis and, 301–303
  foreign body in air or food
    passages and, 294–296
  foreign body in nose or ear
    canal and, 296
  infection and, 303–309
  trauma and, 297–301
Ovarian cancer, 344
Ovarian cyst, 204
Overdose (*see* Poisoning and
    overdose)
Ovral (*see* Ethinyl estradiol)
Oxalates, in plants, 496–500

Oxygen, partial pressure of
    (*see* Partial pressure of
    oxygen)
Oxygenation
  acute respiratory failure and,
    85–86
  anaphylactic shock and, 384
  bronchial asthma and, 379
  carbon monoxide poisoning
    and, 91–92
  cardiogenic pulmonary
    edema and, 23
  central retinal artery
    occlusion and, 317–318
  cyanide poisoning and, 480
  decompression illness and,
    417
  epiglottitis and, 363
  hypovolemic shock and, 5
  myocardial infarction and,
    19
  neurological emergencies
    and, 124
  noncardiogenic pulmonary
    edema and, 88
  pulmonary aspiration and,
    90
  toxic inhalation and, 92–93
  trauma and, 11

P

Pacemaker
  external
    cardiogenic pulmonary
      edema and, 24
    premature ventricular
      contractions and, 35
    sinus bradycardia and, 33
  malfunction of, 25–26
  premature ventricular
    contractions and, 35
  ventricular asystole and, 49
Paint gun injuries, 273

Palate, Kaposi's sarcoma and, 330
Palmaris longus, 260, 261
Palmar space infection, 227
Pancreatic cancer
    antidiuretic hormone and, 339
    thrombosis and, 344
Pancreatitis, 175
Pancuronium
    muscular paralysis and, 438–439
    pediatric dosage of, 372
Papain, 295
Papilledema, 150
Paracetamol overdose, 476–477
Parainfluenza virus, 362
Paraldehyde
    alcohol abuse and, 126
    convulsive disorders and, 152
    dialysis and, 456
    metabolic acidosis and, 53
    seizures in child and, 361
Paramethasone, 382
Paranasal sinus fracture, 291
Paraphimosis, 197–198
Parathion overdose, antidote for, 449
Parathion poisoning, 466
Parathyroid hormone, 69–70
Parenchyma fracture, 186
Parkland formula, 410
Paronychium, 226–227
Paroxysmal atrial tachycardia, 29
Paroxysmal nocturnal dyspnea, 22–23
Paroxysmal supraventricular tachycardia, 27–29
Partial pressure
    of alveolar oxygen, 85

    of arterial carbon dioxide
        in cerebral herniation, 333
        in head injuries, 159
        in metabolic acidosis, 53–54
        in respiratory acidosis, 52
        in respiratory alkalosis, 55
    of arterial oxygen, in respiratory acidosis, 52
    of carbon dioxide
        in bronchial asthma, 378, 379, 381
        and formulas, 85
        in pulmonary aspiration, 89
    of oxygen
        in bronchial asthma, 379
        in carbon monoxide poisoning, 91
        in endotracheal intubation and mechanical ventilation, 86
        and formulas, 85
        in lung contusion, 111
        in noncardiogenic pulmonary edema, 88
        in pulmonary aspiration, 90
        in pulmonary embolus, 75
        in respiratory acidosis, 52
Partial status epilepticus, 149
Partial thromboplastin time
    coagulation pathway disorders and, 351, 355
    heparin and, 77
    septic shock and, 9
    thrombophlebitis and, 237
Pasteurella multocida, 218, 219
PAT (*see* Paroxysmal atrial tachycardia)
Patella
    chondromalacia of, 254

Patella *(cont.)*
  dislocation of, 252
  fracture of, 251–252
Pavulon *(see* Pancuronium)
PCP *(see* Phencyclidine)
Peanuts in airway obstruction, 294
Pectus carinatum, internal cardiac massage and, 41
Pediatric emergencies, 357–376
  appendicitis and, 375–376
  asthma and, 364
  battered child and, 371
  bronchial asthma and, 378
  bronchiolitis and, 364–365
  cardiopulmonary arrest and, 365–366
  croup and, 362–363
  dehydration and, 358–360
  diabetes and, 366–368
  drug dosages in, 371–373
  epiglottitis and, 363–364
  fever and, 357–358
  foreign bodies in gastrointestinal tract and, 376
  gastrointestinal tract bleeding and, 375
  incarcerated hernia and, 374
  infectious diseases and, 368–371
  intussusception and, 374
  pyloric stenosis and, 373–374
  seizures and, 360–362
  torsion of testis and, 374–375
Pediazole *(see* Erythromycin/sulfisoxazole)
Pedicle flap in hand injuries, 273
Pediculosis, 400

PEEP *(see* Positive end-expiratory pressure)
Pelvic inflammatory disease, 173, 202–204
Pelvis
  injuries of, 256–257
  radiation and, 340
Pemphigus vulgaris, 401
Penicillin
  bites and, 218
  caustic ingestion and, 297
  impetigo and, 400
  meningitis and, 335
    pediatric, 368, 369
  nasal pack and, 303
  otitis media and, 306–307
  peritonsillar abscess and, 305
  pneumococcal pneumonia and, 78–79
  pulmonary aspiration and, 90
  scarlet fever and, 397
  staphylococcal scalded skin syndrome and, 403
  streptococcal pneumonia and, 79
  syphilis and, 402
  tooth abscess and, 311
  urticaria and, 403
Penicillin G
  central nervous system infection and, 132
  eye injuries and, 320
  gonococcal dermatitis and, 394
  meningococcemia and, 396
  mushroom poisoning and, 494
  pharyngitis and, 304, 305
  pneumonia and, 370
Penicillin V
  dermatologic disorders and, 390

impetigo and, 400
pneumonia and, 369–370
tonsillitis and pharyngitis
and, 370
Penis injuries, 189–190
Pentazocine
antidote for, 449
noncardiogenic pulmonary
edema and, 87
Pentobarbital overdose, 467
Peptic ulcer, 173
Perforating injuries of eye,
320
Perfusion scanning in
pulmonary embolus, 76
Pericardial effusion
cancer and, 343
needle aspiration and,
113–115
Pericardial tamponade
cardiac arrest and, 40
symptoms of, 99–100
Perinephric abscess, 192
Peripheral vascular
emergencies, 229–239
aortic aneurysm and,
237–239
arterial embolization and,
233
arterial ischemia and,
229–230
arteriosclerosis obliterans
and, 234
trauma and, 230–233
venous disease and,
234–237
Peripheral veins in
hypovolemic shock, 5
Perirectal abscess, 181–182,
228
Peritoneal lavage in abdominal
injuries, 178
Peritonsillar abscess, 305
Permanganate ingestion, 465

Peroneal muscle, spinal cord
levels and, 161
Pesticide poisoning, 466–467
Petit mal seizure, 149
Petroleum ingestion, 450
pH
bronchial asthma and, 379
metabolic acidosis and,
53–54
metabolic alkalosis and, 56
respiratory acidosis and, 52
respiratory alkalosis and, 55
salicylate overdose and, 460
Phalangeal fracture of foot,
256
Phalanx, infection of, 225
Pharyngitis, 303–305
in child, 370
Phenacetin
hemolytic anemia and, 348
overdose of, 443
antidote for, 449
Phenazopyridine
antidote for, 449
cystitis and, 192
Phencyclidine
convulsive disorders and,
150
nystagmus and, 157
overdose of, 443, 456,
472–475, 521–522
violence and, 502, 523
Phenergan (*see* Promethazine)
Phenhydrazine, 348
Phenistix test, 458
Phenobarbital
alcohol abuse and, 126
convulsive disorders and,
151–153
pediatric, 361
overdose of, 467, 468
activated charcoal and,
450
diuresis and, 456

Phenobarbital *(cont.)*
  pediatric dosage of, 372
  phencyclidine overdose and,
    474
Phenothiazines
  chemotherapy and, 341
  overdose of, 443
    antidote for, 448
    dialysis and, 457
    syrup of ipecac and, 450
    stimulant overdose and,
      521
    syndrome of inappropriate
      secretion of antidiuretic
      hormone and, 339
    torsade de pointes and, 38
Phenoxymethyl penicillin
  pharyngitis and, 304, 370
  pneumonia and, 369–370
    pneumococcal, 79
  tonsillitis and, 370
Phentolamine, 372
Phenylbutazone, 377
Phenylephrine
  paroxysmal supraventricular
    tachycardia and, 28
  pediatric dosage of, 372
  tricyclic antidepressant
    overdose and, 472
Phenylethylamine, 493
  mistletoe and, 497
Phenytoin
  convulsive disorders and,
    151, 152
  head injuries and, 158
  overdose of, 443
    activated charcoal and,
      450
    hemoperfusion and, 457
  paroxysmal atrial
    tachycardia and, 29
  pediatric dosage of, 372
  phencyclidine overdose and,
    474

premature ventricular
    contractions and, 36–37
  torsade de pointes and, 39
  tricyclic antidepressant
    overdose and, 472
Phlebotomy in cardiogenic
    pulmonary edema, 24
Phosgene poisoning, 92
Phosphate in hypercalcemia,
    73
Phosphorus in hypercalcemia,
    73
Physostigmine
  as antidote, 447
  atropine-containing plants
    and, 493
  cardiac arrest and, 39
  mushroom poisoning and,
    494
  tricyclic antidepressant
    overdose and, 471
Phytotoxins in plants, 498, 500
PID (*see* Pelvic inflammatory
    disease)
Pilocarpine
  angle-closure glaucoma and,
    318
  antidote for, 448
Piloerection, epinephrine and,
    436
Pilonidal cyst, 228
Piperazine overdose, 469
Piperidine overdose, 468
Pit vipers, 484–486
Placenta previa, 207–208
Plantar reflex in spine injuries,
    161
Plant toxins, 492–500
  commonly ingested,
    496–499
Plasma loss in hypovolemic
    shock, 4
Plasminogen activator, tissue-
    type, 20

Plaster cast (*see* Cast)
Plaster splint (*see* Splint)
Plastic in eye, 316
Plastic surgery instruments,
    facial injuries and, 275
Platelet count in septic shock,
    9
Platelet disorders, 351
Pleural fluid accumulation,
    94–95
Pneumococcus
    central nervous system
        infection and, 132
    pediatrics and
        meningitis in, 368, 369
        otitis media in, 370
        pneumonia in, 369
    pneumonia and, 78–79, 369
    sickle cell disease and, 348
    sinusitis and, 309
Pneumocystis carinii
    acquired immunodeficiency
        syndrome and, 326,
        327
    pneumonia and, 83
Pneumomediastinum
    pneumothorax and, 107
    tracheal or bronchial
        rupture and, 111
Pneumonia, 78–83 (*see also*
    Pneumonitis)
    acquired immunodeficiency
        syndrome and, 326, 327
    bronchial asthma and,
        381–382
    in child, 369–370
Pneumonitis (*see also*
    Pneumonia)
    chemical, 92
    radiation and, 340–341
Pneumopericardium, 107
Pneumoperitoneum, abdominal
    injuries and, 177, 178,
    179

Pneumothorax, 103–109
    cancer and, 344
    decompression illness and,
        417
    hemothorax and, 110
    intercostal nerve block and,
        433
    open, 105–106
        symptoms of, 99, 106–107
        treatment of, 109
    scapula injuries and, 242
    symptoms of, 99
Poisindex, 451, 492
Poisoning and overdose,
    441–500
    acetaminophen and,
        476–477
    animal venoms and,
        484–489
    arthropod bites and,
        489–491
    attempted suicide and, 445
    caustic burns and, 465–466
    ethylene glycol and,
        482–484
    hydrocarbons and,
        464–465
    identification of, 443–445
    iron and, 462–464
    kerosene and, 464–465
    lead and, 460–462
    management of, 445–458
    mercury and, 477–479
    methanol and, 482–484
    mushrooms and, 491–492
    noxious gases and, 479–482
    organophosphates and,
        466–467
    paracetamol and, 476–477
    plants and, 492–500
        commonly ingested,
            496–499
    psychotropic drugs and,
        467–476

Poisoning and Overdose
(cont.)
from regional anesthesia
blocks, 434
rodenticides and, 500
salicylates and, 458–460
signs and symptoms of,
442–443
Polyglycolic acid, 278
Polypeptides in plants, 493
Polypropylene sutures
eyelid and, 284
facial injuries and, 275
skin and, 278
Polystyrene sulfonate, 66
Polyvalent antivenin, 489
Pontine lesions, 123
pupils and, 156
Pontocaine (*see* Tetracaine)
Popliteal artery injury, 251
Positive end-expiratory
pressure
bronchial asthma and, 381
lung contusion and, 111
noncardiogenic pulmonary
edema and, 88
pulmonary aspiration and,
90
toxic inhalation and, 93
Positive-pressure ventilation
flail chest and, 102–103
pulmonary aspiration and,
90
toxic inhalation and, 93
Posterior fossa tumor, 146
Posterior tibial nerve block,
432, 433
Postictal state, 149
Postpartum depression, 523
Postpyodermal
glomerulonephritis, 400
Potassium
dialysis and, 456
hyperglycemia and, 128, 129

hyperkalemia and, 64–67
hypokalemia and, 67–69
metabolic alkalosis and, 56
mistletoe poisoning and, 497
paroxysmal atrial
tachycardia and, 29
pediatrics and
dehydration in, 359
diabetic ketoacidosis in,
367
Potassium chloride
alkaline diuresis and, 455
hypokalemia and, 68
Potassium cyanide overdose,
448
Potassium permanganate, 296
Povidone-iodine (*see* Iodine)
Pralidoxime, 449, 467
Pramoxine, 183
Prednisolone
bronchial asthma and, 382
contact dermatitis and, 392
Prednisone
anaphylactic shock and, 386
bronchial asthma and, 382,
383
drug eruption and, 393
erythema multiforme and,
394
herpes zoster and, 399–400
lye burn and, 465
pemphigus vulgaris and, 401
toxic epidermal necrolysis
and, 403
Pre-eclampsia, 209
Pregnancy (*see also* Obstetric
disorders)
bleeding in third trimester
of, 207–209
cardiac arrest resuscitation
and, 42
cystitis in, 191
ectopic, 200–201
German measles and, 397

herpes genitalis and, 207
metronidazole and, 205
military antishock trousers
and, 7
postpartum depression and,
523
rape and, 211–212
tetracycline in, 394
Preload manipulation in
cardiogenic shock,
21–22
Premarin, rape and (*see*
Estrogen, rape and)
Premature ventricular
contractions, 35–37
isoproterenol and, 34
Priapism in spine injuries, 160,
161
Primaquine
hemolytic anemia and, 348
overdose of, 451
PR interval
atrioventricular block and,
33–34
paroxysmal supraventricular
tachycardia and, 27
premature ventricular
contractions and, 35
Probenecid
gonococcal dermatitis and,
394
pelvic inflammatory disease
and, 203
pharyngitis and, 304
Procainamide
atrial fibrillation and, 32
mistletoe poisoning and, 497
multifocal atrial tachycardia
and, 30
pediatric dosage of, 372
premature ventricular
contractions and, 36
psychiatric disorders and,
511

torsade de pointes and, 38,
39
ventricular fibrillation and,
48
ventricular tachycardia and,
37–38
Wolff-Parkinson-White
syndrome and, 28, 29
Procaine penicillin
lead poisoning and, 461
peritonsillar abscess and,
305
pharyngitis and, 304, 305
pneumococcal pneumonia
and, 79
scarlet fever and, 397
Procarbazine hydrochloride,
342
chemotherapy and, 342
Prochlorperazine
chemotherapy and, 341
headache and, 143
Proctitis, acquired
immunodeficiency
syndrome and, 329
Prodrome, 142, 143
Profundus tendon, 260, 262
Prolixin, overdose of (*see*
Fluphenazine, overdose
of)
Promethazine
bronchial asthma and, 381
sedation and, 437
vertigo and, 147
Pronestyl (*see* Procainamide)
Proparacaine
eye irrigation and, 315
foreign bodies in eye and,
316, 317
Proplex (*see* Prothrombin
complex)
Propoxyphene
cardiac arrest and,
39

Propoxyphene *(cont.)*
  noncardiogenic pulmonary
    edema and, 87
  overdose of, 442
    antidote for, 449
    dialysis and, 457
Propranolol
  aortic aneurysm and, 238
  atrial flutter and, 31
  atrioventricular block and,
    34
  headache and, 143
  hypertensive
    encephalopathy and,
    135
  mushroom poisoning and,
    495
  paroxysmal atrial
    tachycardia and, 29
  paroxysmal supraventricular
    tachycardia and, 28
  pediatric dosage of, 372
  premature ventricular
    contractions and, 36
  sinus bradycardia and, 33
  syncope and, 138
  thyroid storm and, 134
  tricyclic antidepressant
    overdose and, 472
  ventricular fibrillation and,
    48
  ventricular tachycardia and,
    38
Propylthiouracil, 134
Prostate cancer, spinal cord
    compression and, 333
Prostatitis, 195
Prosthetic valve, abscess and,
    221
Protection in psychiatric
    emergencies, 502–504
Proteus, 8
Prothrombin complex, 355

Prothrombin time
  coagulation pathway
    disorders and, 351, 355
  coumadin and, 77
  septic shock and, 9
Protopam chloride *(see*
    Pralidoxime)
Pseudodementia, 526
Pseudohyponatremia, 64
Pseudohypoparathyroidism,
    70
Pseudomonas
  pneumonia and, 81
  septic shock and, 8, 9–10
Pseudomonas aeruginosa,
    meningitis and, 336
Psilocin, 495
Psilocybin, 495
PSVT *(see* Paroxysmal
    supraventricular
    tachycardia)
Psychiatric emergencies,
    501–527
  attempted suicide and, 445
  diagnostic categories and,
    508
  differential diagnosis and,
    524–527
  drug abuse and, 519–522
  life-threatening conditions
    and, 522–524
  mental status examination
    and, 504–507
  nonorganic psychoses and,
    515–518
  nonpsychotic disorders and,
    518–519
  organic mental disorders
    and, 508–515
  physical protection and,
    502–504
  physical protection in,
    502–504

Psychoactive substance-
    induced organic mental
    disorders, 514
Psychogenic vertigo, 145
Psychomotor status, 149
Psychotic disorders, 508–518
    differential diagnosis of, 524
    nonorganic, 515–518
    organic, 508–515
Psychotropic drugs
    mental disorders induced
        by, 514
    overdose of, 467–476
PT (*see* Prothrombin time)
PTH (*see* Parathyroid
    hormone)
PTT (*see* Partial
    thromboplastin time)
Pulmonary arteriography in
    pulmonary embolus,
    76–77
Pulmonary aspiration, 89–90
Pulmonary burns, 408–409
Pulmonary contusion in flail
    chest, 103
Pulmonary disorders
    chemotherapy and, 341,
        342, 343–344
    sickle cell disease and, 349
Pulmonary edema
    military antishock trousers
        and, 7
    noncardiogenic, 87–89 (*see
        also* Noncardiogenic
        pulmonary edema)
    opiate overdose and,
        475–476
    pit vipers and, 486
Pulmonary embolus, 75–78
    cancer and, 343
    cardiac arrest and, 40
    decompression illness and,
        417

thrombophlebitis and, 235
Pulmonary wedge pressure in
    cardiogenic shock, 21
Pulsating hematoma, 230
Pulse
    hypovolemic shock and, 4
    syncope and, 137
Pulsus paradoxus, 113
Pupils
    head injuries and, 156, 158
    neurological emergencies
        and, 123
PVCs (*see* Premature
    ventricular
    contractions)
P wave
    atrial fibrillation and, 31
    atrial flutter and, 30
    electromechanical
        dissociation and, 49
    hyperkalemia and, 65
    multifocal atrial tachycardia
        and, 29
    pacemaker malfunction and,
        25
    paroxysmal supraventricular
        tachycardia and, 27
    ventricular tachycardia and,
        37
Pyelonephritis, 192
Pyloric stenosis, 373–374
Pyridium (*see*
    Phenazopyridine)
Pyridostigmine overdose, 448
Pyridoxine, 495

Q

QRS complex
    atrial fibrillation and, 31
    electromechanical
        dissociation and, 49
    hyperkalemia and, 65

QRS Complex *(cont.)*
  hypothermia and, 414, 415
  pacemaker malfunction and, 25
  paroxysmal supraventricular tachycardia and, 27
  premature ventricular contractions and, 35
  torsade de pointes and, 38
  tricyclic antidepressant overdose and, 471
  ventricular tachycardia and, 37
QT interval
  hypercalcemia and, 72
  hyperkalemia and, 65
  hypocalcemia and, 70
  hypokalemia and, 68
  lithium overdose and, 470
  torsade de pointes and, 38
Quadriceps muscle, spinal cord levels and, 161
Quinacrine, 348
Quinidine
  atrial fibrillation and, 32
  mistletoe poisoning and, 497
  overdose of, 456
  paroxysmal atrial tachycardia and, 29
  premature ventricular contractions and, 36
  psychiatric disorders and, 511
  sinus bradycardia and, 33
  torsade de pointes and, 38, 39
  Wolff-Parkinson-White syndrome and, 29
Quinine
  hemolytic anemia and, 348
  overdose of, 456
Q wave, myocardial infarction and, 18

R

Rabies, 219–224
  prophylaxis for, 222–223, 224
Racemic epinephrine *(see Epinephrine)*
Radial artery anatomy, 260
Radial head fracture, 247
Radial nerve
  anatomy of, 262
  axillary block and, 429
  injury of, 245
  sensation and, 265
Radial nerve block, 426, 428
Radiation
  effects of, 340–343
  spinal cord compression and, 334
Radioactive fibrinogen scanning, 236
Radiographic contrast studies *(see Contrast studies)*
Radius fracture, 248–249
Rales in cardiogenic pulmonary edema, 23
Rape, 210–212
Rash *(see also Dermatologic disorders)*
  fever and, 394–398
  serum sickness and, 387
Rattlesnakes, 484, 485
Rectal examination, 14
Rectal prolapse, 183–184
Rectal sphincter tone in spine injuries, 160, 161
Red blood cells
  anemia and, 346–348
  sickle cell disease and, 349
Reflexes in spine injuries, 161
Refractory ventricular fibrillation, 115, 116

Regional anesthesia, 419–433
  local infiltration block and,
    419–420
  nerve blocks and, 420–433
    (*see also* Regional
    nerve blocks)
Regional nerve blocks,
    420–433
  head and neck and, 420–423
  lower extremity and,
    431–433
  upper extremity and,
    423–431
Regional Spinal Cord Center,
    163–165
Regitine (*see* Phentolamine)
Reglan (*see* Metoclopramide)
Renal colic, 195–196
Renal function tests in
    metabolic acidosis, 54
Renal injuries, 185–188
Reserpine
  psychiatric disorders and,
    511
  thyroid storm and, 134
Resins in plants, 498–500
Respiratory acidosis, 51–53
Respiratory alkalosis, 55–56
  bronchial asthma and,
    378
  hypovolemic shock and, 5
  noncardiogenic pulmonary
    edema and, 88
Respiratory emergencies,
    75–95
  acute respiratory failure and,
    83–86
  effusion and, 94–95
  empyema, 94–95
  hemoptysis and, 93–94
  hemothorax and, 94–95
  noncardiogenic pulmonary
    edema and, 87–89

  pleural fluid accumulation
    and, 94–95
  pneumonia and, 78–83
  pulmonary aspiration and,
    89–90
  pulmonary embolus and,
    75–78
  smoke inhalation and, 91–93
Respiratory failure
  cancer and, 343
  diazepam and, 151
Respiratory infection (*see*
    Upper respiratory tract
    infection)
Respiratory rate in
    hypovolemic shock, 5
Respiratory system (*see also*
    Airway management;
    Breathing)
  anaphylactic shock and, 384
  burns of, 93
  hypovolemic shock and,
    4–5
  narcotics and, 437
  neurological emergencies
    and, 124
  regional anesthesia toxicity
    and, 434, 435
Restraints in violence, 503
Restrictive lung disease, 341
Resuscitation
  after cardiac arrest, 40
  monitoring of, 12–13
Retinal artery occlusion,
    317–318
Retinal detachment, 323–324
Retrograde
    cystourethrography,
    178
Rewarming
  frostbite and, 413
  hypothermia and, 414–415
Rheumatic fever, 303

Rheumatic valve, abscess and, 221

Rib fracture, 100–101
    scapula injuries and, 242

Rickettsiae, 8

Rifampin
    central nervous system infection and, 132
    meningococcemia and, 396
    psychiatric disorders and, 511

Ringworm, 398

Rinne test, 300

Robaxin (*see* Methocarbamol)

Rodenticide poisoning, 500

Rodents, rabies and, 219, 223

Roentgenograms (*see* X-rays)

R-on-T phenomenon in premature ventricular contractions, 35

Roseola infantum, 395, 396–397

R-R interval
    atrial fibrillation and, 32
    atrioventricular block and, 34

Rubella, 395, 397

Rumack-Matthew nomogram for acetaminophen poisoning, 478–479

Rupture of varicosities, 234–235

S

Sacral sensory function, 14

Safety pins in airway obstruction, 294

Sagittal sinus thrombosis, cancer and, 337–338

Salicylates (*see also specific agent*)
    gastrointestinal hemorrhage and, 180

noncardiogenic pulmonary edema and, 87
    overdose of, 443, 458–460
        determining level of, 444
        dialysis and, 456
        diuresis and, 456
        hemoperfusion and, 457

Saline, abscess and, 225

Salmonella
    acquired immunodeficiency syndrome and, 329
    diarrhea and, 176
    sickle cell disease and, 348

Salt
    heat cramps and, 412
    heat exhaustion and, 412

Saponins in plants, 498, 499

Scabies, 401

Scalp, nerve blocks and, 422

Scapula injuries, 242–243

Scarlet fever, 395, 397

Scars, 279

Schiotz tonometer, 314

Schizophrenia, 515–516
    dementia and, 514
    differential diagnosis of, 525
    phencyclidine overdose and, 475
    stimulant overdose and, 521

Sciatic nerve block, 431, 432

Sciatic nerve injury, 250

Scopolamine, 147

Scrotum
    incarcerated hernia and, 374
    injuries of, 190

Seat belts, laryngeal trauma and, 298

Secobarbital overdose, 467

Second-degree burns, 407, 408

Sedatives, 436–438
    bronchial asthma and, 381
    local infiltration block and, 420
    overdose of, 443

violence and, 503–504
Seizures, 149–153
  cancer and, 333
  in child, 360–362
  eclampsia and, 209
  head injuries and, 158
  myocardial infarction and,
    18
  regional anesthesia toxicity
    and, 434
Semustine, 342
Sengstaken-Blakemore tube,
  180
Sensation, hand injuries and,
  265–266
Septal dislocation, 291
Septal hematoma, 300
  facial injuries and, 291
Septic shock, 8–10
  causes of, 1
  clinical findings in, 3
Septra (*see* Trimethoprim/
  sulfamethoxazole)
Serentil, 468
Serous otitis media, 305–306
Serum electrolytes (*see*
  Electrolytes)
Serum osmolality
  formula for, 128
  hyperglycemia and, 128
  metabolic acidosis and, 54
  methanol poisoning and,
    482–483
Serum sickness, 387–388
Shigella
  acquired immunodeficiency
    syndrome and, 329
  diarrhea and, 176
Shingles, 399–400
Shivering in heat stroke, 413
Shock, 1–10
  anaphylactic, 384–387
  cardiac tamponade and, 113
  definition of, 1–3

electric, 410–411
hemothorax and, 110
hypovolemic, 4–7
renal injuries and, 187
septic, 8–10
spinal, 10
tension pneumothorax and,
  106
Shoulder dislocation,
  243–244
SIADH (*see* Syndrome of
  inappropriate secretion
  of antidiuretic
  hormone)
Sickle cell disease, 346–348,
  349
Sigmoidoscopy
  acquired immunodeficiency
    syndrome and, 327
  fecal impaction and, 181
Sigmoid volvulus, 171–172
Signs
  Beevor's, 162
  Chvostek's, 70
  doll's eye, 123, 156
  Homans', 236
  positive Babinski reflex and,
    123–124, 157
  Trousseau's, 70
  Westermark's, 76
Silk, 278
Silver nitrate
  epistaxis and, 302
  fissure in ano and, 183
Silver sulfadiazine in thermal
  burns, 408
Simple pneumothorax, 103,
  104
  symptoms of, 106
Sinus bradycardia, 32–33
Sinusitis, 308–309
Sinus tachycardia, 26
Sinus thrombosis, cancer and,
  337–338

Sitz bath
  fissure in ano and, 183
  perirectal abscess and, 182
  thrombosed hemorrhoids
      and, 183
Skeletal disorders in sickle cell
      disease, 349
Skin
  disorders of (*see*
      Dermatologic disorders)
  shock and, 2–3
    anaphylactic, 384
    hypovolemic, 2, 5
    septic, 2, 8
  sickle cell disease and, 349
  suture materials for,
      278–279
Skin graft in hand injuries, 273
Skull fracture, 157
Skull x-ray in head injuries,
      158–159
Slicing wounds, 280–281, 282
Sling, scapula injuries and, 242
Small bowel obstruction,
      167–172
Smoke inhalation, 91–93
Smoking, aminophylline and,
      380
Snakebite, 484–489
Snellen eye chart, 313
Sodium
  calculation of deficit of, 359
  dehydration in child and,
      359–360
  hypernatremia and, 57
  hyponatremia and, 60
Sodium amobarbital, 153
Sodium amytal, 153
Sodium bicarbonate
  alkaline diuresis and, 455
  cardiac arrest and, 47
  in child, 366
  diabetic ketoacidosis in
      child and, 367–368

electromechanical
      dissociation and, 49
  hyperglycemia and, 128–129
  hyperkalemia and, 66
  hypernatremia and, 57
  iron poisoning and, 462
  metabolic acidosis and,
      54–55
  metabolic alkalosis and, 56
  methanol poisoning and,
      483
  respiratory acidosis and,
      52–53, 53
  salicylate overdose and, 460
  tricyclic antidepressant
      overdose and, 472
  ventricular asystole and, 49
  ventricular fibrillation and,
      48
Sodium iodine, 134
Sodium nitrite
  as antidote, 448, 449
  cyanide poisoning and,
      480–481
  noxious gas poisoning and,
      480
  overdose of, 442–443
Sodium nitroprusside
  antidote for, 448
  aortic aneurysm and, 238
  hypertensive
      encephalopathy and,
      134–135
  overdose of, 480
  pediatric dosage of, 372
  phencyclidine overdose and,
      474
Sodium thiosulfate
  as antidote, 448
  cyanide poisoning and, 481
Soft-tissue infections, 213–228
  abscess and, 221–228
  traumatic wounds and,
      214–221

Soft-tissue trauma, oral, 309–310
Solid viscus rupture, 176–179
Solu-Cortef (*see* Hydrocortisone)
Solu-Medrol (*see* Methylprednisolone)
Somatic preoccupations, 505
Sorbitol, 451
Spectazole (*see* Econazole)
Spectrophotometer in lead poisoning, 461
Spermatic cord torsion, 196–197
Sphygmomanometer in intravenous regional anesthesia, 430
Spider bites, 489–491
Spinal cancer, meningitis and, 336
Spinal cord compression, cancer and, 333–334
Spinal cord levels
    muscles and, 161
    sensory levels and, 162
Spinal immobilization, 13, 160, 164, 165
Spinal injuries, 160–165
Spinal shock, 10
    clinical findings in, 3
Spinal tap (*see also* Cerebrospinal fluid)
    acquired immunodeficiency syndrome and, 327
    central nervous system infection and, 130
    cerebrovascular accident and, 136
    convulsive disorders and, 150
    encephalitis and, 337
    fever in newborn and, 357
    headache and, 143

meningitis and, 335
    pediatric, 368
    seizures in child and, 361
Spine board, 160, 165
Spirochetes in syphilis, 402
Spironolactone, 65
Spleen injuries, 177–178
Splenomegaly, 344
Splint
    acromioclavicular separation and, 244
    bone and joint trauma and, 242
    diaphyseal fracture and, 251
    elbow dislocation and, 246–247
    hand injuries and, 248, 270
    humerus and, 245
    radial head fracture and, 247
    tooth avulsion and, 291
    wrist injuries and, 248
Spontaneous abortion, 201–202
Sprained ankle, 254–255
Sputum
    bronchial asthma and, 381–382
    gram-negative pneumonia and, 80
    Haemophilus pneumonia and, 80
    Legionnaire's disease and, 82
    Mycoplasma pneumonia and, 81
    pneumococcal pneumonia and, 78
    staphylococcal pneumonia and, 79
    streptococcal pneumonia, 79
    viral pneumonia and, 82
SS disease (*see* Sickle cell disease)
SSSS (*see* Staphylococcal scalded skin syndrome)

Staphylococcal scalded skin
  syndrome, 402–403
*Staphylococcus (see also
  Staphylococcus aureus)*
  epiglottitis and, 363
  hordeolum and, 324
  impetigo and, 400
  meningitis in child and, 369
  pneumonia and, 79
  sickle cell disease and, 348
  toxic shock syndrome and,
    10
Staphylococcus aureus
  bites and, 218, 219
  meningitis and, 336
  toxic epidermal necrolysis
    and, 402
  wound infections and, 216
Stasis dermatitis, 392
Status epilepticus, 149–153
  nonconvulsive, 149
Steam inhalation, 408–409
Stelazine, 469
Stellate laceration, 280, 282
Steroids *(see also
  Corticosteroids)*
  adrenal crisis and, 132, 133
  anaphylactic shock and,
    385–386
  atopic dermatitis and,
    389–391
  bronchial asthma and,
    380–381, 382, 383
  brown recluse spider and,
    491
  caustic ingestion and, 297
  contact dermatitis and, 392
  croup and, 362
  drug eruption and, 393
  erythema multiforme and,
    394
  esophageal burn and, 465
  gastrointestinal hemorrhage
    and, 180

  head injuries and, 159
  herpes simplex keratitis and,
    323
  herpes zoster and, 399–400
  mushroom poisoning and,
    494
  ophthalmologic emergencies
    and, 314
  pemphigus vulgaris and, 401
  psychiatric disorders and,
    511
  pulmonary aspiration and,
    90
  septic shock and, 10
  serum sickness and, 388
  stasis dermatitis and, 392
  total eosinophil count and,
    379
  toxic epidermal necrolysis
    and, 403
  uveitis and, 323
Stethoscope in arterial
  ischemia, 229
Stevens-Johnson syndrome,
  393, 394
Stimulant overdose, 521 *(see
  also specific stimulant)*
STK *(see Streptokinase)*
Stomach evacuation, 446–450,
  452–453
Stomatitis, 311–312
Stool culture in diarrhea, 176
Strangulation in intestinal
  obstruction, 171
Streptococcus
  bites and, 218
  central nervous system
    infection and, 132
  epiglottitis and, 363
  impetigo and, 400
  meningitis and, 368
  pharyngitis and, 303, 304,
    370
  pneumonia and, 79

scarlet fever and, 397
tonsillitis and, 370
Streptokinase
myocardial infarction and, 20
pulmonary embolus and, 77
Stress cystogram, 189
Stroke, 136
myocardial infarction and, 19
Stroke volume in cardiac tamponade, 113
Strychnine overdose
activated charcoal and, 450
dialysis and, 456
gastric lavage and, 450
ST segment
myocardial infarction and, 18
pulmonary embolus and, 75–76
Stupor
alcohol abuse and, 125–127
central nervous system infection and, 130–132
cerebrovascular accident and, 136
endocrine dysfunction and, 132–134
evaluation of, 117, 120
hepatic failure and, 130
hyperglycemia and, 127–129
hypertensive encephalopathy and, 134–135
hypoglycemia and, 129
uremia and, 129
Sty, 324
Subarachnoid hemorrhage
convulsive disorders and, 150
headache and, 142
Subclavian artery injury, 230

Subcutaneous emphysema
laryngeal trauma and, 298
pneumothorax and, 107
simple, 106
tracheal or bronchial rupture and, 111
Subcutaneous tissue suture, 278, 280
Substance abuse (*see* Drug abuse)
Succinylcholine
muscular paralysis and, 438
pediatric dosage of, 372
Sucking chest wound (*see* Pneumothorax, open)
Suicidal risk, 522
mental status examination and, 506
poisoning and overdose and, 445
Sulfa
cystitis and, 191
hemolytic anemia and, 348
Sulfacetamide
bacterial conjunctivitis and, 323
corneal abrasion and, 320
hemolytic anemia and, 348
Sulfamethoxazole
cystitis and, 191
hemolytic anemia and, 348
Sulfamethoxazole/trimethoprim (*see* Trimethoprim/ sulfamethoxazole)
Sulfisoxazole
cystitis and, 191
otitis media in child and, 370
Sulfones, 348
Sulfuric acid, 296
Sulfur oxide poisoning, 92
Superficial cervical plexus block, 422–423

Superficialis tendon, 260, 262
Supracondylar fracture
    of femoral shaft, 251
    of humerus, 245–246
Supraorbital nerve block, 421,
        422
Suprapubic cystostomy, 196
Supratrochlear nerve block,
        421, 422
Suture techniques in facial
        injuries, 278–279, 281
Swath dressing
    humerus and, 245
    scapula injuries and, 243
    shoulder dislocation and,
        244
Sweat gland infections, 228
Sweating
    heat stroke and, 412
    myocardial infarction and,
        18
Symphysis fracture, 289
Synalar (*see* Fluocinolone
        acetonide)
Syncope, 137–139, 145
Syndrome of inappropriate
        secretion of antidiuretic
        hormone, 338–339
Syphilis, 401–402
    rape and, 211
    urinary tract infections in
        men and, 194
Syrup of ipecac, 447–450
    activated charcoal and, 450
    iron poisoning and, 462
    salicylate overdose and, 459

T

Tachycardia
    cancer and, 343
    in cardiogenic pulmonary
        edema, 24
    epinephrine and, 379, 436

hypokalemia and, 68
    septic shock and, 8
Tachypnea
    asthma in child and, 378
    hypovolemic shock and, 4–5
    septic shock and, 8
Takayasu's disease, 139
Talofibular ligament injuries,
        254–255
Talwin (*see* Pentazocine)
Tangential speech, 505
Tannic acid, 309
Tattoo, accidental, 294
Tea bags, 309
Teeth (*see* Tooth)
Temporomandibular joint
        disorders, 312
TEN (*see* Toxic epidermal
        necrolysis)
Tendon injuries of hand, 272
Tennis elbow, 247–248
Tenosynovitis, 227
Tension headache, 142, 143
Tension pneumomediastinum,
        111
Tension pneumothorax,
        103–105
    cardiac arrest and, 40
    obstructive shock and, 1, 3
    open pneumothorax and,
        109
    symptoms of, 99, 106
    treatment of, 109
TEPP poisoning, 466
Terbutaline
    bronchial asthma and, 379,
        382
    psychiatric disorders and,
        511
Testis
    injuries to, 190
    torsion of, 196–197,
        374–375
Tetanus immune globulin, 214

Tetanus prophylaxis, 214–215
  abdominal gunshot wounds
    and, 179
  facial injuries and, 276
  frostbite and, 414
  open fractures and, 15
  thermal burns and, 406
Tetanus toxoid, 214, 215, 220
Tetracaine
  epistaxis and, 301
  eye irrigation and, 315
  foreign bodies in eye and,
    316, 317
Tetracycline
  Bartholinian abscess and,
    207
  bites and, 218
  bronchial asthma and, 382
  cystitis and, 191
  dermatologic disorders and,
    390
  epididymitis and, 195
  gonococcal dermatitis and,
    394
  Mycoplasma pneumonia
    and, 81
  pelvic inflammatory disease
    and, 203
  prostatitis and, 195
  sinusitis and, 309
  syphilis and, 402
Thalamic lesions, 123
Theophylline
  aminophylline and, 380
  overdose of
    activated charcoal and,
      451
    determining level of, 444
    dialysis and, 456
    hemoperfusion and, 457
Thermal burns, 405–410
Thiamine
  neurological emergencies
    and, 121, 125

Wernicke-Korsakoff
    syndrome and, 520
  Wernicke's encephalopathy
    and, 127
Thiazide diuretics
  hypercalcemia and, 72
  hyperkalemia and, 66
  hypertensive
    encephalopathy and,
    135
Thiethylperazine maleate, 341
Thigh
  femoral nerve block and,
    431, 433
  regional nerve blocks and,
    431–433
  sciatic nerve block and, 431
Thioctic acid, 494
Thioridazine, overdose of, 468
Thioridazine overdose
  antidote for, 448
Thiosulfate as antidote, 448
  cyanide poisoning and, 481
Thioxanthines, overdose of,
  469
Third-degree burns, 407, 408
Thoracic aortic aneurysm,
  237–238
Thoracic aortic injuries, 230
Thoracic injuries, 97–116
  airway management in,
    97–99
  breathing evaluation in, 99
  circulation evaluation in, 99
  diagnosis and treatment of,
    100–116
    aorta and great vessels
      injuries and, 112–113
    cardiac tamponade and,
      113–115
    diaphragmatic rupture
      and, 112
    flail chest and, 101–103
    hemothorax and, 110–111

Thoracic injuries *(cont.)*
  lung contusion and, 111
  myocardial contusion and, 113
  pneumothorax and, 103–109
  rib fracture and, 100–101
  thoracotomy and, 97, 115–116
  tracheal or bronchial rupture and, 111–112
  initial evaluation in, 99
Thoracic spinal cord levels, 161–162
Thoracostomy, tube, 107–111
Thoracotomy
  cardiac arrest and, 41
  cardiac tamponade and, 115–116
  hemothorax and, 111
  thoracic injuries and, 97
Thorazine *(see* Chlorpromazine)
Thought broadcasting, 505
Thought process assessment in mental status examination, 505–506
Throat infections, 303–305
Thrombocytopenia
  cancer and, 344
  coagulation disorders and, 351
  septic shock and, 9
Thrombocytosis
  cancer and, 344
  false potassium levels and, 67
Thrombolytic therapy
  myocardial infarction and, 20
  pulmonary embolus and, 77
Thrombophlebitis, 235–237

Thrombosis
  in cancer, 337–338
  cancer and, 344
  hemorrhoids and, 183
  pulmonary embolus and, 75
Through-and-through lip laceration, 283
Thyroid hormone in myxedema coma, 133
Thyroid medication, sinus tachycardia and, 26
Thyroid storm, 133–134
Thyrotoxicosis, 31
Tibial muscle, anterior, spinal cord levels and, 161
Tibial nerve block, 432, 433
Tibial shaft fracture, 254
Tidal volume in hypovolemic shock, 5
Tigan *(see* Trimethobenzamide hydrochloride)
Timber rattlesnake, 485
Tissue-type plasminogen activator, 20
TMJ disorders *(see* Temporomandibular joint disorders)
Tobacco, premature ventricular contractions and, 36
Tobramycin, 9
Tolnaftate, 398
Toluene overdose, 452, 454
Tongue
  injuries of, 281–283
  mandibular nerve block and, 420
Tonometry, 313–314
Tonsillar herniation, 122
Tonsillitis, 370
Tooth
  avulsion of, 291, 310
  caries and, 311
  injuries of, 310–311

mandibular nerve block and, 420

Topicort (*see* Desoximetasone)

Torecan (*see* Thiethylperazine maleate)

Torsion of spermatic cord, 196–197, 374–375

Total eosinophil count, 378–379, 383

Tourniquet
anaphylactic shock and, 384–385
axillary block and, 429, 430
bloodless field and, 270
coral snake bite and, 487, 488
false calcium levels and, 73
intravenous regional anesthesia in lower extremity and, 431
noncardiogenic pulmonary edema and, 89
vessel injury and, 232

Toxalbumins in plants, 500

Toxic abnormalities in cancer, 338–340

Toxic epidermal necrolysis, 402–403

Toxicity (*see* Poisoning and overdose)

Toxicology screen
metabolic acidosis and, 54
neurological emergencies and, 124

Toxic shock syndrome, 10

Toxoplasma gondii, 337

tPA (*see* Tissue-type plasminogen activator)

Tracheal intubation (*see also* Endotracheal intubation; Nasotracheal intubation)
cardiac arrest resuscitation and, 44–45

phencyclidine overdose and, 474
spine injuries and, 163

Tracheal rupture, 111

Tracheostomy
epiglottitis and, 363
laryngeal trauma and, 299
tracheal or bronchial rupture and, 111

Tracheotomy in caustic ingestion, 297

Traction
elbow dislocation and, 246
facial bone injuries and, 291
femoral shaft fracture and, 251
shoulder dislocation and, 243
wrist and hand injuries and, 248

Tranquilizer overdose, 468–469

Transtentorial herniation, 122

Transverse carpal ligament, 260, 262

Trapdoor wound, 281

Trapezius muscle, spinal cord levels and, 161

Trauma care, 11–15
airway management in, 11
breathing and ventilatory exchange in, 11–12
circulatory evaluation in, 12
clothing and, 13
extremity injuries and, 14–15
intubation in, 13
neurological monitoring in, 13–14
resuscitation monitoring in, 12–13
spinal immobilization in, 13

Trendelenburg position in neurological emergencies, 125

Triamcinolone
  dermatologic disorders and,
    391
  trochanteric bursitis and,
    251
Triamterene, 65
Triceps muscle, spinal cord
  levels and, 161
Triceps stretch reflex, 161
Trichloroacetic acid, 302
Trichloroethane overdose,
  452, 454
Trichloroethylene overdose,
  452
Trichomonas vaginalis, 200,
  205
Tricyclic antidepressants
  cardiac arrest and, 39
  overdose of, 443, 470–472
    activated charcoal and,
     451
    dialysis and, 457
    hemoperfusion and, 457
  premature ventricular
    contractions and, 36
  torsade de pointes and, 38
Tridesilon (*see* Desonide)
Trigeminal nerve block,
  420–423
Trilafon, 469
Trimethobenzamide
  hydrochloride, 341
Trimethoprim in cystitis, 191
Trimethoprim/
  sulfamethoxazole
  cystitis and, 191
  otitis media and, 307, 371
  prostatitis and, 195
  pyelonephritis and, 192
  sinusitis and, 309
Trismus, peritonsillar abscess
  and, 305
Trochanteric bursitis, 250–251

Trochar, pneumothorax and,
  109
Trousseau's sign, 70
Tuberculosis, 87
  meningitis and, 131
Tube thoracostomy
  hemothorax and, 110–111
  pneumothorax and,
    107–109
Tubocurarine, 438
Tubo-ovarian abscess, 204
Tucks pads, 183
T wave
  hyperkalemia and, 65
  hypokalemia and, 68
  lithium overdose and, 470
  pacemaker malfunction and,
    25
  potassium replacement and,
    69
  premature ventricular
    contractions and, 35
  pulmonary embolus and, 76
  torsade de pointes and, 38
Tylenol (*see* Acetaminophen)
Tyramine, 493, 497

U

Ulcer
  duodenal, 375
  gastrointestinal hemorrhage
    and, 181
Ulnar artery, 260, 262
Ulnar fracture, 248
Ulnar nerve, 262
  anatomy of, 260
  damage to, 269
  sensation and, 265
Ulnar nerve block, 425, 427
Ultrasound
  arterial ischemia and, 229
  ectopic pregnancy and, 201

placenta previa and, 208
renal colic and, 196
torsion of spermatic cord
and, 197
Uncal herniation, 122
Unconsciousness (*see*
Consciousness)
Unipolar depressive disorder,
516
Untidy wound of face, 278
Upper airway burns, 408
Upper extremity
injuries of, 242–250
regional nerve blocks and,
423–430
Upper respiratory tract
infection
benign positional vertigo
and, 146
bronchial asthma and,
381–382
viral conjunctivitis and, 322
Urea, atopic dermatitis and,
389
Ureaplasma urealyticum, 194
Uremia, 129
Ureteral injuries, 188
Urethral colic, 195–196
Urethral injuries, 189
pelvis injuries and, 257
Urethritis in men, 192–194
Urinalysis
cystitis and, 191
renal injuries and, 187
Urinary catheter,
contraindications to use
of, 12
Urinary output
hypovolemic shock and, 5
resuscitation monitoring
and, 12
Urinary retention, 196
herpes genitalis and, 206

Urinary tract
infections and, 193
injuries of, 257
obstruction of, 195–196
sickle cell disease and, 349
Urine pH in salicylate
overdose, 460
Urography, 188
Urticaria, 387, 403
Uveitis, 323
U wave in hypokalemia, 68

V

VA (*see* Ventricular asystole)
Vagal nerve
paroxysmal supraventricular
tachycardia and, 27
radiographic contrast
material and, 386–387
Vaginal bleeding, 200
Vaginal discharge, 200
Vaginitis, 204–206
Vaginosis, 205–206
Valisone (*see* Betamethasone)
Valium (*see* Diazepam)
Varicella, 398
Varices
esophageal, 180
rupture of, 234–235
Variola, 395, 396
Vascular disorders
cancer and, 337–338
coagulation and, 351
as emergencies, 229–239
(*see also* Peripheral
vascular emergencies)
sickle cell disease and, 349
syncope and, 139
Vascular headaches, 141, 143
Vascular injuries
hand and, 272
tibial shaft fracture and, 254

Vaseline, atopic dermatitis and, 389

Vasoactive agents, septic shock and, 10 (*see also* Vasopressors)

Vasocon (*see* Naphazoline)

Vasodilators, 414

Vasopressin
gastrointestinal hemorrhage and, 180
syndrome of inappropriate secretion of antidiuretic hormone and, 338

Vasopressors
anaphylactic shock and, 385
barbiturate overdose and, 468
hypovolemic shock and, 7
septic shock and, 10
thyroid storm and, 134

Vasovagal syncope, 139

Vecuronium, 439

Velpeau (*see* Swath dressing)

Venography in thrombophlebitis, 236

Venoms
animal, 484–489
spider bites and, 489–491

Venous disease, 234–237

Venous stasis
pulmonary embolus and, 75
thrombophlebitis and, 235

Ventilation
in child, 365
mechanical (*see* Mechanical ventilation)

Ventilation-perfusion scanning, 76

Ventilatory exchange in trauma, 11–12

Ventricular asystole
cardiac arrest and, 48–49
electric shock and, 411
hyperkalemia and, 65

hypothermia and, 415

Ventricular fibrillation
cardiac arrest and, 47–48
electric shock and, 411
hyperkalemia and, 65
hypothermia and, 415–416
premature ventricular contractions and, 35
thoracotomy and, 115, 116

Ventricular tachycardia, 37–38
premature ventricular contractions and, 35

Verapamil
atrial fibrillation and, 32
atrial flutter and, 31
paroxysmal supraventricular tachycardia and, 27
pediatric dosage of, 372

Versed (*see* Midazolam)

Vertebral bodies, spinal cord levels and, 162

Vertebrobasilar artery insufficiency, 146

Vertigo, 145–147

Vestibular neuronitis, 146

VF (*see* Ventricular fibrillation)

Vinblastine, 339

Vincristine, 339

Violence in psychiatric emergencies, 502–504

Viruses
conjunctivitis and, 322
meningitis and, 131
pneumonia and, 82–83
noncardiogenic pulmonary edema in, 87
septic shock and, 8
vestibular neuronitis and, 146

Viscus rupture, 176–179

Vision loss in central retinal artery occlusion, 317

Vistaril (*see* Hydroxyzine)

Visual acuity in ophthalmologic emergencies, 313
Vital signs, shock and, 2–3
 hypovolemic, 2, 4
 septic, 2, 8
Vitamin C (*see* Ascorbic acid)
Vitamin D in hypocalcemia, 69, 70
Vitamin K
 mushroom poisoning and, 494
 warfarin poisoning and, 500
Vitreous hemorrhage of eye, 323
Volar carpal ligament, 260, 262
Volar pad infection, 225–226
Volkmann's ischemic contracture, 245–246
Vomiting, induced (*see* Emesis)
von Willebrand's disease, 353–355
V-Q scanning (*see* Ventilation-perfusion scanning)
V-shaped laceration, 280, 282
VT (*see* Ventricular tachycardia)

W

Warfarin overdose, 500
Warming
 frostbite and, 413
 hypothermia and, 414–415
Water
 heat cramps and, 412
 heat exhaustion and, 412
 hypernatremia and, 57
 hyponatremia and, 60
 hypovolemic shock and, 4
Water pressure injuries, 416–417

Weber's test, 300
Wenckebach atrioventricular block, 33–34
Wernicke-Korsakoff syndrome, 520
Wernicke's encephalopathy, 127
Westermark's sign, 76
Wheezing in bronchial asthma, 378
White blood cell count
 fever in newborn and, 357
 meningitis and, 335, 336
 septic shock and, 9
Wild animals, rabies and, 219, 222
Window edema, 242
Wire brush, inground foreign material and, 284
Wiring of facial bone injuries, 291
Wolff-Parkinson-White syndrome
 atrial fibrillation and, 31, 32
 paroxysmal supraventricular tachycardia and, 27, 28–29
Wood alcohol (*see* Methanol)
Wound infections, 215–217
WPW syndrome (*see* Wolff-Parkinson-White syndrome)
Wrist
 anatomy of, 260, 261
 dorsum of, 260–261, 263
 injuries of, 248–250
 radial aspect of, 261–262, 264

X

Xeroform
 inground foreign material and, 285

Xeroform *(cont.)*
  thermal burns and, 408
X-rays
  abdominal (*see* Abdominal
      x-ray)
  acromioclavicular separation
      and, 244
  ankle injuries and, 255
  bone and joint trauma and,
      241–242
  caustic ingestion and,
      297
  cervical spine
    head injuries and, 159
    spine injuries and, 163
  chest (*see* Chest x-ray)
  epiglottitis and, 363
  facial bone fractures and,
      285

  foreign body in air or food
      passages and, 295
  head injuries and, 158–159
  knee injuries and, 253
  orbital
    eye injuries and, 320
    foreign bodies and, 316
Xylene overdose, 452, 454
Xylocaine (*see* Lidocaine)

Y

Yeast vaginitis, 205
Yersinia, 176

Z

Zovirax (*see* Acyclovir)
Zygomatic fracture, 287–288,
      292